My Marriage
Bliss vs Curse
An Anthology of 108 Co-Authors

Compiled by
ABHISHAIK CHITRAANS | RAINU MANGTANI

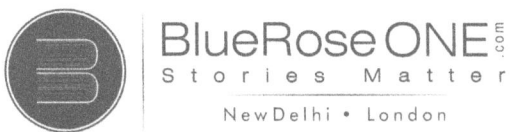

BLUEROSE PUBLISHERS
India | U.K.

Copyright © Abhishaik Chitraans 2024

All rights reserved by author. No part of this publication may be reproduced, stored in a retrieval system or transmitted in any form or by any means, electronic, mechanical, photocopying, recording or otherwise, without the prior permission of the author. Although every precaution has been taken to verify the accuracy of the information contained herein, the publisher assumes no responsibility for any errors or omissions. No liability is assumed for damages that may result from the use of information contained within.

BlueRose Publishers takes no responsibility for any damages, losses, or liabilities that may arise from the use or misuse of the information, products, or services provided in this publication.

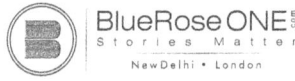

For permissions requests or inquiries regarding this publication, please contact:

BLUEROSE PUBLISHERS
www.BlueRoseONE.com
info@bluerosepublishers.com
+91 8882 898 898
+4407342408967

ISBN: 978-93-6261-512-1

Cover Design: Sadhna Kumari
Typesetting: Pooja Sharma

First Edition: December 2024

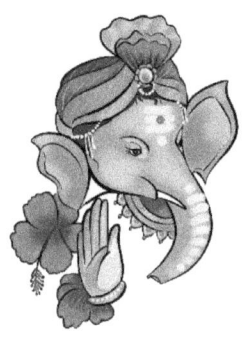

एकदंताय विद्महे, वक्रतुण्डाय धीमहि, तन्नो दंती प्रचोदयात्।।

My Marriage : Bliss vs Curse

An Anthology of 108 Co-Authors

A collection of articles/ poems/ suggestions/ opinions/ inspirational and unheard real life stories of married and unmarried individuals on the same Topic with different Individual Title

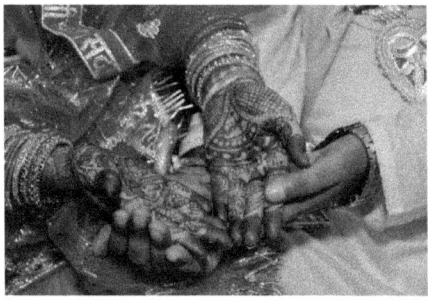

Compiled by

Internationally Renowned Author Couple

Rainu Mangtani
Abhishaik Chitraans

(ईष्ट कृपा एवं गुरु आशीष)

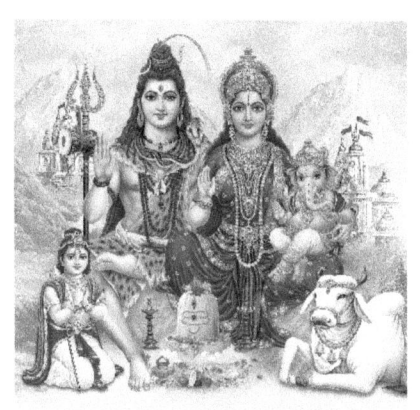

|| प्रार्थना ||

त्वमेव माता च पिता त्वमेव, त्वमेव बन्धुश्च सखा त्वमेव।

त्वमेव विद्या च द्रविणं त्वमेव, त्वमेव सर्वम् मम देवदेवं॥

|| महा मृत्युंजय मंत्र ||

ॐ त्र्यम्बकं यजामहे सुगन्धिं पुष्टिवर्धनम्।

उर्वारुकमिव बन्धनान् मृत्योर्मुक्षीय मामृतात्॥

|| नवग्रह मंत्र ||

ॐ ब्रह्मा मुरारी त्रिपुरांतकारी भानु: शशि भूमि सुतो बुधश्च।

गुरुश्च शुक्र शनि राहु केतव: सर्वे ग्रहा शांति करा भवंतु॥

Disclaimer

The stories and perspectives presented in **'My Marriage : Bliss vs Curse'** are the personal reflections, experiences and opinions of the individual co-authors. This anthology does not intend to provide professional advice or counselling on relationships or marriage. Each contribution is a unique narrative, shaped by the author's own journey, cultural background and life experiences.

Readers are encouraged to approach the content with an open mind, understanding that every marriage is distinct and what is shared here may not apply to all situations or reflect the views of every reader. Any actions taken based on the content of this anthology are the sole responsibility of the reader. If you are seeking guidance or support in your personal relationships, please consult a qualified professional counsellor/ advisor.

The publisher, compilers and co-authors are not responsible for any actions or consequences that result from reading this anthology. This book is meant to be a source of insight and reflection not a definitive guide on marriage or marital relationships.

|| ॐ ||

Dedication

To everyone who has dared to say "I do."

This anthology is dedicated to the brave hearts, who have ventured into the sacred and unpredictable journey of marriage – to those who have tasted its sweetness and to those who have faced it's challenges.

To the married couples, who have found joy in each other's arms, to those who have weathered storms and to those who have gracefully let go – your own stories are the essence of this book.

To our 108 co-authors, thank you for your honesty, courage and willingness to share your personal/ unheard truths of marital life's journey. Through your voices, we celebrate the highs, acknowledge the lows and honour the complexities of the marital bond and to our readers, may you find comfort, understanding and perhaps a piece of your own story within these pages.

With deepest gratitude,

To the journey of love, fight and togetherness – in all its forms

|| ॐ ||

Preface

Marriage is a journey – often celebrated, sometimes questioned and always evolving. It is a tapestry woven from moments of joy and sorrow, triumph and defeat, understanding and confusion. In **'My Marriage : Bliss vs Curse',** we set out to explore this ancient yet ever-changing institution through the eyes of 108 courageous co-authors, who have dared to share their own truths of life and marital life as well.

This anthology is not a fairy tale. It is a candid exploration of what it means to commit to another person, to embrace both the beauty and the chaos that comes with living side by side. The stories found here do not shy away from the raw, unvarnished moments of life – the misunderstandings, the disappointments, the heartbreaks – nor do they diminish the sweetness of companionship, the deep bonds of friendship and the powerful moments of connection that make marriage a source of profound joy.

We often hear that marriage is a union of two souls, yet the reality is far more complex. It is a dynamic dance, where love and pain, laughter and tears, victory and struggle coexist, each shaping the other. This book is an invitation to witness that dance, to engage with the raw truths that make up the marital journey and to find resonance in stories that reflect the universal and deeply personal experiences of marriage.

As you turn the pages of **'My Marriage : Bliss vs Curse',** we invite you to set aside judgment, open your heart and immerse yourself in the wisdom, pain, humour and grace that each story has to offer. Whether you are newlywed, long married, divorced or somewhere in between. This anthology is a testament to the power of love, the endurance of the human spirit and the courage. It takes to be vulnerable in the face of uncertainty.

We hope that within these pages, you will find stories that resonate with your own journey, challenge your perceptions and perhaps even offer a moment of clarity or comfort. This book is for anyone who has loved, lost, hoped and endured – and for those who continue to believe in the transformative power of human connection.

Welcome to **'My Marriage : Bliss vs Curse'** – a collection of voices that remind us all that marriage, in its many forms, is a journey worth understanding.

|| ॐ ||

Acknowledgement

Creating **'My Marriage : Bliss vs Curse'** has been a journey as profound and complex as the very subject it explores. This anthology would not have been possible without the contributions, insights, and courage of many individuals, to whom we are deeply grateful.

First and foremost, a sincere thanks to our 108 co-authors. Your willingness to share your stories – stories of love, struggle, sacrifices, growth and endurance – has been the foundation of this book. Each of you has offered a piece of your heart, revealing the beauty and challenges of marriage with authenticity and vulnerability. Your diverse experiences have enriched this collection and provided a tapestry of perspectives that will resonate with readers from all walks of life.

To our families, friends and colleagues thank you for your unwavering support and patience throughout the creation of this book. Your encouragement, understanding, and belief in the importance of this project have kept us going.

Lastly, to every individual who has been a part of the journey of marriage – whether you have found joy, faced challenges or simply navigated the ordinary moments – you are the inspiration behind this anthology. This book is a tribute to the strength, resilience and profound humanity found within the bond of partnership.

Thank you, from the depths of our heart, to everyone who made **'My Marriage : Bliss vs Curse'** a reality. This book stands as a testament to the complexity of love and the enduring spirit of those, who continue to believe in its power.

With regards and heartiest gratitude,
Abhishaik Chitraans & Rainu Mangtani

|| ॐ ||

Contents

Foreword by Nivedita Basu..1

Foreword by Sidhharrth S Kumaar 3

Foreword by Sneha..5

Abhishaik Chitraans (Compiler) 14

Rainu Mangtani (Compiler) 16

1. Intense Love Beyond Words (Compiler's Pen) 17
2. Abhilasha Bhatnagar
   The Pieces Not Meant to Fit Together 20
3. Acharya Madhu B Chawla
   Bond to be Free 23
4. Aditya Ujjwal
   Why Do Marriages Fail? 26
5. Aekta Doshi
   Marriages are Made in Heaven 29
6. Akanksha Rebecca George
   Forever Us 32
7. Amrit Kaur
   Lifetime Partnership or Agreement 35
8. Anita Gupta
   Relationships are Divinely Destined 38
9. Anu Chauhan
   Love is Never Enough 41
10. Anuradha Bijawara
    My Marriage Was, Is and Will Be 43
11. Archana Nadella
    An Experiential Journey 45
12. Archana Nair
    In the Garden of Togetherness 47
13. Aruna
    A Delicate Balance Between Joy and Sorrow 50
14. Avneet Chaudhary
    Unique Sense of Companionship and Partnership 52
15. B D Surana
    Way to Family System 55
16. Baljit Jaggi
    Mr. & Mrs. Perfect to Help Each-Other 58

17.	Bhavana M Patle How I See a Marriage	61
18.	Binita Nandi Under One Sky	64
19.	C. P. Belliappa A Tight Rope Walk	67
20.	CA Meenaz Cyrus Surty Grief to Gratitude	69
21.	Deepa Jain Psalm of Life	72
22.	Deepti Sood From Wife to Wonder Woman	74
23.	Divvya A Singh Wedded Bliss or Near Miss	76
24.	Dr. A S Poovamma Marriage is a Part of Human Journey	80
25.	Dr. Agalya VT Raj Navigating the Peaks and Valleys of Wedded Life	82
26.	Dr. Anisha Mahendrakar Fate's Chains	84
27.	Dr. Ellakkiyaa Sankar Embracing Individuality in Togetherness	87
28.	Dr. Heena P Finding Strength in Adversity	89
29.	Dr. K.G.Veena A Bond of Mutual Respect	91
30.	Dr. Mahima Mohit Dand Our Story from Chennai to Hubli	93
31.	Dr. Mehjabeen The Life Journey of a Couple	96
32.	Dr. Navjot Kaur A Testament of Unwavering Support and Motivation	99
33.	Dr. Noothan Rao Wedding Day vs Married Life	102
34.	Dr, Priti Doshi Dual Opinion in One	105
35.	Dr. Priyadarshini MM Connect the Disconnect	107
36.	Dr. Shalini Garg The Sacred Union of Shiva and Shakti	109

37.	Giresh LD Chawda The Unique Journey of Marriage : Life From Imperfect to Perfect One	112
38.	Harishita (Vicky Chauhan) A Pathway to Transform Yourself	115
39.	Harsatvir Kaur Tips for Healthy Married Life	117
40.	Himani Bajaj Colors of Life	120
41.	Himani Verma Tradition Meets Modern Love	123
42.	Isha Singh Embracing the Imperfect Beauty of Marriage	125
43.	Jiggna B Bhatt The Blessings instead of Curse	127
44.	Kala Malpani Balancing Dualities in Marriage	129
45.	Kalpana Priyadarshi A Lifetime Companionship	132
46.	Kanan Jolly Bliss if you Notice	135
47.	Kanchan Lakhwani Are All The Mothers-in-law Devils?	137
48.	Kavitha Bhutada A Dance Between Heaven and Hurdles	140
49.	Keerthika Best Friends for Life	143
50.	Kiran Yadav The Journey	145
51.	Lalit Sharma Shaadi Ka Laddoo	148
52.	Leena Lalwani A Beautiful Relationship	150
53.	Lipiie Banerjjee A Story of Endurance and Bliss	153
54.	Madhu Soni The Knot That Binds	156
55.	Manissha Shah Marriage is a Learning, to Enjoy the Differences	159
56.	Mayur Ghate The True Essence of Married Life	162

57.	Mehul Gupta The Double-Edged Sword	164
58.	Mini Baijal My Marriage – My Lifeline	167
59.	Neelam Khemani Marriage is a Blissful Curse	169
60.	Neena Puri Nagpal Marriage Through My Eyes	171
61.	Neetu A Beel Tides of Togetherness Embracing Growth in Marriage	173
62.	Neha Piyush Nashine Bliss or Curse – Depends on In-Laws	175
63.	Nidhi Chugh The Dual Nature of Marriage	178
64.	Nimishaa Mathur Learn from Mistakes	181
65.	Nitender Mann A Journey of Support and Stability	184
66.	Om Prakash Priyadarshi A Self Registered Bond of Trust	186
67.	Pooja Gulati Marriages are Made in Heaven	189
68.	Pooja Saxena Balance of Personal Aspirations and Family Duties	191
69.	Pragya Sharma Love, Laughter and a Merrily Ever After	193
70.	Priyaa Chauhan A Union of Bliss and Challenges	195
71.	Priyanka Sapraa Every Heart Sings a Song	197
72.	Prof. Sarojini Gupta Biddanda A Beautiful Married Life	200
73.	Promila Devi Sutharsan Huidrom The Eternal Connection	202
74.	Punam Vishwkarma A Bond of Love	204
75.	Radhika Devgan Composed of a Single Soul Inhabiting Two Bodies	207
76.	Raghunandan Chowdarapu (Raghu NC) The Joy of Wedded Life	209

77. Rahul Churi
    Marriage is a Toss 211

78. Reva Sarangal
    Marriage is a Boon 214

79. Rita Sehgal
    Journey To Bliss.. 217

80. Rohan Jain
    The Epitome of Love and Togetherness... 220

81. Rohet B Kummbar
    Marriage Can Become an Obstacle to the Spiritual Path 222

82. Romi Maakan
    A Blessing Disguised as a Curse 224

83. Sadhana Athinamilagi
    Tying the Knot: The Ebb and Flow of My Marriage 227

84. Sapna Gaurav Gupta
    Embracing My True Self 229

85. Sharlet Seraphim
    A Journey of Acceptance 232

86. Sheetal Pratik
    A Beautifully Created Real Bliss 234

87. Shelaj Kant
    Freedom in Relationship 237

88. Shelly Arora
    A Beautifully Created Real Bliss 240

89. Shetall G Desai
    Husband is a Powerful Pillar 243

90. Shikha Meher
    Will Meet Again… 245

91. Shipra Goswami
    Our Marital Journey 247

92. Shweta Singh
    When Handled Right, A Dynamic, Else A Dynamite... 250

93. Sri Rajeshwari Devi
    Sapthapadi... 253

94. Sudha Krishnan
    The Seven Sacred Vows of Unity and Love... 256

95. Suvigya Seraphim Raj
    Union of Two Souls Embracing Each Other's Imperfections 258

96. Suyog Patil
    Children vs Marriage Wed-Lock 260

97. Tanvee Kakati
    A Bliss or Burden? 263

98. Tejjal Bhanshalii
    From Despair to Healing : Embracing Obstacles as Blessing 266

99. Trina Kanungo
    Arranged Marriage : An Unexpected Recipe for My Life 268

100. Uman Hooda
     Essential base of Life and Happiness 270

101. Vaishali S Iyer
     A Beautiful Journey of Learning 273

102. Veena Chugh
     Marriage : The Gamble of Love 276

103. Veenu Mehendiratta
     A Journey of Efforts and Blessings 279

104. Vijay Jain
     The Blissful Beginnings 283

105. Vijayshri Panchikal
     An Unique Experience of Joy & Sorrow 286

106. Viji S
     Clues to be a Cheery Couple 288

107. Vinieta
     Marriages are Made in Heaven 290

108. Vishal Sachdev
     The Bliss Called Marriage 294

Blurb 297

Gratitude to Readers 298

Kindly Connect with Us 299

List of Books 300

Foreword by Nivedita Basu

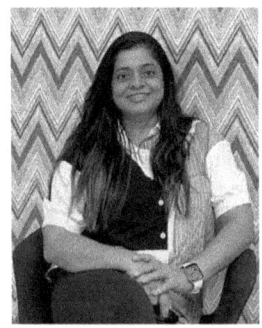

Marriage – such a simple word, yet so complex in its meaning. It carries the weight of tradition, the promise of companionship, and the challenge of navigating life's unpredictable journey hand in hand. When I was asked to write this foreword for **'My Marriage : Bliss vs Curse'**, I was instantly drawn to the idea of an anthology that doesn't shy away from the dual nature of this sacred institution. It is an honour to introduce a book that so openly explores the highs and lows, the love and pain, the bliss and challenges of married life.

This anthology of 108 voices is not merely a collection of stories, but a reflection of what it means to be human – to connect, to endure, to grow. Each narrative is a testament to the courage it takes to commit to another person, to weather the storms and to savour the joyful moments that make it all worthwhile.

I have always believed that the most powerful stories come from a place of truth. In **'My Marriage : Bliss vs Curse'**, the contributors have bared their souls, allowing us to witness their deepest fears, their greatest joys and everything in between. These stories are raw and real, full of the vulnerability that comes with sharing one's own experiences. They are not about perfection, but about the authentic realities of relationships—the small victories, the painful compromises, and the unexpected blessings.

For anyone, who has ever been in a relationship, this book will resonate deeply. For those who are married, it will offer a sense of solidarity and understanding. And for those who are curious about the nature of marriage, it will provide a window into the realities that lie behind the ceremony. This anthology is not about offering solutions or prescribing ideals; it is about sharing human experiences with all their imperfections and beauty.

I hope you find in these pages a sense of connection, a feeling that you are not alone in your journey. Whether you are in a marriage that feels like bliss or one that has tested your limits, may this collection serve as a reminder of the enduring strength of the human spirit and the incredible capacity of love to heal, inspire and transform.

Congratulations to all 108 contributors/ co-authors, who had the courage to share their stories and to **Mrs. Rainu Mangtani** and **Mr. Abhishaik Chitraans** who have collected that wonderful articles/ stories that show the different aspects of married life, beautifully woven these diverse voices together. I am truly honoured to be a part of this remarkable project.

With best regards and blessings,

Nivedita Basu

Writer, Creative Director, Producer

Nivedita Basu is a well-known figure in the Indian Television Industry. She is living a happy married life with her caring husband Mr. Yadunath Bhargavan (Advocate) and also a lovely mother of a cute baby girl Oyshee Yadunath Karimbil. She has made a significant mark as a Producer, Creative Director and Content Developer. Over the years, she has worked on several popular TV shows and projects, playing a key role in shaping content for Indian television audiences.

Currently, as the Vice President of content, business alliances at **Atrangii Group** and owns a celebrity cricket team namely **Kolkata Baabu Moshayes** on the television reality show Box Cricket League.

Nivedita Basu is responsible for overseeing the creative direction, content development and programming strategies for the channel. Her background in the entertainment industry and experience with successful TV productions makes her a notable figure in the industry.

॥ ॐ ॥

Foreword by Sidhharrth S Kumaar

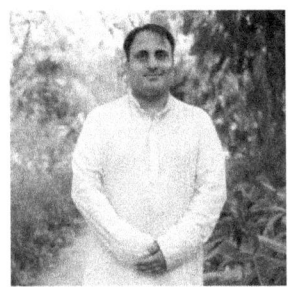
For millennia, human interactions have revolved mostly on marriage as an institution. This is the best kind of cooperation, the one we think will help us across the ups and downs of life. What then occurs when the reality of marriage deviates from our ideal vision? **'My Marriage : Bliss vs Curse'** boldly enters this area and presents 108 different points of view that expose the intricacies of one of the most personally intimate yet generally shared events of life.

Neither is this anthology a warning tale of doom nor a sugar-coating of matrimony. It finds a careful balance, honoring the pleasure of company without sacrificing the times that could seem more like a curse than a gift. And this is the beauty of this collection—it enables you to view marriage as a real, breathing organism that develops, falls, and sometimes soars rather than through a prism of perfection.

This book's quality that it doesn't pretend there is one "right" approach to negotiate marriage appeals to me. Rather, it presents an experiential tapestry. These tales serve as a reminder that every marriage has unique set of difficulties, successes, and lessons; no two are the same. Certain stories will be familiar to you, like a mirror reflecting your own path; others may provide insights into the marriages of others, maybe inspiring you to say, "I never considered that."

These pages will provide a welcome honesty—an openness about the challenges that occasionally cause us to doubt the fundamental basis of our relationships and the successes that justify all the effort. This book emphasizes how marriage is significantly more than the fairytale ends we see on television. It's about the daily, the ordinary, the magical, and the times between when we have to constantly decide to remain dedicated to one another.

This book might not offer somebody seeking a blueprint on how to make a marriage work exact step-by-step directions, which is a wonderful thing. Rather, it provides something far more worthwhile—wisdom. From those who have seen both the delight and the grief, the laughter and the tears, and still find value in the trip, the kind of wisdom that results from living experience.

'My Marriage : Bliss vs Curse' honors the complexities of marriage. It not only depicts what happens when everything goes according but also shows compassion for what happens when things go wrong, when the fractures surface, and when couples have to face difficult problems squarely. And in doing this, we are reminded that often the strength and lifetime of a partnership are defined by these very challenging but vital events.

Let yourself be receptive to the many experiences found on these pages as you travel over 108 viewpoints. You could find comfort, support, and perhaps the drive you need to keep working through your own relationships. This book does not pretend marriage is easy; marriage is not easy. It does, however, demonstrate how one of the most fulfilling relationships we will ever know may result from love, patience, and a readiness to grow.

So back off, plunge in and let these tales develop right around you. **'My Marriage : Bliss vs Curse'** has something to offer everyone, an invitation to explore the highs and lows, the bliss and the curses, and finally, the unbreakable links that make marriage a trip worth traveling—regardless of how long you have been married or how recently you are starting to consider the concept.

With Love Light and Blessings,

Sidhharrth S Kumaar

Founder, NumroVani

Sidhharrth S Kumaar is a biopharma strategy consultant transformed into Astro Numerologist, Life & Relationship Coach, Energy Healer, Music Therapist and Brand Growth Consultant with a proven experience of around a decade.

He is the Founder & Chief Happiness Officer at **NumroVani,** who is on a mission to improve the happiness quotient in life by leveraging his proprietary 3P formula i.e. Proactive, Preventive and Personalized based on synergistic combination of Astrology, Numerology and Vedas with Modern Science.

He is known for innovations in baby name, wedding astrology and astrology for business. He has published 20+ research papers, 2 Books, and 20+ Research Guest Lectures at UGC- approved universities and has guided numerous people and brand in their growth journey. He also has one published patent in his credit and has guided people from all walks of life to become their best version.

Sidhharrth is also a TEDx Speaker (Youngest Numerologist globally to be one), Josh Talks Speaker, Fit India Champion and an avid writer on the subject. He has been felicitated with many recognitions, including the Times 40 U 40, ET Wedding Leader Award, Times of India Leaders of Tomorrow Award and Ayushcon Excellence Award.

|| ॐ ||

Foreword by Sneha

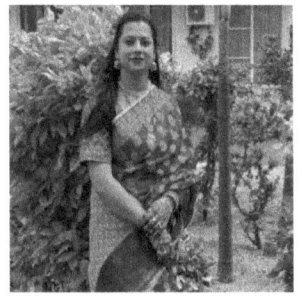

One word that has the weight of countless feelings aspirations and promises is marriage. Though as unique as every pair who enters its holy tie, this union is as old as time itself. In **'My Marriage : Bliss vs Curse'**, you're not only reading stories; you're entering a world where the complexity of love, friendship and the unavoidable obstacles of life are exposed with unvarnished truthfulness and gentle contemplation.

The capacity of this anthology to address every phase of married life really speaks to me. From the times of pure delight when two souls seem to dance in perfect unison to the times when the dance stumbles and life's challenges front stage. It doesn't hold back when showing marriage as it is: a complex mix between wishes achieved and dreams postponed, between happiness and struggle.

With 108 points of view, we see the ups and downs of marriage from moments of joy to the challenges that test us. **Mrs. Rainu Mangtani** and **Mr. Abhishaik Chitraans** have brought together this collection of stories/ articles that show both the happiness and struggles of marriage. These 108 stories/ articles help us understand how love, patience and resilience shape our relationships every narrative acts as a mirror reflecting the highs and lows of relationships to which everyone may identify. These stories encourage us to see, to feel, and to consider; they do not teach or criticize. They gently remind us that often in marriage as in life, we negotiate the toughest storms by means of endurance, forgiveness and a strong will to love.

The honesty of this anthology is what appeals most about it. It does neither minimize marriage to constant conflict nor show it through rose-colored glasses. Rather, it catches the core of what marriage is—a dynamic trip that demands much of us yet pays off in ways we cannot usually forecast. It's about realizing that the curse and the bliss are often entwined and learning how to negotiate that conflict can help you to make the trip very worthwhile.

'My Marriage : Bliss vs Curse' will speak to you whether your marriage is fresh, you travel frequently in the realm of wedlock, or you are someone considering the secrets of this age-old institution. Though most significantly they will cause you to reflect carefully on the continuing power of love and the strength needed to sustain it. These stories will make you laugh, they will make you cry.

Let yourself relate to the universality of these experiences as you flip every page. This collection reminds us greatly that in the complexity of marriage we frequently discover our actual selves and celebrates the victories and hardships of love.

Thus, start this road and enjoy every narrative. These pages represent life itself rather than only a mirror of marriage.

With the best wishes

Sneha

Founder, GrowthBeats Communications

Sneha is a management professional with around half a decade experience into People Management transformed into a relationship coach with proven experience of around half a decade in the same. She is Founder of **GrowthBeats Communication**s and Managing Chairman of **Haneeka Foundation**, where she devotes her time to women empowerment by facilitating health and education for girls and women all across globe. Sneha is also a mother of cute baby girl **Haneeka S Sandilya.**

॥ ॐ ॥

|| ॐ भूर्भुवः स्वः तत् सवितुर्वरेण्यं भर्गो देवस्य धीमहि धियो यो नः प्रचोदयात् ||

Marriage is an art of turning challenges into stories of resilience, where every sacrifice deepens the bond and every struggle fuels enduring inner love and growth.

– Rainu Mangtani

Marriage is a union of two souls, yet the reality is far more complex. Actually, it is a union of two families as well as culture with a dynamic dance of two individuals, where love and pain, laughter and tears, victory and struggle coexist, each shaping the other.

– Abhishaik Chitraans

|| ॐ ||

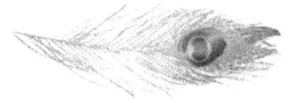

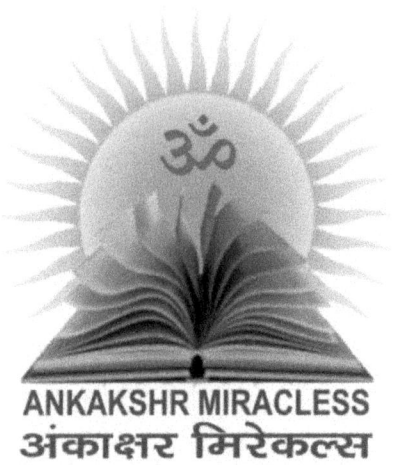

ANKAKSHR MIRACLESS
अंकाक्षर मिरेकल्स

The Institute of Occult Sciences, Spiritual Activities and Research
Regd. by Ministry of MSME, Govt. of India
ISO 9001:2015 Certified
IVAF & AAA (USA) Recognized

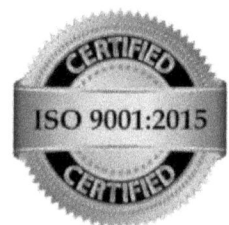 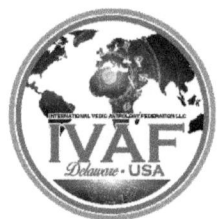

IVAF : International Vedic Astrology Federation (USA)
(An American Organization of Research)
AAA : Astrological Academic Alliances (USA)
(The World's Best International Astrology Forum

www.abhishaikchitraans.com

The Family of Visionary Co-authors

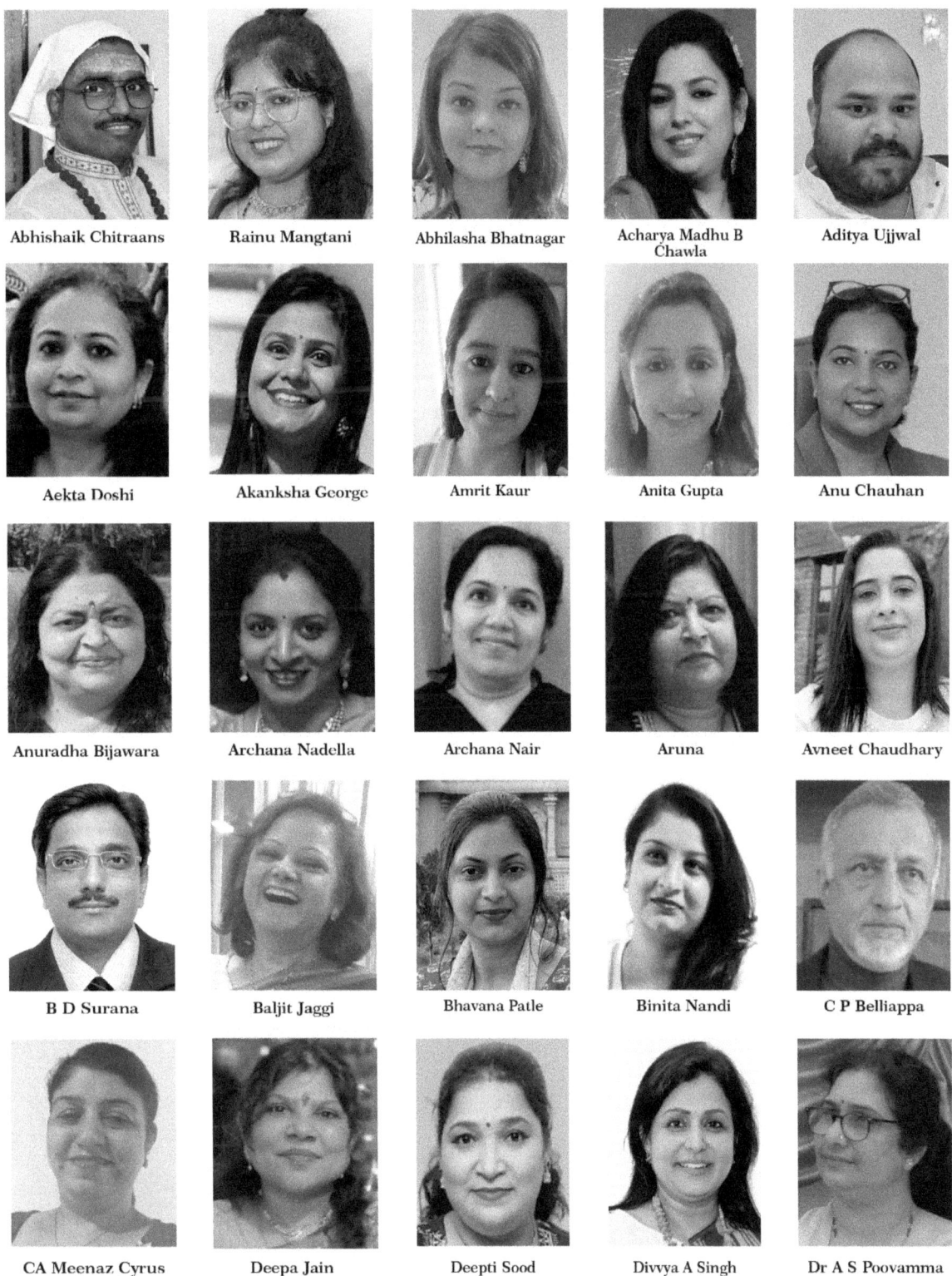

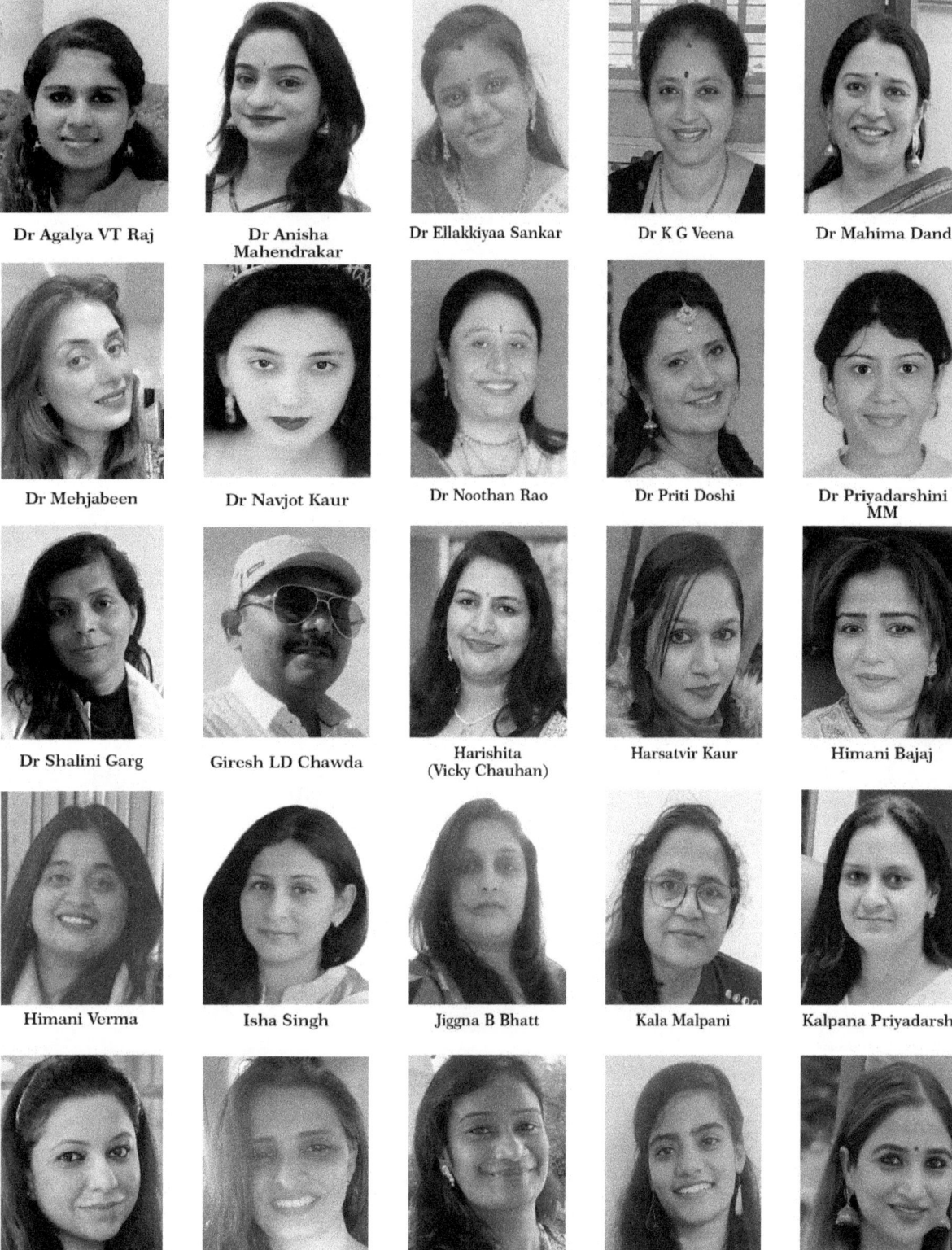

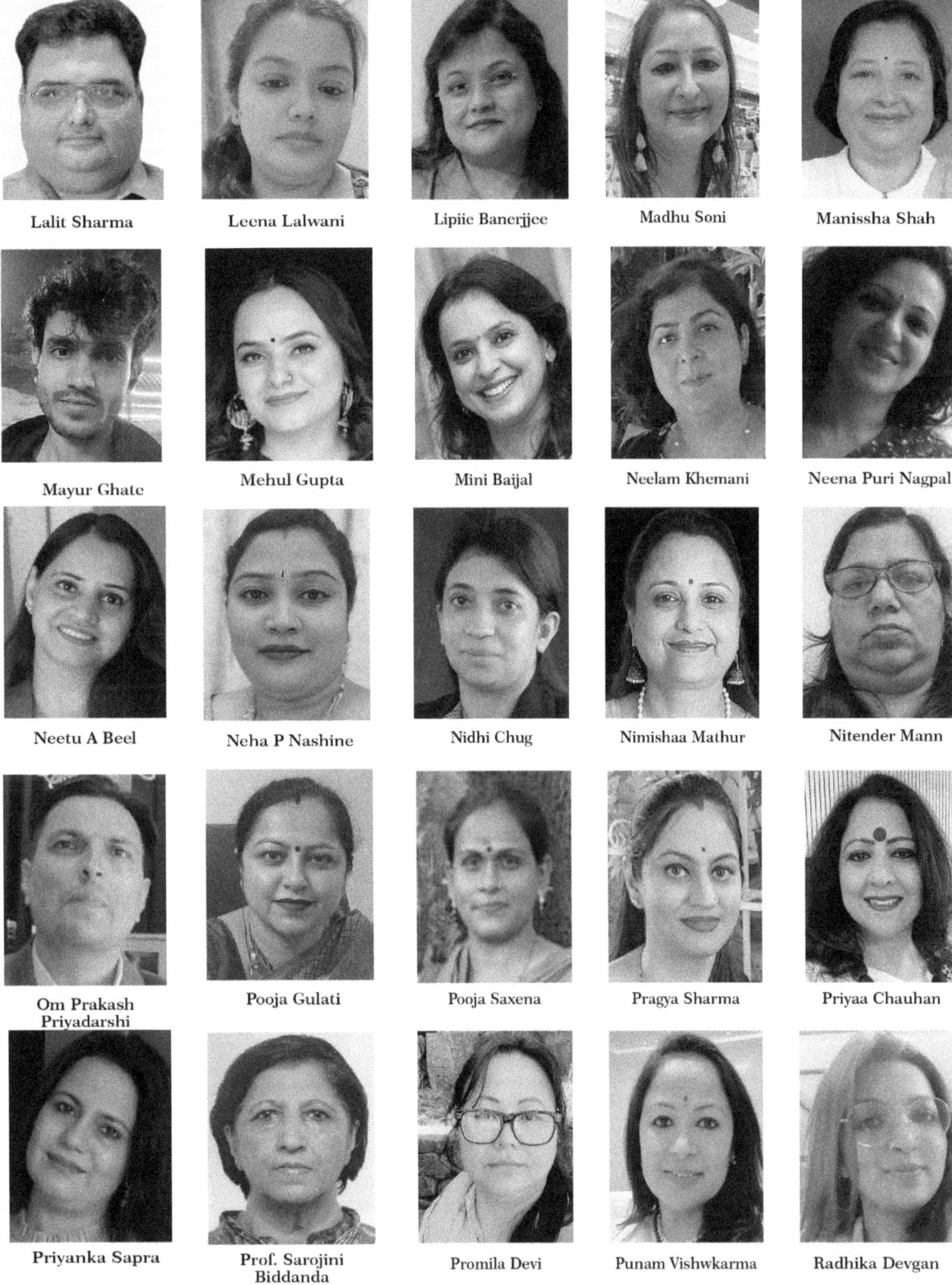

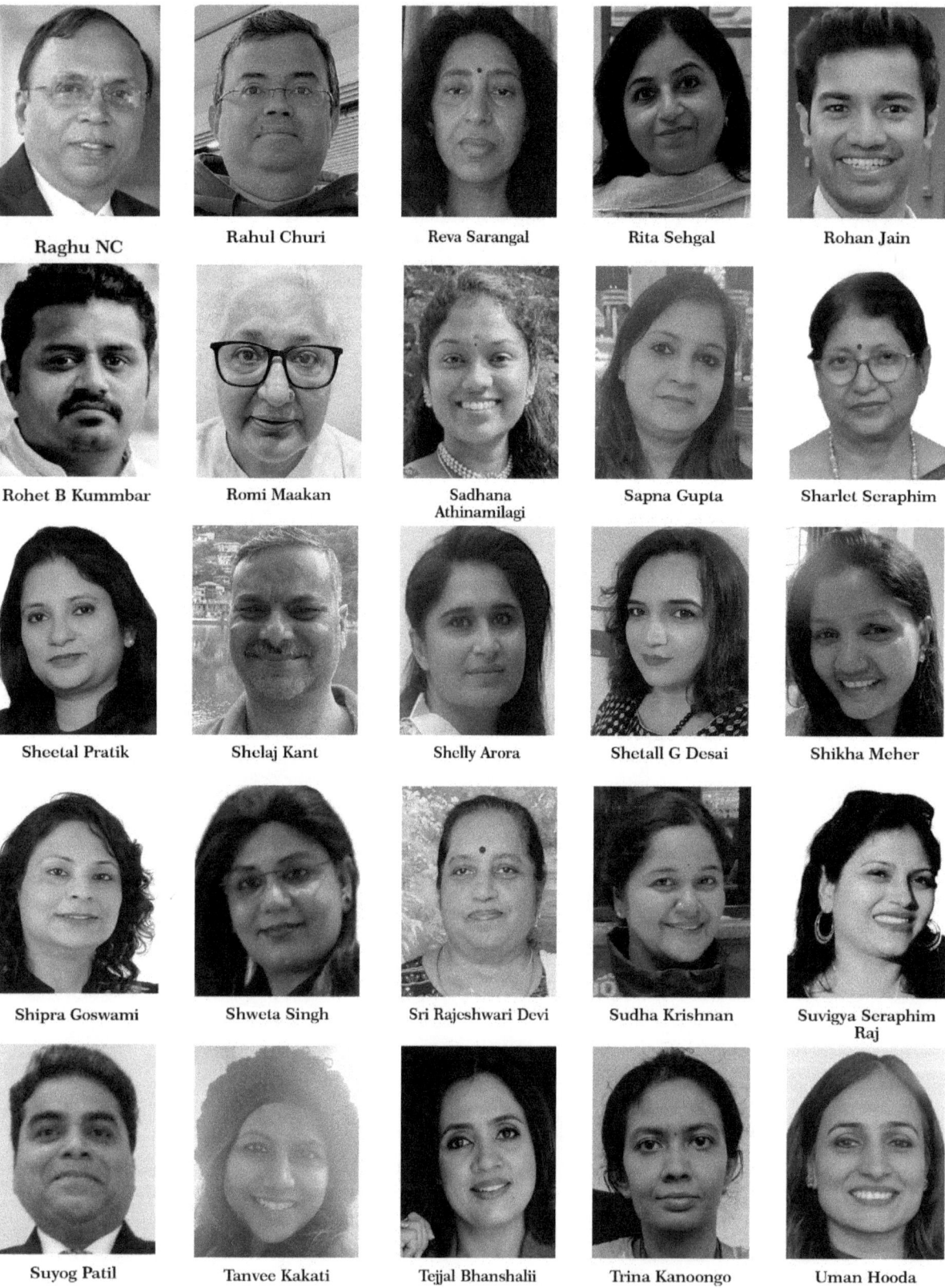

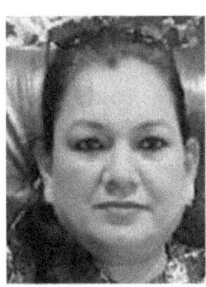 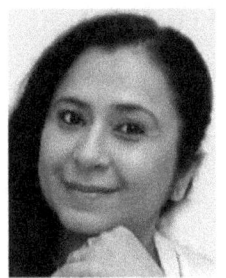 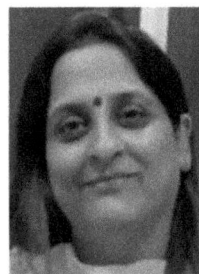 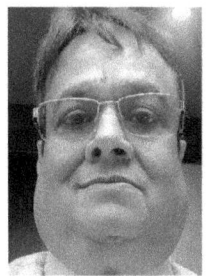 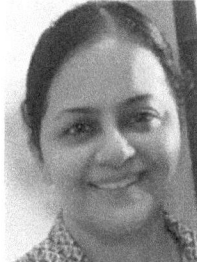

Vaishali S Iyer   Veena Chugh   Veenu Mehendiratta   Vijay Jain   Vijayshri Panchikal

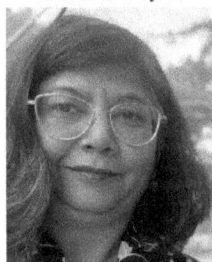 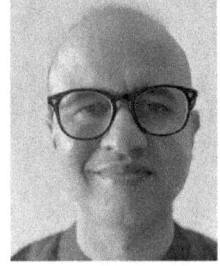

Vinieta   Vishal Sachdev

|| ॐ ||

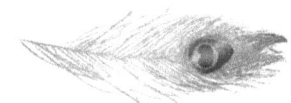

Abhishaik Chitraans

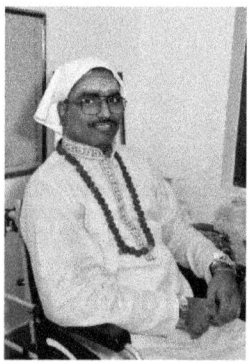

Abhishaik Chitraans is a distinguished numerologist, educator and internationally renowned published author, poet, expert columnist, philosopher as well as the visionary Founder and CEO of **Ankakshr Miracless,** *The Institute of Occult Sciences, Spiritual Activities and Research,* an institution registered by the Ministry of MSME, Government of India and certified with ISO 9001:1015. Recognized by IVAF (International Vedic Astrology Federation) & AAA (Astrological Academic Alliances), USA. *Ankakshr Miracless* stands as a testament to Abhishaik's commitment to advancing numerology on a global scale. He is celebrated as the only numerologist worldwide to develop over five unique numerological formulas, combining the principles of BODMAS (mathematics) and physics to calculate life paths through date of birth. His contributions have set a new standard in numerology and his research has been published in over 10 international journals and prominent astrological magazines, including presentations at UGC-approved universities.

With three master's degrees in Commerce (M.Com.), Economics (M.A.) and Business Administration (MBA), Abhishaik brings a profound understanding of both academia and practical expertise. His professional journey spans more than a decade in high-level finance roles, including as Deputy General Manager of Accounts, Banking & Finance and an Internal Auditor with a top-10-ranked shipping cargo company in Africa and the Gulf region. However, his career took a remarkable turn in 2009, when he was diagnosed with *'Transverse Myelitis',* an untreatable condition that has left his lower limbs paralyzed. Despite this, he continues to excel and inspire, earning the moniker **'The Bed Traveller'** for his resilience and dedication to his life's mission.

In addition to his professional achievements, Abhishaik has become a Certified Professional Teacher, with a significant educational impact. He has guided over 1,000 Students/ Clients across 10+ countries, offering insights and consultations in numerology that span the globe. His published works include more than 30 articles on numerology and name numerology across leading magazines and online platforms.

Abhishaik's excellence and dedication have been widely recognized with numerous awards:

- World Record Holder for an International Poetry Anthology on Zodiac Signs
- First Prize in a state-level article writing competition by PCRA in Uttar Pradesh

- Excellence in Numerology & Research by ISA
- Jyotish Gaurav, Astro Diamond, Manavta Ratn, Vishisht Hindi Sewi, Sahitya Alankar Samman, Thai Sri Buddha Maharshi Award and Maharshi Agasthya Award etc.

Abhishaik Chitraans exemplifies resilience, knowledge and global influence in numerology, continually enriching the field with ground-breaking insights, innovative methodologies and a passion for transforming lives.

|| ॐ ||

Rainu Mangtani

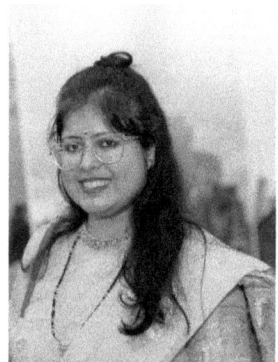

Rainu Mangtani, fondly known as *'The Versatile Iconic Personality'*, is a distinguished figure whose accomplishments span diverse fields, including banking, literature, content creation, and motivational speaking. A certified numerologist and graphologist with M.Com and IIBF Certification as a Digital Banker, Rainu has over six years of experience in the banking and insurance sectors, specializing in digital products for international clients and NRIs. Her professional expertise is matched by her impressive literary journey as a self-published and internationally recognized author, co-authoring over 25 books and compiling six anthologies that have highlighted over 500 voices.

Renowned for her dynamic presence, Rainu has graced multiple magazine covers, establishing herself as a true icon. She has been awarded titles such as *'Youth Icon'* by the Governor of Maharashtra and Asia's Top 30 Leading Women. She is an Expert Columnist, Best Author of the year 2022, Model Icon, Social Activist, World Record Holder, Perfect Author of year 2022, Best Content Writer of year 2023, Vlogger, The Celebrity Queen 2023, Brand Ambassador, Crown Girl, Speaker: Swell cast (Voice Over Artist). She's also the recipient of the prestigious National & International Dr APJ Abdul Kalam Awardee and got participation certificate for contributing her story to the world of cinema. As a finalist for CT Miss India International 2022, adding another dimension to her impressive repertoire recognized as *'The Celebrity Queen'*, a model and an inspirational figure.

Her works, ***The Height of Life in 24 Rains, Today's Corporate World (A Robotic Mechanism of Youth)*** and ***Ladder of Success,*** reflect her commitment to inspiring others

Rainu Mangtani is also a celebrated podcaster on **Ankakshr Miracless'** YouTube channel, a vlogger and an influential voice in the content creation realm. She uses this platform for empowerment and change, making her a beloved figure and an enduring *'Crown Girl'* in the public eyes.

|| ॐ ||

Intense Love Beyond Words
Blend of Humor and Realism

Compilers' Pen :

In *My Marriage : Bliss vs Curse,* celebrated authors Rainu Mangtani and Abhishaik Chitraans, a renowned as well as National and International Award-Winning Personalities, husband-and-wife duo, where the husband is Certified Master Numerologist, Internationally Renowned Published Author, Columnist, Motivational Speaker and Relationship Counsellor, who has transformed the lives of many global individuals and corporate business houses and his wife is Celebrity Queen, Ex. Banker, Internationally renowned author , Youth Icon Awarded by Honorable Governor of Maharashtra and much more offer readers an honest and thought-provoking journey through the complexities of *Married Life.*

Known for their profound insights into relationships, the compilers draw upon personal experiences and extensive research to present the dual nature and ups & downs of marriage. Their work masterfully explores both the blissful aspects of love, companionship and growth as well as the challenging facets like misunderstandings, compromises and conflicts that can test even the strongest bonds. Through relatable anecdotes and heartfelt reflections, they invite readers to contemplate their own experiences and find a deeper understanding of the commitment and resilience needed to sustain a fulfilling marriage.

Abhishaik Chitraans, a spirited soul from Bareilly (U.P) and **Rainu Mangtani**, a vivacious Mumbaikar are a match made in the Universe, tied together in love and companionship since June 2023. Their story began as two distinct worlds-colliding — Abhishaik's calm, introspective nature perfectly balancing Rainu's zest for life. Their lives have intertwined beautifully, combining the serenity of Abhishaik's spiritual mind-set with Rainu's vibrant personality. Since that fateful day they wed, they've woven a life that brims with love, laughter and a shared dedication to their work and beliefs. Their love is so profound that no argument ever holds them apart for long; when one is upset, the other finds a way to bring back joy, a testament to their unbreakable bond.

In February 2024, they made their mark at **World Book Fair**, Pragati Maidan, New Delhi, unveiling their much-acclaimed book, ***Deep Secrets of Name***, which explores advanced name numerology. The book captivated readers, offering insights into how names shape destinies, reflecting their dedication to spirituality and the occult sciences. United by their faith in God Shiva and Goddess Parwati, Abhishaik and Rainu embrace life's highs and lows with deep devotion and grace, bringing this spirit to their work at **'Ankakshr Miracless'**, *The Institute of Occult Sciences, Spiritual Activities and Research*, where, they guide others toward inner peace, balance, self-discovery, enlightenment and help individuals globally align with the universe's rhythm.

The newly married couple came up with the series of Anthology, where their first book with **51 co-authors** titled as '***Women Empowerment & Economic Developments***' was another hit and many more are on the way… As devout followers of God Shiva, Abhishaik and Rainu channel their faith into the work.

The couple also manages a popular YouTube channel namely **'Ankakshr Miracless'**, sharing knowledge and insights into numerology, spirituality and occult sciences, inspiring many to explore their inner selves through podcasts, reviews/ feedbacks and recording of online meetings and classes as well. Their passion for nurturing young talent led them to establish the **'Write-To-Earn'** community, where writers/ poets/ composers are rewarded for their contributions, fostering a space for creativity with a nominal annual registration as membership.

Living in a warm and close-knit joint family, Abhishaik and Rainu thrive in an environment that celebrates togetherness, wisdom and respect. Their story is a testament to love's power to elevate and transform a journey, where they evolve side by side, inspiring others and leaving a meaningful legacy for the future with eternal love, devotion and motivation.

Their journey isn't just one of personal fulfilment, but of community, faith and the beauty of togetherness. Their bond radiates love, proving that true partnerships grow through every shared vision, every laugh and every moment of unshakable faith in each other.

Marriage is the connection of two souls and which actually becomes one, when they get married. This Bonding has to be like where one feels thirsty for water, the other gets to know about his/ her thirst. So, we can say that this love is so intense, deep and above all it is beyond the words. This union goes far beyond the physical – It's a deeper emotional and spiritual connection that asks each partner to grow and adapt. When a marriage is seen as a journey of shared souls, it elevates both partners, transforming individual lives into a shared legacy of mutual respect, patience and boundless love. In this way, marriage remains one of life's most profound adventures, an experience that is indeed, as the quote goes, "beyond words."

In *My Marriage : Bliss vs Curse,* Abhishaik Chitraans and Rainu Mangtani illustrate that true marital happiness is a journey of resilience, understanding and unwavering love. They show that while marriage brings moments of unparalleled bliss, it also tests partners with challenges that can feel overwhelming. Yet, by embracing each other's flaws, supporting growth and prioritizing communication, couples can transcend struggles to find lasting harmony. Their story is a reallife example to the idea that marriage with all its ups and downs is ultimately a powerful and transformative partnership, where love deepens through shared experiences and mutual respect, but what is the actual reality behind their own Love-Story and Life's Challenges?

Stay tuned to read soon…

'With a blend of humor and realism, My Marriage : Bliss vs Curse is a powerful read that sheds light on the nuances of marital happiness and hardship.'

|| ॐ ||

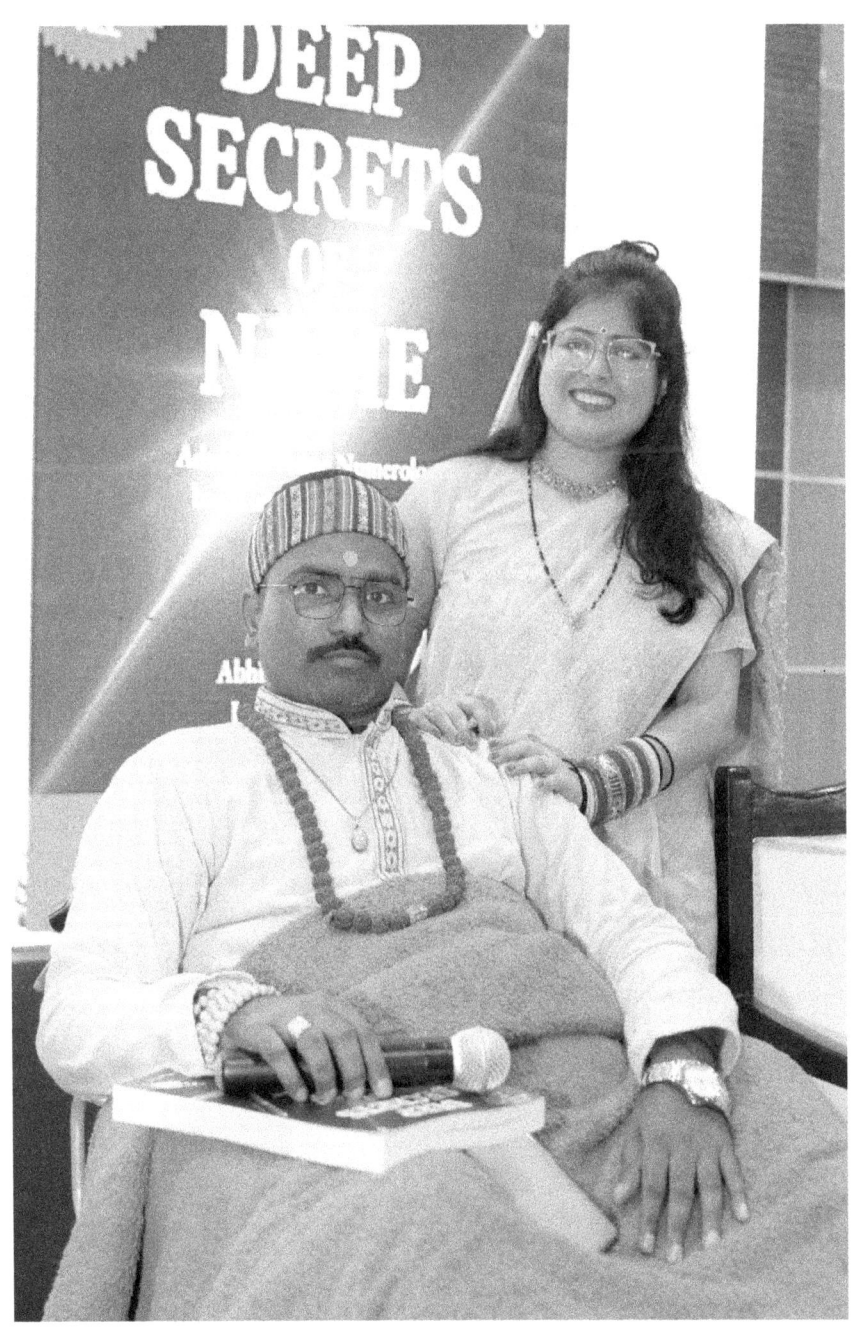

The Pieces Not Meant to Fit Together

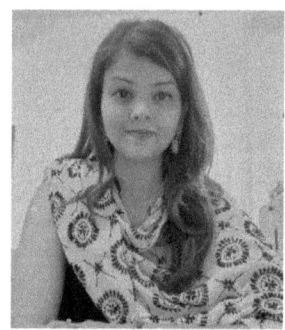

Author's Name	:	Abhilasha Bhatnagar
Qualification	:	M.Sc (Mathematics), M.Tech(IT), MCA, B.Sc Mathematics (Hons), B.Ed, CTET Qualified
Current Profession	:	Mathematics Facilitator
Age	:	38 years
E-mail ID	:	**bhatnagarabhilasha.17@gmail.com**
City/ Country	:	**Gurugram, India**

Abhilasha Bhatnagar is known for her strong academic achievements and creative talents, which highlight her dynamic personality and dedication to making a positive impact in education and culture. With triple Masters degrees in Mathematics (M.Sc.), Information Technology (M.Tech IT) and Computer Applications (MCA), along with a B.Ed. and CTET qualification, she exemplifies a deep commitment to education and continuous learning.

Her professional journey includes notable roles such as Lecturer at a college affiliated to IP University, Delhi and currently a Mathematics Facilitator, where she brings her expertise to inspire and educate students. Abhilasha is not only a proficient educator but also a budding author. She is also a recipient of the Global Teacher Award in 2021 by AKS Education Awards.

Her expertise extends beyond traditional teaching methods; she has been acclaimed as the "Online Teaching Supremo 2021" by Harper Collins, highlighting her innovative approach to digital education.

Outside academia, she is a multifaceted personality, having been crowned "Mrs. Congeniality 2015". She is also a travel enthusiast, who loves exploring new places and cultures.

Keywords : Coexistence, Divorce, Family Dynamics, Memorable, Personal Trauma, Turmoil

Marriage is an important life event that represents the union of two people in a legally recognized partnership. Marriage is like two sides of a coin, with both pleasant and unpleasant moments, coexisting in a delicate balance. Just like a coin, both sides are essential. Without one, the other loses its value. Embracing this dual nature, and actively working towards maintaining a healthy balance, a couple can lead a fulfilling and enduring relationship.

Rumi, an IT Professor and Sujoy, a young software engineer got married in an arranged marriage setup with the blessings of both families. Their marriage was filled with a mixture of both emotions, encompassing moments of joy, love and connection, as well as phases of conflict, misunderstanding and personal sacrifices. The adverse phases worked as a test of commitment, while the blissful moments brought them closer together and strengthened their bond. But in their share, blissful moments were fewer, yet each one was cherished deeply for its rarity and significance. They had frequent and intense fights over small issues as Sujoy was very short tempered and Rumi was way too emotional. This continued for more than 7 years, but one fine day, Sujoy decided to move out of this relationship, believing it would be better for him, Rumi and Swapn, as he thought the frequent fights between Rumi and him were taking a toll on Swapn and affecting his childhood adversely. Although Rumi was never in favor of his decision, she reluctantly agreed for the sake of her husband's peace of mind and with the belief that it would truly bring peace to her son's childhood.

Swapn, their 5-year-old son, was a bright and curious child with a sensitive nature. He inherited Rumi's intelligence and Sujoy's knack for technology, often showing a keen interest in gadgets and computers even at his young age.

However, Sujoy's decision to move out left Swapn feeling uncertain and vulnerable. He was deeply affected by the sudden change in his family dynamics, struggling to understand why his father is no longer living with them. Rumi moved to a smaller rented apartment with her parents because she could no longer afford the old one along with Swapn's school fees and daily expenditures. Rumi had been a housewife for the past 6 years after leaving her job when she became pregnant with Swapn. She also restarted her career as a school teacher after a 6-year break, which was stressful in addition to the personal trauma she was going through. This was because Sujoy had stopped all financial assistance for Rumi and Swapn from his side. But her parents offered her all the financial and emotional support she needed to normalize her life again.

After a year, Sujoy ceased all communication with Rumi and Swapn. Rumi also found peace in her life after the daily fights and turmoil, gradually adjusting to her new reality and focusing on rebuilding her and Swapn's lives. Nearly a year later, she bravely filed for divorce, sending papers to Sujoy's last known address. It took almost 2 years in court, countless emotional struggles, and a strong determination to dissolve their 7-year-long marriage, which had been built on the fragile foundation of an arranged setup and strained by frequent conflicts. Rumi was granted full legal custody of her son by the court of law.

For Rumi, this marriage was a mix of joy and sorrow, yielding the cherished love of her son, newfound independence and the social judgment of being labeled a divorcee. In moments of solitude, she reflects on the complexities of her journey, balancing the blessings and challenges that define her path forward. Rumi and Swapn were now living independently, fulfilling their dreams of traveling to new places together, enjoying peaceful weekends, going on dinner outings, taking ice cream drives, and making each moment memorable for both. They held a belief in their hearts that wherever Sujoy was, he too was at peace, enjoying his personal and professional life with satisfaction.

Whether this marriage turned out to be more blissful or a curse for Rumi, Sujoy and their son Swapn is ultimately left to the perspective of each reader. Sometimes the pieces of a puzzle we believe will form a beautiful picture are not meant to fit together.

Bond to be Free

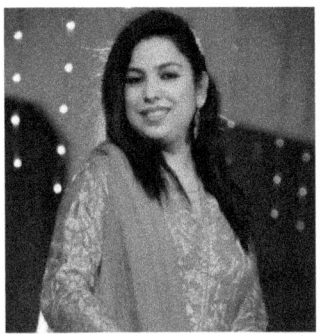

Author's Name	:	Acharya Madhu B Chawla
Qualification	:	M.B.A, MA in Astrology. Pursuing PHD
Current Profession	:	Numerologist & Astrology Consultant
Age	:	40 years
E-mail ID	:	**madhuchawlajpr@gmail.com**
City/ Country	:	**Jaipur, India**

Acharya Madhu B Chawla is a Renowned Astro-Numerologist from Jaipur Rajasthan, India, who specializes in using numerology to help individuals achieve their personal and professional goals. She has done her MBA. After that she has done Diploma from TISS-Mumbai on Child Protection & Diploma in CSR from Ministry of Corporate affairs. She had worked for 10 Years with NGOs & closely work & raise funds for many organizations & she was a trainer also. In 2016 she founded "Jeevan Sparsh Ngo" as she is keen interest & rich experience in development sector. She is into occult sciences since 2002, when she did Grand Master in Reiki in 2002. She has done Acharya (MA Astrology) and now Pursuing Phd In Astrology. She has great knowledge in different modalities like Numerology, Astrology, Vastu, Reiki.

She has mentored hundreds of students worldwide. She offers personalized consultations and coaching sessions to clients all over the world.

Acharya Madhu B Chawla believes that numbers are powerful tools for self-discovery and personal growth and she is dedicated to helping her clients unlock their full potential using the principles of numerology.

Keywords : Acceptance, Love, Respect, Responsibility, Silence

Everyone wants to be in a happy marital relationship. However happiness is not something, which makes marriage the most beautiful. Marriage can be beautiful, when both partners understand each other, love each other and most importantly respect each other, irrespective of the differences. It's really hard to find perfect partners and perfect relationships in any relationship, especially in martial relations.

I believe marriage is moreover a lifelong commitment, responsibility and equal partnership to carry responsibility for domestic things, as well as mutual respect and acceptance. It has always been seen that both men and women are different. Psychologically if you see both carry different perspectives to look up something. Men always have male ego, strong, dominating and aggressive behaviour. But if we talk about females they are emotional, sensitive and caring. This nature is because of male and female has different personality, but problems occur in relationships, when they don't accept each other's differences and start behaving in a particular way. They want to change each other rather than accepting them as they are.

Many times I have seen in the relationship they don't even communicate properly so that they can understand each other's point of view. The communication gap is the most dangerous thing in the relationship. Gradually they start assuming about each other and start making wrong perceptions. A healthy communication over a dinner date or during some personal time is very important. Many couples don't spend personal time with each other and gradually it turns into misunderstanding, communication gap, lack of acceptance and false beliefs etc.

In a relationship it's so important to listen to each other properly and try to help each other to make happy. Sometimes I have seen people are not in listening mode, they always want to speak rather than listening to each other. So gradually their conversation turns into arguments and gradually fights.

The next important thing I have observed is rather than convincing each other they try to dominate each other and try to impose things, gradually they start blaming others and relationships turn into separation.

Marriage is indeed a beautiful relationship and bonding if both partners have decided to love each other, forgive each other on small-small mistakes rather than blaming others and if anyone of them has made a mistake unconsciously so try to correct it, or forgive each other as we do with our children, rather than blaming. During my marriage, my guruji once told me, in a marriage relationship it works "when you see yourself in others eye" (एक दूसरे में खुद को देखना). And accept other people's mistakes as yours, as if we commit any mistake we forgive ourselves, so we should also ignore the partner's mistake rather than arguing or humiliate. One most important point I have observed if both partners are friends and carry good friendship, friendship is the pillar which carries fun, sharing, bonding etc. Then relationship can be long lasting, but for that they must spend quality time with each other. So it would be easier to live in a long lasting relationship. One last and most important thing which always saved my relationship is *silence*. In any relationship, when one partner gets angry or shout other one always should be calm & silent, so that it will never turns into arguments, disrespect, shouts and it will definitely help to save the relationship…this is the **Mool Mantra** to save the relationship- **"Silence"**

As in this era I have seen more broken relationships, separations and unhappy married' life. A little bit more understanding, acceptance, friendship and most importantly love can save them.

॥ ॐ ॥

Why Do Marriages Fail?

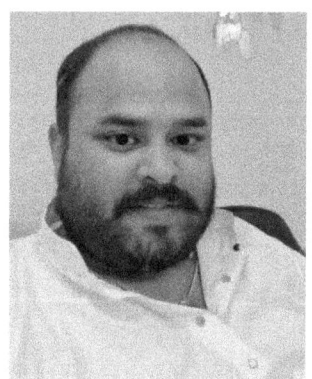

Author's Name	:	Aditya Ujjwal
Qualification	:	BBM, Masters in Astrology and Vastu
Current Profession	:	Businessman, Consultant
Age	:	31 years
E-mail ID	:	**adityaujwal7@gmail.com**
City/ Country	:	**Bangalore, India**

Aditya, hailing from Chapra, Bihar, holds a Bachelor's in Business Management (BBM) and a Master's Degree in Astrology and Vastu, showcasing his deep-rooted interest in spiritual sciences. Currently, he is expanding his knowledge by studying Numerology and Graphology. In addition to his academic pursuits,

Aditya is also a successful entrepreneur, running his e-commerce business, M/s Aditya Enterprises, which exports products internationally. His diverse expertise and entrepreneurial spirit make him a unique voice in the fields of spirituality and business.

Keywords : Commitment, Understanding, Value, Grihastha Ashram, Communication

To explore whether marriage is bliss or a curse, it's essential to understand what marriage truly means. It's more than a word from the dictionary; it's an institution rich in tradition, emotion, and responsibility. While we often think of marriage as joyous occasions filled with celebrations, laughter, and love, marriage goes far beyond the wedding day. It's about the shared life that follows. In this article, I will explain how my own marriage has been a true source of bliss.

For me, marriage has been a blissful journey. My spouse and I united under the wisdom and guidance of our elders, who laid the foundation for our union based on values, culture and tradition. In today's world of technology and artificial intelligence, these values have helped us build a strong, successful marriage.

Marriage is not just a one-time event—it's a journey of understanding each other and growing together. Coming from similar cultural backgrounds, our transition was smooth and we became each other's support system. Over time, we've drawn inspiration from our grandparents' and parents' strong relationships. They taught us the importance of loyalty and devotion, which became the bedrock of our own union. Our Hindu deities—Sita-Ram, Shiv-Parvati, Lakshmi-Narayan—serve as guiding lights, symbolizing the perfect love and partnership we strive to achieve. These ideals, passed down through generations, shape and strengthen our marriage every day.

Marriage at the right time brings stability and purpose to life. It provides a partner who genuinely supports you in tough times and celebrates with you in successes. In a world where fake friendships and superficial connections are common, a spouse is the one person who truly stands by you, wanting the best for you. I live by a simple rule taught by my Guru: We are here to play our role in life, and we must perform our duties diligently. As husband and wife, our role is to support each other and our families, which is the essence of **Grihastha Ashram**, the household stage of life in Hindu philosophy.

Why some see Marriage as a Curse ?

In my opinion, marriage is bliss when rooted in values and traditions. But why do some see it as a curse? The problem doesn't start after marriage; it often begins in adulthood. When individuals have multiple relationships or affairs before marriage, they lose the sense of stability and loyalty. It's like eating outside food regularly—you become accustomed to the excess and can't appreciate the simplicity of home-cooked meals. In relationships, some people lose the ability to appreciate a simple, stable marriage. The issue lies not with marriage itself, but with the absence of values like **Sanyam** (self-control), which can spoil everything.

Another reason people may view marriage as a curse is the influence of social media and unrealistic portrayals in movies. Marriage is about far more than fulfilling material desires—it's about being there for each other in every situation. Unfortunately, today's world often prioritizes wealth, status, and external pleasures over emotional connection. This mindset leads to dissatisfaction and infidelity, as people seek out others who can offer more. The interference of third parties, whether friends or family, can also damage relationships if not managed carefully.

In some cases, people lose the essence of marriage by neglecting traditional practices. Modern weddings that dismiss sacred customs—such as vegetarian food, refraining from alcohol, choosing auspicious times, and involving priests—often lead to superficial unions that don't last. The sanctity of marriage lies in these values, which ground the couple in their spiritual and cultural heritage.

How to make Marriage Blissful ?

To transform marriage into a source of bliss, we must in still core values from childhood. Children should be taught the importance of relationships and how to live with **Sanyam** (self-discipline). Shiva and Shakti, for example, represent the oneness and balance in marriage. When Sati Mata self-immolated after her father disrespected Shiva, it showed her deep love and dedication to her husband. This kind of devotion is vital in marriage, where individuality becomes secondary to partnership.

Consider the story of Maa Parvati's meditation to marry Shiva. When Narad Ji tested her by speaking negatively about Shiva and praising Narayana, Maa Parvati was unwavering in her dedication. She wanted only Shiva, despite the imperfections Narad Ji mentioned. This is the level of commitment needed for a marriage to succeed. True partnership thrives when both partners are dedicated to each other, regardless of external challenges.

Take another example from **Valmiki Ramayana**. When Lord Ram was exiled to the forest for 14 years, he instructed Maa Sita to stay behind and care for his family. Maa Sita swiftly responded that it was her duty to be with him, whether in the palace or the jungle. For her, being with her husband was heaven, and without him, even the palace would feel like hell. This unwavering love and devotion are the keys to a blissful marriage.

In conclusion, marriage can only become a curse if it is devoid of values and genuine commitment. It's not about being rich or poor examples like Bill Gates or celebrities like Hrithik Roshan show that wealth doesn't guarantee a successful marriage. True bliss in marriage comes from dedication, respect and following the path of **Dharma**, while nurturing values from childhood and marrying at the right time. When both partners are aligned in purpose, supporting each other through every challenge, marriage becomes one of life's greatest blessings, a source of stability, joy and fulfilment.

Marriages are made in Heaven
Is it Twin Flame, Soulmate or Karmic?

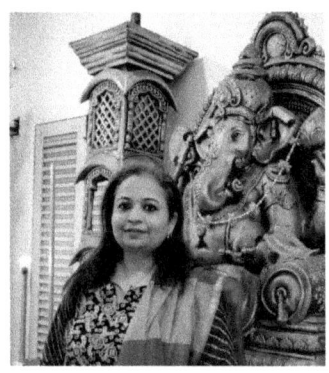

Author's Name	:	Aekta Doshi
Qualification	:	Home Science
Current Profession	:	Consultant and Counselor
Age	:	47 years
E-mail ID	:	**aad700@gmail.com**
City/ Country	:	**Mumbai, India**

Aekta Doshi has studied in Home Science followed by Diploma in Fashion Designing. She had been working in a Leading Garment Export house as a Merchandiser, but her family life & her passion for teaching made her an Entrepreneur and had established her Preschool Nursery for 6 years but due to health challenges it discontinued. After a break of 2 years she re-established her freelance academy namely **"Edify Education"** which trains Teachers through her experiences and prepare them to apply or establish their own academy. She also works as a Consultant in setting up Preschool Nursery & activity centre. She is a Graphologist, Handwriting expert and has authored cursive writing books for a publishing house and mentored to conduct Handwriting Competitions. Her passion for learning has driven her in the field of Occult Science. She is a Certified Numerologist, Bach Flower therapist, Tarot Card Reader, crystals and a remedial Vastu consultant and many more modalities as such for the betterment of the society.

Keywords : Family Behavior, Mutual Respect, Trust, Adaptability, Compromise

We don't choose our Parents, siblings neither our relatives but our life partner is Chosen by our own wish. Marriage is union of two hearts and soul. It's nature of being blissful or curse largely depends on how the couple mysteriously manages for their dichotomy. Various factors plays a significant role which comprises of individual Karma, your companionship and to support each other dreams, family behavior and stability, to manage conflict and stress, emotional and financial differences, Mutual respect towards each other, compromise, commitment to mutually grow, respecting each other independence, accepting the differences, adaptability, unresolved conflicts, love, trust and intimacy.

I am blessed to live in country like India and born in Gujarati family where seeds of marriage are rooted in the girls mind at a very early stage .at the tender age of 6 years I had fasted, followed puja rituals and ate unsalted food for 4 days followed by staying awake overnight and the last day which is celebrated by gifting articles to those who have followed this fast it is called "Morakaat" this is followed to owe a good life partner same way there are many such rituals & festivals which wives does for her husband like Jaya Parvati, Diwasa, Vaat Savitri Poornima, Karva Chauth, but no such customs mentioned for Husbands. And occasion of daughter's wedding is the most integral part for the family members. When a girl is grown up she is prepared to do household work, cooking and basic sacrifices.

The generation has changed now the priorities are different for the Genzee girls; they have started building up their career and are getting more of financial independent.

Why did this happen? One of the reason is they must have observed their mothers or any other female sacrificing the entire life taking for the family but still being financially dependent on their husband and not being praised by their spouse or the family members. Some people criticize or complain about the generation now; but I would say aren't we responsible to demotivate them to get married.

As I said earlier a girl starts dreaming about her spouse and things goes smoothly they find appropriate life partner lot of celebrations and expenses in wedding, photography, make up, clothes, food & ceremonies but does this solve the purpose of long term marriage? In my opinion Marriage is just not between two people, there are two different families involved in it. In India basically everyone prefers to get married in the same community, caste or religion and Love Marriage or inter caste marriage is a taboo. In Gujarat, basically everyone prefers to look for social status first and then financial status. May be any part of the world, I can't personally share my opinion since I haven't observed about it .In love marriages both the partners know each other but in arranged marriage it is very important for the family members to help the couple settle well. A girl never forgets 2 things in her life, one is how she is been treated in her 1st year of marriage and how is she been treated during her first child pregnancy. In my opinion when a girl after her marriage starts staying with her husband's family, it is a mere responsibility of the in-laws to cooperate well and help her to settle and adapt in the new surroundings. but the mentality was not like that earlier they expected the newly wed bride to take up household responsibility only to cook food, sacrifice in her dreams, tolerate unnecessary mood swings or ego of the family members, takes permissions for every little things, even to meet her parents, her friends whom the girl has spent her entire childhood with these are small matters, but when they don't understand the feelings then the marriage can turn out to be a major curse. Since I am a Bach flower therapist, I have heard many cases with emotional issues which can be easily resolved.

"When a Man truly loves his Wife, she becomes his weakness and when a Woman truly loves his Man, he becomes his strength. This is called Exchange of Power"

Title of the book is very beautiful; and I really appreciate the initiative about the book where we are free to share our opinions and I hope if this article which I have expressed in the form of two stories helps to improve some ones thinking pattern or any one's life, it would be a blessing to me.

Marriage is a very beautiful relationship out of all the relationships because it is chosen by you; your life partner can be your best friend, adapt to each other likes and dislikes, give freedom of their space, don't try to change them, respect each other and trust each other. Efforts should be from both the partners. Set your boundaries and limitations of tolerance of behaviors, before it turns to be disaster. It should not be termed as compromise, but it should be in the form of understanding; because it won't make any difference to all the external factors i.e. the friends, family or relatives, but if your partner is affected it is you who are the sufferer and vice versa. Stop the things before it's too late and the life can be very beautiful. If there are challenges try to resolve at its best. Separation is the most crucial emotion specially, if you have Children instead cursing each other try to find solution to the problems. Hire, Fire and Promote you are the own boss of your life.

Your marriage will be considered successful when your Children will be willing to get married seeing you as a Lovely Couple.

|| ॐ ||

Forever Us
A Thriving Marriage

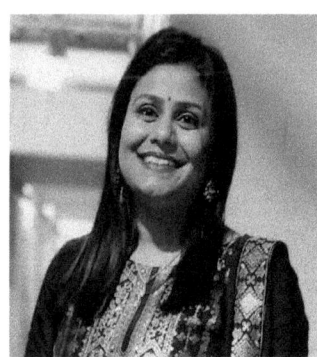

Author's Name	:	Akanksha Rebecca George
Qualification	:	B.Com., M.B.A.
Current Profession	:	Teacher, Avocational Writer
Age	:	36 years
E-mail ID	:	…
City/ Country	:	**Ghaziabad, India**

Akanksha Rebecca George is a wife and a mother of a boy. She is an orator and avocational writer. She has done her Bachelor of Commerce from Delhi University and completed her Master in Business Administration in Finance from SRM University.

After working a couple of months in the finance department of a prestigious organization, she realized her passion of imparting knowledge to others and her oratory skills. She started working as a corporate and soft skill trainer and then moved on to guide the children as per the education system. She is still working on molding the minds of children for a bright and fruitful life.

Keywords : Appreciative, Beautiful Union, Disagreement, Nurture, Respect

Marriage: Bliss or Curse? The question everyone is always confused about.

For some it's a blessing, which has made their life journey worthwhile and for some it's a bane in their life and for some it's both.

So first let's understand what is marriage? Basically, marriage is a beautiful union between two matured adults, who agree to take each other's responsibilities in all circumstances. It's solely an individual decision based on their emotional, social, economic, psychological and physical needs. These needs also vary as we grow.

As a child when I was in school, I never wanted to marry, when I started college, I began to give it thought and fantasized about the beautiful white gown I would wear and walk down the aisle with white and pink rose decoration, candles lit everywhere. Later when I started working, my friends were getting married, parents pressure, interaction with many suitable prospects, I realised that the real world is different from my fantasy world. I was very nervous and stressed out. After all it was about my entire life. I wanted a partner who was well settled with six figure salary, understanding, loving and caring. There was a time, when I was so exasperated, I agreed to get married to any 'TOM DICK AND HARRY' my family wanted. But there is a saying 'Marriages are made in Heaven', so was mine.

Out of nowhere, in 2014, I received an anonymous bouquet of red roses and a card on Valentine's Day with only a mobile no. mentioned. All my friend and I were very thrilled and excited to find this mysterious anonymous sender. We tried to contact the person using different numbers but didn't get any response. I thought someone must have been fooling around with me and closed the chapter. But later in the evening when I was on my way back home, I received the call from the same number, I was little scared but at the same time curious to know about my admirer. I answered the call not knowing that this anonymous caller would be actually my future life partner. And yes, now I am here, happily married to this anonymous bouquet sender from past 10 years.

So, if you ask me if marriage a 'Bliss' or 'Curse', I would definitely go with the former. Marriage is not a 3 hours movie wherein you fall in love, live with love and die in love. But it's a life long journey that thrives on love, commitment, trust, respect and communication. It is a relation of give and take.

When I said I am happily married and my marriage is a blessing, I didn't mean that we never had disagreements and conflicts with each other. We had our share of problems. Some major one being financial crunches, different work role at home and outside, clashes in upbringing of our child, prioritizing patriarchal family. There are many situations where we didn't see eye to eye at all. Many circumstances made us believe that it is best for us to part ways and make a clean break. Still, we both held steadfast to each other and plan to do that always.

My secret to a happy married life is the analogy of garden? I simply love it and connect it to my marriage. Just like you sow seeds in garden and patiently wait for it to bloom while tendering and nurturing it timely. In relationship too when you sow seeds of love, kindness and appreciation and nurture them with your actions and words, it thrives and grows to a beautiful garden. But you have to find right balance of attention and input. Over tend them, you will drive the person away and under tend them and your relation will wither and die.

With this analogy, I also learnt some more important points to nurture my relationship:

1. Be patient and persistent to build a strong relationship.

2. Be present wholly without any distraction to show love and kindness.

3. Be supportive and understanding to build confidence in each other

4. Communicate, be open and be honest to each other to build an emotional connection

5. Empathize, be appreciative and grateful to earn to respect

There is no perfect marriage. No one is perfect, we all have flaws. It is how you accept the differences and respect each other's individuality. Remember we must live by example. We get what we give!!! So, judge less, give more and love endlessly. Respect and gratitude are the foundation of marriage. Appreciation, empathy and communication is the network for thriving a healthy relationship.

॥ ॐ ॥

Lifetime Partnership or Agreement

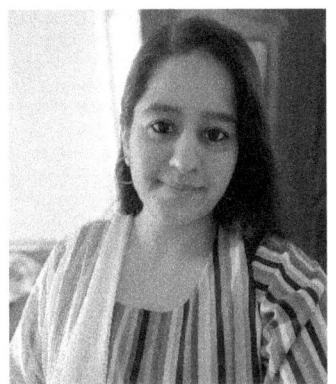

Author's Name	:	Amrit Kaur
Qualification	:	Diploma in Positive Mental Health
Current Profession	:	Tarot Card Reader & Vastu Consultant
Age	:	27 years
E-mail ID	:	**amritkaurmaan41@gmail.com**
City/ Country	:	**Pune Maharashtra, India**

VGM, Acharya Amrit Kaur, a 27-year-old author from Pune, Maharashtra, is a Professional Tarot Card Reader & Life Coach with over five years of experience. In 2024, she became the first youngest Vastu Grand Master & Vastu Acharya in Pune. She also won the **Indian Icon** of the Year award 2024 for becoming the best Vastu Consultant, Tarot Card Reader and Life Coach in Maharashtra.

Keywords : Freedom of Life, Compromise, Awareness, Perfect Partner, Decision Making

Marriage is a sign of partnership, not of compromise. Finding a good life partner has become a big question these days, hasn't it? Whether to opt for an arranged marriage or a love marriage is confusing! However, in my opinion, it is not a difficult task. Choose a partner, but don't forget to prioritize yourself, because we have never given ourselves priority and have always made decisions under the pressure of others. So, what difference does it make whether it is our family, relatives, society, or anyone else involved? If this continues, marriage, whether it is love or arranged, can become a blessing or a curse.

Is Marriage Compulsory?

The decision to marry or not should be a personal choice, free from any coercion. It is not true that if you don't marry, you won't achieve anything, and if you do, you'll gain everything. Is age increasing? Are others getting married? Do you need to start a family? Is it a societal norm to marry? One should never marry based on these thoughts. More important than name, bloodline or family is your mindset, behavior and conduct, which will provide the next generation with discipline, strength, knowledge and power.

Marriage is Bliss, if You Have a Life Partner

If one person alone is stronger than a hundred, they are called a life partner. This person will stand by your selflessly and will aspire to elevate you to greater heights. You and your self-respect will be top priorities for them. A life partner never worries about what family, relatives, neighbors, society or others will say; such a marriage is a blessing.

Marriage is a Curse, if You Have a Life Agreement

Where one person alone bears the burden of everything, you will find a life agreement. It includes fulfilling selfish desires, heeding society's expectations, demeaning loved ones, misunderstanding your dreams, and signs of being bound by constraints. Your freedom will be snatched away and you will feel suffocated in this relationship. Such a marriage is not a blessing but a curse.

Does a Perfect Partner Exist? How Do I Know?

No one is perfect in this world, but in my opinion, there are seven qualities. If you don't underestimate them, you can become a good life partner for someone else, or you can find a perfect life partner instead.

1. Practical

To run a marriage, it is very important to have practical bonding, because it demonstrates your thinking and how you can support each other.

2. Mental

It is essential to have mental stability in relationships because it fosters emotional balance, enabling mutual understanding and providing support during challenging situations.

3. Physical

Creating a physical bond is not necessary just for physical relationships; your physical health also holds significant importance. Your diet, strength, and overall health indicate a strong connection in any marriage.

4. Spiritual

Knowledge of spiritual matters is also necessary for you. It will guide you through future difficulties so that you can navigate through challenging situations, failures, and guilt.

5. Emotional

Strengthening emotional bonding is essential to understanding each other because it keeps relationships fear-free, builds psychological strength, and helps in understanding each other.

6. Materialistic

Being materialistic is also necessary to support each other because whether or not one exists, 90% of life's problems are solved through money.

7. Support

Trust, power and positive support have always been given importance in marriage because our confidence, dedication and steadfast perspective bring lifelong happiness in married relationships.

Now, What about Family, Neighbors, Relatives & Society?

People often say, "What will people say?" is the biggest disease. Every time we took a step for ourselves, society, family, relatives and others questioned us. If this continues, your life will become a puppet in the hands of others. While parents and relatives are our well-wishers, there are also enemies in the form of societal pressures, making life a gamble. The current generation gap is causing bitterness in family environments, where understanding each other properly is becoming difficult. If you remain mentally, practically and emotionally stable, your married life will certainly be a blessing, not a curse.

|| ॐ ||

Relationships are Divinely Destined

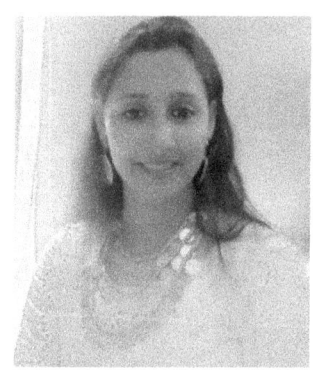

Author's Name	:	Anita Gupta
Qualification	:	M.A, B.Ed.
Current Profession	:	PYP Educator
Age	:	43 years
E-mail ID	:	**anitya1008@gmail.com**
City/ Country	:	**Gurgaon, India**

Anita Gupta, an IB PYP Educator at Delhi Public School, Ghaziabad Society, holds a Master's degree in Sociology from Banaras Hindu University along with a Bachelor of Education (B.Ed.) with extensive experience spanning over 15 years in teaching across various schools in Varanasi and Gurgaon. She is also trained in Nursery Education and proficient in educational technology. Anita is devoted to Lord Krishna and holds strong beliefs in spirituality.

Keywords : Marriage, Unique, Couple, Relationship, Well-being

Family Hardships :

"Marriages are said to be made in heaven, but I've been amazed to witness such unique relationships."

I come from a family where relationships were unconventional. My father married two women and regrettably, I was the daughter of his second wife. This uncommon family dynamic led to extensive hardship and disgrace for my mother, my brother and me. Remarkably, despite the complexities, we all lived together with love and warmth, a bond that persists even though my father is no longer with us. In this complex family structure, there were both positives and negatives, but I deeply admired my father's courage in facing societal and familial challenges. Yet, my sister's marriage and personal experiences made me skeptical of matrimony. By the time I turned 28, several marriage proposals had come and gone, none of which felt right. Many rejected me solely because of my lineage, adding to my disillusionment and depression.

My Awakening

I hit rock bottom, losing nearly 15 kilograms in weight, when my father suffered a debilitating stroke and was hospitalized for a month. His condition shook me awake, compelling me to care for him and to also start caring for myself. I resolved to rebuild my life and my spirit.

Pre-wedding nerves

Months later, a marriage proposal came through a relative. Despite my initial lack of hope, I agreed due to my father's health. Aditya, the prospective groom, was someone I had minimal contact with before agreeing to marry. We met in July and were engaged by October, during which time we barely communicated.

On our engagement day, overwhelmed by memories of past disappointments, I was nervous and tearful. Aditya's gentle request for my phone number provided a glimmer of relief. From that moment, he patiently and steadily comforted me, revealing his gentlemanly demeanor and family values. Despite of my initial fears, Aditya turned out to be genuine, contrasting sharply with my previous experiences.

Post-marriage Challenges encountered

We married on March 8th. Leaving my family behind was emotionally wrenching, but Aditya held my hand throughout, comforting and supporting me. His family, though conservative, also welcomed me with warmth. Adjusting to life in Delhi and finding a job were daunting tasks, but Aditya stood by me unwaveringly. Together, we faced challenges and nurtured our relationship with devotion and support. Aditya transformed my view of marriage from a **Curse to a Blessing** and I have found profound love and happiness with him.

In July of the same year, my father passed away and I was completely shattered. Despite the overwhelming grief and loss, Aditya stood firmly by my side. He provided unwavering support and took care of me with exceptional compassion and understanding during this difficult time. His presence and care were a source of immense comfort and strength, helping me navigated through the pain of losing my father. Aditya's steadfast support further solidified our bond, demonstrating his unwavering commitment and love.

Securing Personal well being

As we all understand, a wedding signifies not just the union of two individuals but the merging of two families. Aditya has proven to be not only a wonderful husband but also a loving father to our two children. Beyond that, he has shown himself to be a cherished son-in-law, a supportive brother-in-law, and more importantly, a caring son and brother within his own family. His role extends far beyond just being a husband to me; he takes immense pride in nurturing our children and ensuring their well-being. His dedication to family extends to his interactions with my extended family, where he has earned admiration and respect for his caring nature and thoughtful gestures.

In every facet of our lives, we exemplify kindness, responsibility, and genuine concern for each-others. His ability to seamlessly blend into and enrich our family dynamics has made him not just a life partner but a cornerstone of love and support in our lives. In conclusion, despite my initial reservations and past hardships, Aditya has become my rock and our marriage has blossomed into a source of joy and fulfillment that I never imagined possible.

|| ॐ ||

Love is Never Enough

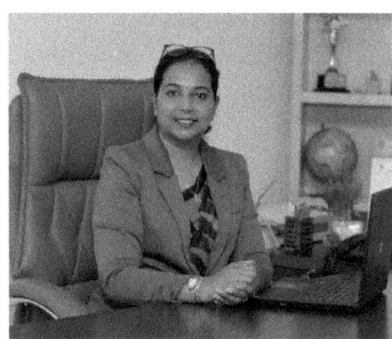

Author's Name	:	Anu Chauhan
Qualification	:	B.Com., M.B.A,
Current Profession	:	Educationist and Trainer
Age	:	41 years
E-mail ID	:	**anuchauhanfp@gmail.com**
City/ Country	:	**Gurugram, India**

Anu Chauhan is an educationist with a specialization in Eary Years with more than 14 years of experience. She is an entrepreneur and running a successful pre-school in the heart of Gurgaon since last 8 years. She holds a Master Degree in Business Management. She has worked with reputed Bank for years and moved to renowned educational institutes after realizing her passion towards learning & development of young learners. She has a passion to empower new parents.

She is a teacher and a trainer empowering Eary Years Educators with the access of new possibilities. She believes that learning is a never ending process and with that passion she is deeply invested in transforming teachers & child development in early years.

Keywords : Bondage, Responsibilities, Partnership, Relationship, Empower

Marriage is an organic way of binding two people together. It is a commitment and a long one. A stepping stone for a larger union where two individuals come together to build a life, to live joyfully and experience everything staying by each other and weaving their life in one.

I get to hear lot of young people these days who are not interested in the institution of marriage and that stir something inside me.

In a normal scenario marriage is considered "negative" by youngsters in todays era as they perceive it something that will take away their freedom. It looks like a bondage or a chain tied up with responsibilities.

It is assumed that when we are young, we do not need anyone. Let's see this from a little different prospective now. "When I am young, I do not need anyone, but when I am weak and old I need a good partner to share my sorrows and pains" In my opinion, a good partnership is formed when you are strong and well. When you are on your highs is the right time to have a partner so that the same person can be with you during your lows. That person who has seen your strength will understand your weaknesses well. Psychologically we all need a companion in our life to share our emotional needs. Its not just physical support but also emotional. A stable life demands a stable life partner.

How to find the right partner :

Marriage is about sharing of space, your true self with someone. There will be situations where the other is overstepping but then you cannot walk out; and vice-versa. There shall be no filters with your partner, but then when you are sharing so many things with the person, you become comfortable in your own true self around them and that is when magic happens. Marriage becomes successful not because of a perfect person or two, but because of integrity. Who you are should not change because of where or with whom you are. It's about when you have established the way of your being, things become easy. Marriage is about give and take where one cannot be a giver all the time. You need compatibility and companionship. Find someone who is reasonably compatible with you. It becomes a beautiful relationship If you love, respect, accept, care for and take responsibility for each other.

Everything that makes a relationship "work" (and by work, I mean that it is happy and sustainable for both people involved) requires a genuine, deep-level admiration for each other. Without that mutual admiration, everything else will unravel.

How will it feel if you are always a giver :

It is said that marriages are made in heaven. But many create a hell out of their marriages! that's because they want to extract out all the happiness through someone who should make a haven for them. If your relationship is about extracting something out of someone, it does not matter in how much time but it will get over soon. So instead make it into an offering to the relationship and see how magic happens.

Few things I vouch for :

The precious the relationship with some is, the more efforts we put to understand them. As in our day-to-day life also, someone becomes closer and dearer only when we understand them well. A friend or a family member becomes close to you when you start understanding their actions during situations. The more you understand each other the better the relationship grows. If you expect the other person to understand you with your limited understanding towards them then conflicts will happen. Marriage is an active partnership. You need to open your heart for a fulfilled relationship in marriage. And for that matter you need to have little reminders here and there to keep loving each other for all the small things. May be that's why we celebrate a reminder of our marriage once a year just to remind ourselves that you two people came together consciously and you have to conduct it consciously too. The mantra is "I water you, you water me. We do not drain each other, we grow together".

|| ॐ ||

My Marriage Was, Is and Will Be

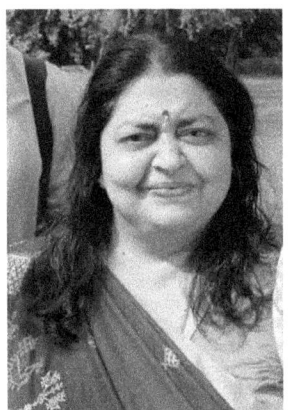

Author's Name	:	Anuradha Bijawara
Qualification	:	Graduate
Current Profession	:	Acupressure Therapist
Age	:	49 Years
E-mail ID	:	**anuradhasree09@gmail.com**
City/ Country	:	**Bangalore, India**

Anuradha Bijawara is a lovable home maker. Passionate story teller and an Acupressure Therapist. She is a B.A. graduate with lots of interest in social work. She has helped her nephew, who is hearing her impaired boy to learn speech and his studies.

After dedicating her 28 years of her family, now wants to pursue her passion. She is also animal lover, especially street dogs and has also adopted 6 dogs in her street and plans to start an NGO for street dogs along with her son, She is an excellent cook also.

Anuradha is a patient listener and extrovert, a reliable friend and is loved by everyone in her neighbourhood.

Keywords : Compromise, Commitment, Compatibility, Communication, Couple

'Respect your Partner & Unbiased acceptance of your partner.'

My marriage is a combination of bliss and curse, so I cannot totally argue, whether it is bliss or curse. Marriage in totality is a blissful living of two different individual under one roof with compromise, respect, commitment and acceptance of your partner as they are. Marriage can be curse, when there is no mutual respect, dominating character of one partner especially Men as they are chauvinists to some issues. That is because in some families boy is brought up to be superior than woman so as their wives. It can even be curse as the lady of the house is in logger head with her in-laws and vice versa.

Whether marriages are arranged by elders or arranged by the couple themselves, the journey of togetherness is same to both the couples.

In Kannada litereature Mahakavi Kuvempu regarded as the national poet and Jnana Peeta awardee has evolved a new conception of marriage called:

Mantra Mangalya (Hymns of Marriage) where a man and a woman are marry by promising themselves to be husband and wife without following the general traditional of marriage.

This oath tells the couple to make an effort to get away from mental and spiritual binding from family & society. Free themselves from superstitious customs and traditions.

The oath also states that there is no particular time to get into wedlock, but whole of your life time is an auspicious journey. The next oath is not to give up each other's individuality and stand up to your rights and your space to live your dreams.

Speak your heart out to anything you feel is wrong in front of your family. There will always be initial disagreement, but acceptance will follow.This systems of Mantra Mangalya is creating waves is some parts of Karnataka (A State in India)

As I mentioned earlier my marriage was a union of two mismatched individuals. I and my husband had nothing in common neither thoughts, taste, hobbies none of them matched only one common thing was the binding of marriage and the oath we took during our wedding while tying the scared thread and Saptapadi ceremony. The mantra which is in Sanskrit while tying scared thread says. Mangalyam Tantunanena (this is a sacred thread) Mama Jevana Hetuna This is essential for my long life).

Kante Badhami subhage (I tie this around your neck O maiden having many auspicious attributes) Twan Jeeva Sarada Satam (May you live happily for hundred years) Over the years both of us compromised for each other and accepted our weakness and never highlighted it front of each other, that is why we were able to sail the cruise of life for 28 years with a huge extended eccentric family with us.

To conclude I would tell that marriage is a communion of two souls who will live together with mutual understanding. The marriage will be curse when we don't understand our responsibilities to treat both the parents as ours and accept each other's families. It would be a curse when you don't trust each other.

So making our marriage a bliss or curse is in our hands. For all the young friends out there practically marriage is a gamble, if u work for it you win. (Bliss) if you lose (curse). Please follow this popular saying in Tamil Marapom Mannipom which means FORGET AND FORGIVE. To top it all the blessing of the SUPREME POWER is very essential

To end I request all the youngesters to follow one simple Mantra told by the groom to bride during wedding rituals in Sanskrit, it says "Dharmecha Arthecha Kamecha Mokshecha Na thi charami (Meaning I promise never to walk away from my spouse for reasons pertaining to my work, my finances, my desires, or spirituality.

|| ॐ ||

An Experiential Journey

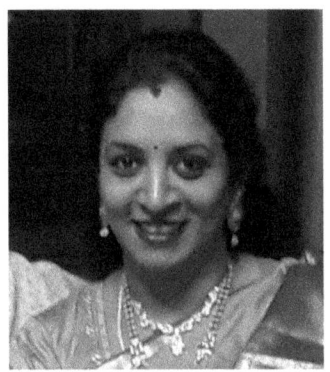

Author's Name	:	Archana Nadella
Qualification	:	B.Com., MBA (General Management)
Current Profession	:	Healer and Therapist
Age	:	49 years
E-mail ID	:	na.archanaa@gmail.com
City/ Country	:	**Bangalore, India**

Archana Nadella is an Internationally Certified Handwriting Analyst & a Graphotherapist. She has done her Graduation in Commerce and Post-Graduation in General Management. She has a worked as admin with few organizations and as a Senior Personal Loan Officer at a renowned MNC Bank.

Archana Nadella, has acquired several skills sets in various healing modalities and been certified as a counselor from few renowned counseling centers. She has closely worked as associates with several other practitioners to adept and strengthen her knowledge. Always have worked one on one personally as she believed in giving complete attention, however with the necessities being dissimilar is now slowly expanding and extending to make a big opening in the field.

Archana Nadella, has trained several individuals to have a tailored personality and healed and counselled several issues.

Keywords : Marriage, Roller Coaster, Rejection, Love, Support

Marriage : Bliss vs Curse is like Knife, Good/ Bad or Money, Good/ Bad

A knife can be used for both good and unwanted reasons, how money in the hands of good people grows to do good and in the hands of unwanted people turns into mafia activities, similarly Marriage when properly executed and endured with proper guidance and aspects it becomes a blissful experience. Too much of anything is bad and that holds right even in marriages too, too much of lenience, too much of rigidity, too much pampering, too stingy, only pampering and no practicality, too much of attitude, too less attitude, etc., all can lead marriage as a curse.

Every blessing ignored becomes a curse, says a great mind and holds good in marriage too. Add a blessing in every aspect, rather than a curse. There is nothing perfect in any relationship for that matter. Just take an imperfect thing and work together to make it perfect.

One may think if the author is so positive about Marriage, she must have had a wonderful marriage, let me interrupt and tell, two different family backgrounds, two different financial status, two different educational backgrounds etc etc etc, a complete **roller coaster** ride, still held on to each other so strongly, guiding each other at the time of distractions, supporting each other by way of compromises, sacrifices, understandings, so many years of married life when I turn back and see, I wonder if it was me who travelled this far…

Started with a complete rejection from my side as I wanted to study further, but he fell topsy turvy at the first sight itself in my photo. We belong to a community huge amount will be asked as marriage gift, but he was least bothered and just wanted me in his life, I took a step ahead to go and convince him why he should not get married to me, I thought he would change his mind as he belonged to a small town, but destiny is so strong that he became much more determined to make this marriage work saying where will he find a girl, who is so open and fearless.

Probably this is why it is said "**MARRIAGES ARE MADE IN HEAVEN**". If I narrate my complete story till now, one can make a juicy movie on it. Lots of mistakes, lots of learnings, lots of Let goes, lots of hurts, lots of healings, still lot to go and looking forward to go till the end of the earth.

From there to here when I turn back and see it looks like someone else's life. He knew how to keep me and knew how to hold me with him this long and made me what I am today. He has chiseled me and carved me to the best of how I could be, when I say He here it's my husband of course, the He, He cannot be in everyone's life personally and He creates more He's like Himself.

Marriage offers an opportunity for personal growth and development, as both partners navigate life's challenges and triumphs together. In a happy marriage, couples create cherished memories and moments that they can back on with fondness.

A good marriage isn't something, which you find, it's something you have to make and keep making it.

Knife can be used to cut vegetables and same knife can be used to take out a life. Similarly, a marriage can be made a bliss or can be turned into curse depending on how we in that relationship. Lust and Love or two different aspects, lust lives shorter, love is eternal. It's all up to us to decide and make a marriage, that is filled with bliss or curse. According to me marriage is a must to have a loving companionship and the experience of eternal love, ultimate goal should be to change the spelling of **Marriage to Love**.

Ultimately, a successful marriage is built on a foundation of trust, communication and mutual respect, creating a supportive and loving environment where both partners can thrive and make **HAPPY MARRIED LIFE**.

|| ॐ ||

In the Garden of Togetherness

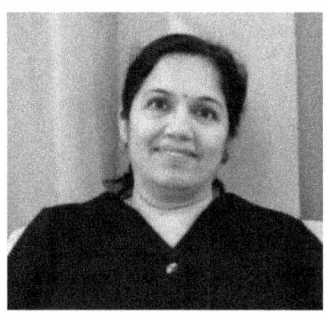

Author's Name	:	Archana Nair
Qualification	:	M.B.A., M.Sc. (Applied Psychology)
		PG Diploma in Counseling
Current Profession	:	Lecturer in Management, Corporate Trainer, Management Consultant, Counseling Psychologist
Age	:	50 years
E-mail ID	:	archana.nairkr@gmail.com
City/ Country	:	Cochin, India

Archana Nair has been teaching Management at the university level since, 1998. She serves as a project guide for management students in undergraduate, postgraduate and M.Phil. courses. She is a member of the Board of Examinations at Universities in Kerala and has published several papers on Integrated Marketing Communication in both international and national journals.

The author also holds M.Sc. degree in Applied Psychology with a Post Graduate diploma in counseling, she has been involved in counseling for over 15 years. Archana is a hypnotherapist and a graphotherapist for the past three years.

As a trainer, she provides training to various corporate offices, teachers, students, and individuals from all walks of life. The author is the Managing Director of TU Consultors Pvt. Ltd, where she supervises market feasibility studies for many FMCG products as a Management Consultant. Archana Nair is one of the leading trainers in NLP and has successfully trained 20 batches of trainees.

Keywords : Tolerance, Adjustment, Forgiving, Soulmate, Life Partner

Fine-tuning our personality often happens during hostel life, where we live with near strangers. Room-mates teach us valuable lessons in sharing, accommodating, adjusting, and forgiving. Tolerance develops when living with another person, regardless of shared interests. Marriage represents a deeper form of sharing, transforming partners into soulmates. While we rarely choose our hostel room-mates, we have the privilege of selecting our life partners. Many notice the physical changes marriage brings, but the true beauty lies in the positive transformations in each partner's mental state. In a marital relationship, synergy occurs as each partner fills in the gaps of the other's mental state, enhancing their overall energy. Whether one partner lacks motivation or needs support, the other can provide the necessary encouragement.

Kishore and Meera met in a training course, began dating and eventually decided to tie the knot. They started their new life with excitement, sharing household responsibilities and enjoying their work. However, things changed when Meera was promoted, requiring her to spend more time at the office. Kishore took on most of the home duties and while he didn't complain at first, Meera sensed he was avoiding her whenever she tried to connect. Months passed without them dining together or having meaningful conversations.

Frustrated, Meera spoke to her manager about getting an assistant to have more family time. When she returned home to share the news, Kishore seemed indifferent. Determined to address their issues, Meera confronted him, leading to a fierce argument. The next morning, she packed her bag and left a note for Kishore, stating she would stay with a friend for a few days.

Meanwhile, Sara's parents were arranging her marriage to John. Although she resisted the alliance, she ultimately married him. Sara soon realized that John spoke little and rarely interfered in her life. His care was evident in his actions—especially when she was sick or caring for her ailing mother—but he never expressed it directly. They seldom dined together or visited friends and family.

As time passed, Sara understood that this was not the life she had expected, feeling disheartened by the lack of love and togetherness, she observed in other couples. One day, feeling hopeless, she left John and returned to her parents.

There, Meera couldn't concentrate on work or engage in activities that once fascinated her. Taking a few days off, she realized she wasn't okay after leaving home. One evening, sitting in a nearby park, she reflected on her life with Kishore, longing for a magician to wave a wand and restore her happiness.

On the other side of the bench sat Sara, contemplating whether to leave her marriage. John called her repeatedly, but she didn't answer. She wanted to decide but felt blocked, wishing for divine guidance.

Suddenly, Meera and Sara felt something shift on the bench and to their surprise, a beautiful fairy appeared! She smiled at them and asked, "Why do you need me, darlings?"

"We need happiness," they replied in unison. The fairy gave them a sympathetic smile and asked, "Why did you leave your spouses?"

"Because he doesn't love me," Meera said softly and Sara nodded.

"Why do you think that? Isn't he giving you freedom? Doesn't he care for your needs? Has he ever hindered your goals or abused you?" Both girls shook their heads.

"I know you have communication issues, but you'll understand each other's unique styles if you pay attention. Don't you feel incomplete without him? Don't you long for him now?" Tears rolled down their cheeks.

"Aah, partners may argue and trust can wane, but love is essential. You must nurture it like a child. Then you'll feel the real happiness."

"Now that you recognize your mistakes, do you want to return home?"

"Yes!" they exclaimed, jumping to their feet.

The fairy smiled and handed them two small packets. "These are magic potions for you and your husbands to drink daily."

"But they're small!" Sara protested.

"Don't worry, my child. You'll discover the recipe with the last dose."

They returned to their spouses and received a warm welcome. From that day onward, both couples began their daily dose of the fairy's potions. They felt happier than ever and life seemed much easier. A week later, when Meera finished her potion, writing appeared on the bottle: "1 spoon of love + 1 spoon of trust + 1 spoon of respect + 1 spoon of communication."

Love, inherent in all humans, starts to reveal itself when a couple decides to marry. If not nurtured, conflicts can cause harm to both partners. While some damage may be irreparable, recognizing love can heal wounds. Ultimately, as children grow independent, only the husband and wife will remain together forever.

|| ॐ ||

A Delicate Balance Between Joy and Sorrow

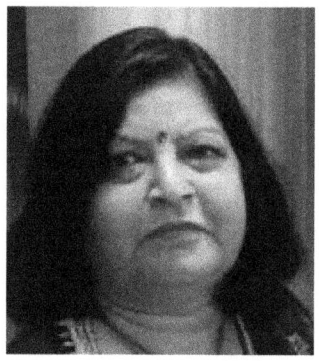

Author's Name	:	Aruna
Qualification	:	B.A., L.L.B
Current Profession	:	Artist and Freelancer
Age	:	64 years
E-mail ID	:	**arunachaudhary19@gmail.com**
City/ Country	:	**Gurugram, India**

Aruna is a multifaceted homemaker, blending her professional expertise as a lawyer with her artistic passion. As a freelancer, she constantly explores new business ideas, driven by her inquisitive nature. A well-traveled soul, she delights in experiencing diverse cultures and cuisines. An avid reader and natural teacher, Aruna's spiritual inclination draws her to the tranquility of nature. She finds immense joy in spreading happiness, using her rich life experiences to motivate and inspire others.

Aruna's unique combination of skills, creativity and positivity makes her a captivating and insightful author, offering a wealth of knowledge and inspiration.

Keywords : Awakened Soul, Fairytale, Marriage, Stark Reality, Wounded Soul

Marriage can be both a curse and a blessing, depending on the individuals involved and their behaviour with each other. For some, marriage brings companionship, support, and a deep sense of fulfilment. For others, it can lead to feelings of confinement and unhappiness. It's essential that both partners in a marriage communicate openly, show mutual respect, and have a willingness to work through challenges together. Ultimately, the impact of marriage on an individual's life varies from person to person.

In my journey through life, I encountered a married couple, Ruchi and Rahul, who discussed everything in detail before their marriage to avoid potential troubles. Their thoughtful approach helped them navigate many issues that commonly arise in marital relationships. From observing their experience, I learned a few key lessons. Both husband and wife should never take each other for granted. While the beginning of a marriage is often filled with love, over time, it becomes crucial to accept each other's merits and flaws. Acceptance of each other as they are is fundamental. Respecting each other's values and giving each other space is vital. Marriage is about give and take, though some conservative families believe only the woman should adjust.

One of my friends, Reena, married Suresh. Initially, they were quite happy, but later Reena couldn't bear the pressure of her job and household responsibilities. She fell into depression. When she confided in me, I advised her to talk to her husband frankly and state all her problems. I encouraged her to stand up for herself and not to behave like a victim. She followed my advice and shared her concerns with her husband, who helped her sort out everything. Today, they are leading a very happy married life, and Reena always thanks me for my support and motivation.

'Marriage can be a bed of roses or a bed of thorns'; it all depends on how the married couple handles their relationship. Marriage is not a fairy tale; it's a stark reality. It is like a rose plant that must be nurtured properly to produce lovely roses that spread their fragrance. Similarly, if married life is nourished properly, it becomes a blessing. However, if the married couple keeps fighting due to false egos, it becomes a curse for them and those connected to them.

Women, in particular, should not always behave like wounded souls but should become awakened souls. One must love oneself before loving others. Life should be lived beautifully and one should pursue hobbies and interests instead of feeling suffocated in marriage. Married couples should support each other while maintaining their private space. Both partners should complement each other rather than compete. Life is beautiful when both partners truly value each other.

Personally, I have taken up gardening and started a freelancing business to support my hobbies, which gives me a lot of mental satisfaction. I have begun to understand human relationships more deeply. Be generous but never become an emotional fool, and learn to say no when necessary. We should thank God for our beautiful lives, which enable us to make choices that bring us joy.

In conclusion, one should enjoy life to the fullest by making meaningful contributions to society. I have learned these lessons from a married couple, Aradhana and Naveen. They helped each other overcome difficulties. Naveen supported Aradhana in completing her studies after marriage and both of them helped those in need. They respected each other's values and lived a happy married life for over fifty years. Marriage is a blessing if the couple enjoys each other's company and a curse if they keep sulking. One must become an awakened soul instead of a wounded soul to truly appreciate and nurture the beauty of marriage.

॥ ॐ ॥

Unique Sense of Companionship and Partnership

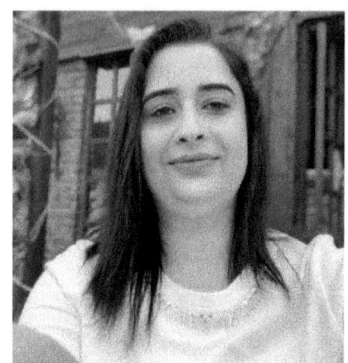

Author's Name	:	Avneet Chaudhary
Qualification	:	B.A., M.B.A. (HR & Marketing)
Current Profession	:	Teacher, Painter, Influencer, Entrepreneur, Homemaker
Age	:	36 years
E-mail ID	:	**avneet6choudhary@gmail.com**
City/ Country	:	**Gurugram, India**

Avneet Chaudhary is self-managed personality. She is a proficient entrepreneur ,painter. Avneet is a dedicated and resourceful homemaker with the passion for creating a warm and organised home environment .She believes that a well managed home is the foundation of a happy and productive family life. Feels great joy nurturing her family and ensuring that home is welcoming space for everyone.

Openness friendliness thoughtfulness emotional stability are features of our personality singing cooking reading are her passion.

Keywords : Marriage, Emotional, Communication, Spiritual, Happiness

Marriage is the best profound source of happiness, offering a unique emotional and spiritual sense of companionship, can go to any extent to support each other. Marriage is a confluence of immense trust and respect between two knitted people. However, if not nurtured, this relationship can become a commencement of great challenge, even a curse.

Marriage binds two soul together, creating a partnership that, when properly understood, becomes a sanctuary. But the journey is not always smooth and external pressures or the involvement of a third party can weaken the bond.

Marriage is a concurrence of two rivers joining together with immense love, trust and dedication are the key. However, negative emotions—anger, pride, ego, regret—can also arise. It's a misconception that loving couples do not face difficult times, when frustration and negative emotions surface, communication can become strained and the loving feelings between partners may begin to fade. During these moments, the strength of the marriage is truly tested.

The role of each partner is crucial. How one responds—by listening and understanding or by ignoring—can determine the relationship's fate. If both partners are emotionally connected and supportive, the marriage can withstand any storm. Emotional intimacy in marriage fosters a sense of security and safety that is difficult to find elsewhere. Sharing life with someone who genuinely cares provides profound satisfaction and emotional support.

Marriage is a shared journey, strengthened by moments of joy, confidence, and spiritual love. Having someone special to share your thoughts and feelings with creates a unique sense of fulfilment, Companionship and partnership. For many having a partner means never facing lives challenges alone fostering a strong sense of belonging and emotional stability.

Love is one of the best feelings in the universe, and when found within marriage, life becomes filled with happiness—a blissful gift. However, maintaining this bliss requires more than just love. Desire and commitment are essential to keep the relationship alive. The day someone says they no longer have time for the relationship, it should be understood that the relationship is in trouble. Desire is crucial to sustain a marriage.

Men and women often have different needs. While men may crave space to handle stress, women often seek intimacy and emotional connection. These differences can create challenges but also enrich the relationship. Understanding and respecting each other's needs is a key to maintaining balance.

Lack of communication is one of the biggest threats to a marriage. It can lead to misunderstandings, blame, anxiety, and resentment. If ignored, these issues can grow into bigger problems, potentially leading to separation. Harmony in marriage is built on open communication and mutual respect. When one partner is weak, the other should offer support, creating a balanced relationship where both know how to care for each other.

Emotional intimacy is vital to a healthy marriage. As people go through different stages of life, their priorities and circumstances change, which can affect the relationship. It is unrealistic to expect that marriage will only bring good times. A marriage that endures bad times often emerges stronger if both partners are committed to staying connected and working through challenges together.

No relationship is without conflicts—whether with parents, friends, or siblings. Yet, we do not sever these ties over disagreements. So why, when it comes to marriage, do some choose to cut each other out of their lives instead of working through their differences? Marriage is not just about the good times; it's about navigating the difficult times together and coming out stronger on the other side.

The greatest curse in marriage, however, is losing a spouse—the one who promised to be your companion for life. This loss can be an unbearable burden, and those who have experienced it know the profound sorrow it brings. In these moments, the absence of a spouse's support can make life incredibly challenging.

Despite the potential challenges, marriage is more a blessing than a curse. When two people are truly in love and committed to each other, they can overcome any difficulty, and their relationship will flourish. In the end, marriage is a journey of two souls who, despite the ups and downs, choose to walk through life together, making it one of the most profound sources of happiness.

॥ ॐ ॥

Way to Family System

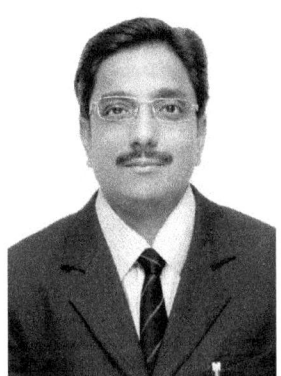

Author's Name	:	B D Surana
Qualification	:	B.Com (Hon) CA (Inter) Certified Graphologist and Counselor
Current Profession	:	HR & Management Consultant, Stock Sub Broker, Trainer, Graphologist, Social Worker
Age	:	58 years
E-mail ID	:	**bdsurana@gmail.com**
City/ Country	:	**Kolkata, India**

B D Surana is SEBI authorised AP. His Education is B.Com (Hons.), CA Finalist, Accounting Certificate from ICAI. Diploma in Counselling & Psychotherapy, MILT Leadership Course, Leadership in Recruitment, Mind Training etc., Advance Level Certification in Graphology, Scientific Logos, Face Reading, Watch Analysis etc.

He is attached with several Professional and Social Organisations like Lions International, holding various important positions and have received many awards and recognitions. He is a life member of JITO, ISTD, NIPM, NHRD, MILT, All India Marwari Sangh, RSFF, Chinmoy Mission and other bodies.

B D Surana is associated with HR Business as Founder & Chief Consultant at Surana Equity Pvt. Ltd. For more than 26 years. (www.hrequity.in)

Keywords : Population, Rituals, Family Values, Expectations, Management

Indian Marriage is one the best rituals in the world. I love marriage functions. Can human population produce cultured citizens without social system in place i.e. marriage (this is my personal opinion). Without marriage whole society will be in the state of situation without imaginations. All cultural, rituals, social system, family values, economic condition, Parenting, nurturing will not be in place. Marriages are legally accepted relationship.

No Maa, No Papa, No Dada, No Dadi, No Nana, No Nani, No Mama and so on. (No Families or family values in in place)

We may debate endlessly on marriage as bliss or curse, but well thought & well planned marriages will be good for us. Here I do not want to be judgemental.

I know couple for last 30 years or more & fortunate enough to attend their 60th marriage anniversary. They are happily married since I am seeing them and listen from family and friends, they are made for each other since first day & now also helping each other at this age also.

I was happily married since 1993 having one lovely daughter. But I got deep shock of death of my lovely wife suddenly due to Covid attack in April 2021. Then after her absence, I realized value of real Marriage. Why marriage is important? Why child & family need both male & female? Both Anima & Animus compliments each other. Whether family can run without male or female is a big question to me. I am facing problem, without female in house, how emotional men becomes weak some times and can't handle family & society expectations.

So, Marriage is bliss till then you manage it very well and good for society and family. On the contrary, it becomes curse, when couples fight since inception of marriage, beat each other, disrespect each other, refuse to listen, do not accept each other or ones families, refuse to adjust, stick to past bad experience/ pain, love & hate relationships or death of any of partner or matter of fact divorce.

After separation most of the life becomes miserable due to property/ financial disputes, child possession/ not possession, society/ family/ personal issues, legal issues, emotional/ psychological turmoil etc. They do not want to go into any relationships of marriage again, because of above or other various other reasons. Although this doesn't set pattern of society or families or individuals.

There are cases where remarriage are good & bonding is good among them. Marriage is a need of both the Individuals, not only one, because both compliment to each other. We have to cultivate the art of maintaining relationships in other words. Marriage is an art of relationship management. Now in this new modern era to make marriage bliss one has to learn this art. It's because we are moving from joint family structure to nuclear family structure. In the past, family members of joint families use to work as marriage counsellors and able to hold marriages through decades because of various systems and power of joint family of sharing of thoughts, helping in rebuilding relationships through proper listening, conflict management etc. Joint families help in emotional support, shared relationships, inculcating "family first not individuals" attitude, close bonds, experience/ tradition sharing etc. Sharing values & caring each one in family is important part of marriage, which we learn from our family culture. If we are moving towards single family structure then one big umbrella is missing to bring each one of us in time of sunshine, rain or togetherness. In single family, we may have some personal independence, greater control of children, more personal time, but we lack whole family support, lack of emotional support, hand holding & conflict resolution.

In this era of fast movement, technological advancement, should not we redefine marriage & development new methods to hold on attitude rather than part our paths and move towards single parenting issues and burn our self & children? Now marriage counsellors can play big role in sustaining marriages.

Let do debate on *My Marriage : Bliss vs Curse*, but end of the day be responsible citizens and learn the art of sustaining marriage, because here we are talking about marriage only. As we enjoy Indian Fat Wedding, let us enjoy our marriage also. Enjoy togetherness it will be a bliss, hate each other it will be a curse. Choice is yours. So, be alert while choosing right partner rather than regret later on in life and create myths about marriage. Be Partner in Bliss not in curse. Let's bless New wed couples for long lasting relationships.

|| ॐ ||

Mr. & Mrs. Perfect to Help Each-Other

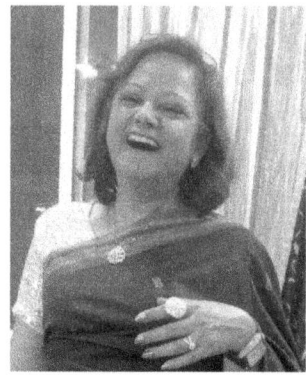

Author's Name	:	Baljit Jaggi
Qualification	:	B. Com, M.B.A,
Current Profession	:	Life Coach & Healer
Age	:	54 years
E-mail ID	:	**winningbells@gmail.com**
City/ Country	:	**Pune, India**

Baljit Jaggi is a budding Author, Certified Coach & a Ho'oponopono Healer, whose mission is to facilitate in transforming 100,000 lives. She has done her Master in Business Administration and Advanced Diploma in Marketing & Sales. She has worked for more than 5 years as Director for an Event Management company providing customized solutions to Top Notch Corporate Houses & also worked as Corporate Trainer for more than 7 years providing training, from Bharat Ratna Organizations like BPCL, NTPC, ONGC to MNCs like Nestle, Coco-Cola, Hindustan Levers Ltd., Honda Motors, HDFC-SLIC to Top National companies like Reliance Infocomm., Maruti Udyog Ltd, SBI, Indian Railways, VSGM and many other.

Also contributed as an Academic Counselor with a MNC for more than 3 years and began her career as a teacher. She has been an avid trekker and a sports lover, dabs her fingers in sketching & painting sometimes and loves cooking occasionally. She is a nature lover plus a kitabi Keera!! Not to mention she is HAPPILY MARRIED too!!

Baljit Jaggi is happily married to Col. K.S Jaggi, who incidentally happens to be a Col. of Indian Army.

> **Keywords :** Fauji Kid, Individuality, Intricacies of In-laws, Is marriage the recipe of fulfillment, Rishtedar Kya Bolenge?

"A Marriage is a union of two people based on Friendship, Mutual Understanding, Respect & Unconditional Love. It is about not looking down at each other but looking at each other."

It's very aptly said that marriages are made in heaven and so…..true is that! But I would go Beyond this statement and say that, Marriages are made in Heaven… Yes…. But consummated, actually lived here on this very Mother Earth and this is where the understanding, caring, partnership, commitment, Love and sense of belonging flows in

This coming from me is Huge, who at one point of time never gave importance to marriage, especially when all my friends, acquaintances, colleagues were tying up the nuptial knot left, right & center. (Happy ones, I believe!) I only had my eyes fixed on my career.

I always believed that women should not only be a daughter, sister, friend, wife or mother but besides that should always have their own identity. It is the independent identity that made me opt for staying single & I didn't regret it then. I felt being single is just a state of being & not a sentence. I had embraced being single over matrimony in my quest for success. I would question, "Is marriage the recipe of fulfillment?"

It is not that I was against the institution of marriage as such, but the compromises & adjustments that a girl has to make after marriage, scared me no end. I being a Fauji officer's daughter, (a typical Fauji kid) and a Fauji officer's sister had seen life & experienced liberation, was not ready to give up my independence. I gave more importance to my career, my individuality. I had worked my butt off to establish my career. I at 27 was the youngest franchise of India's top notch MNC, followed by being a corporate trainer conducting workshops for Maha Ratna, Nav Ratna Organizations, Top National companies and MNCs. I eventually turned into a successful entrepreneur, as an Event Manager who would clinch orders in tons along with my brother, (with whom I made a great team). We were thriving professionally.

Being an old timer, came from a school of thought that if you earn well, have a house of your own (not your parents), can afford all luxuries & amenities of life then you don't really need to be married. Little did I realize how materialistic I was??

My parents accepted my decision, (half-heartedly though). My mom felt bad that her daughter had not tied the knot…so much so that she avoided going to family functions fearing ki rishtedaar kya bolenge? Ki Beti ki Shaadi ab tak kyo nahi kari? She would even duck the Fauji reunions, irrespective of the fact that the Faujis are very broadminded people and have a very unique outlook towards life.

I remember when my Fauji Bro. used to come on leave, we would have chats on pros & cons of marriage at length, whilst on long morning walks, which used to be invariably inconclusive.

I finally tied the knot with my husband who happened to be an Army officer. My husband being a typical Bombayite and that too from SOBO, Colaba, after seeing my palatial bungalow was like – How will you adjust in a small flat like mine? After marriage, we stayed with the family for approx. a month to bond & understand "The so-called intricacies of In- Laws!" My Father-In – Law was like a Devta, who would address everyone with ji, so it was Baljit ji for me. My Ma-In-Law lives life Queen Size. My Bro-In-Law made me feel so much at home (because he himself was never at home, as he is settled abroad) & my Co- Sister has been like a sister, which I never had, as we are 3 siblings & I am the only sister to my 2 elder brothers. I felt so much blessed to be a part of this family. My husband is a gem of a guy. The principle that governs the family is to "Live & Let Live", without muddling into each other's lives. But yes…. Always ready to help each other, when needed.

Marriage is for keeps. what is important is to marry the right person. It's definitely a gamble…. A gamble, to not know, if you would sail through or hit the rock bottom. Luckily the gamble has paid off for me. Today, after 17 years of Marriage I am now convinced that he has been "Mr. Right" for me, considering that we are a Shaadi.com alliance followed by 6 months of courtship of short & sweet letters & tele-calls from Campbell Bay, (the Southernmost tip of India) to an elite town in Punjab. Marriage is great, when the spouse becomes your strength, & is always there to back you up with love, support & understanding.

So Yeah, Marriage is definitely a Bliss. A bliss overflowing with Unconditional Love, Peace and Happiness. Immense Gratitude to the Divine Power, The Supreme Power, The WAHEGURU for our union!! I wonder how true is the Saat janam ka Bandhan? but I definitely would like HIM to be my friend & life partner in agla janam as well! I for one can say with firm conviction that I am in a Happy space, in blissful state! However, it needs to be understood no marriage is perfect but one has to endeavor to make it Great, if not perfect.

I take pride in sharing my past, present and vow to facilitate in transforming millions of lives through my coaching & healing modalities with blessings of my Gurus!! I really appreciate Abhishaik ji and Rainu ji for taking an initiative to present 108 views in this Anthology Book to encourage the future generations of our society.

॥ ॐ ॥

How I See a Marriage
Goal: Bliss over Curse

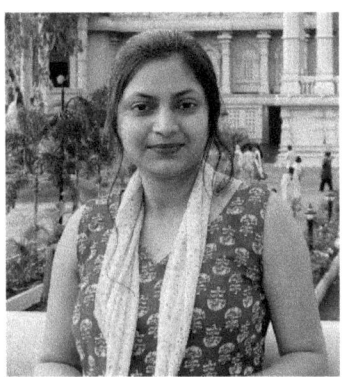

Author's Name	:	Bhavana M Patle
Qualification	:	B.B.A., M.B.A. (HR)
Current Profession	:	Data Analyst, Content Writer
Age	:	24 years
E-mail ID	:	**bhavi1111patle@gmail.com**
City/ Country	:	**Nagpur, Maharashtra, India**

Bhavana Patle is a Certified Data Analyst and Data scientist. She is a budding poet she wrote poems in Marathi and Hindi, English as well on love, spirituality, fun, self-love & care etc. she is writing articles on self-awareness, ancient taboos for women's or individual persons mental health & care. She is also interested in Psychology and Numerology, Yoga/Exercising, Reading.

Bhavana Patle is professionally working as Team Lead & Data Analyst in Government organization known as Mahatma Jyotiba Phule Training and Research Institution (MAHAJYOTI), Nagpur. She is Fun Loving, Spiritual and kind Person Also Started Travelling in Maharashtra, many more to Explore. She Participated in Career Counselling Programs with Colombia Maxim Institutions, Digital marketing programs.

Keywords: Attachment, Empathy, Faith, Myth, Peace

Now a days '**Marriage**' Actually means living together but, in my dictionary, it has different meaning it's a mutual growing of two persons may be they think opposite, their aura is opposite, may be their profession, culture is opposite but only because of love and attachment they are staying together in each other's heart & life.

Trusting each other and trust is not only represented by loyalty but also glimpse of empathy in everything, in every action partner has to know what the next step of other one. Controlling each other is not going to work forever if you want to be forever with your partner then feel freedom with each other.

This is different thing also I can talk here about **Myth of the fairy-tale marriage** is carries magic that magic is only 'faith', faith is going to take place reaction Peace. i.e. Marriage/ Relationship +faith = Peace of Souls.

Marriage Starts with Love and Purity, but may be ends or pauses somewhere with negativity, toxicity, unrealistic overthinking etc.

Let's discuss bliss over curse:

Bliss :

- Companionship brings sharing joy and challenges, Partnership carries emotional, mental sometimes financial Support.
- Love and intimacy provide a stable environment for emotional connection between partners
- Family and Children can be a source of great happiness
- Some personal space in marriage is necessary to knowing ourselves first then we can understand another one.
- Nowadays Couples often ignores development communication and conflict-resolution skills but is necessary in fairy-tale marriage.

Curse :

- In marriage Sometimes it feels like restricting, limiting but it is common because of this some may feel trapped or suffocated by the constant presence of another person.
- If Conflicts or Problems not managed well, these lead to stress and unhappiness. For example : Differences in thoughts, financial issues Communication styles, Lack of awareness, Different priorities, Emotional intelligence, Past experiences etc.
- In Growing apart interest of some couple may change over time sometimes because of compatibility. Personalities, Interest can change, but we have to accept rule of nature is CHANGE/GROWTH
- Failure of Relation starts from generation to generation according to me societal and familial pressure, Unrealistic expectations, and cultural norms/recognition this always creates disappointments between partners.

For achieving bliss over curse partner needs to understand each other not only by common aspects, but also they have to care about each other's soul/aura. It doesn't matter what's happening around you, hug each other's problems solve or analyse mutually and maturely. In marriage loving each other is basic need it will improve bond.

Controlling or pressurising each other will not work forever if you want to be together with your partner then feel freedom with each other's. (He or she deserves to be feel free forever).It is frustrating when one of them making effort to understand their partner, but that effort is not being reciprocated.

It is important to communicate openly and honestly with your partner about what you feel, express your thoughts and emotions let him/her understand you & vice versa. Encouraging, valuing your partner is also very important. Try till end if it's really not working then lastly you go for do or die means stay or leave because in all of these mainly important thing according to me is individual. Self-love or care is also important.

May be if you want to try Counselling or therapy it can be also helpful for improving relationships.

I think *"My Marriage: Bliss vs Curse",* this is deep and interesting topic to express marriage thoughts, I am not married, but because of this topic I studied lots of books about marriage, this is pride and grateful awareness in the society. Thanking God, founder, co-founder, compiler, each and every connecting soul for giving me the chance to write among 108 eminent co-authors.

In healthy, happy marriage Focus on communication, mutual respect and growth, Cultivate a more realistic and compassionate understanding of love and partnership but marriage perspectives is different in different personalities.

Perfect partner will choose love over hate/ complaint, discussion over argument, sometimes space over domination or anger, compromising over separation, peace over curse, when He or She is really in happy marriage.

At the end, I can say marriage is beauty of soul which represents purity and sweetness.

"विवाह आत्मा की वह सुंदरता है, जो पवित्रता और मधुरता का प्रतिनिधित्व करता है"

|| ॐ ||

Under One Sky

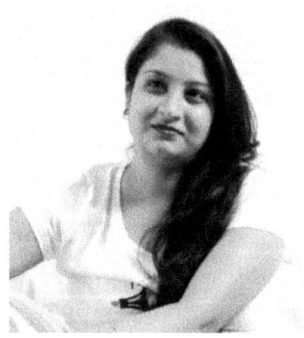

Author's Name	:	Binita Nandi
Qualification	:	M.Sc.
Current Profession	:	Career Strategist and Life Coach
Age	:	43 years
E-mail ID	:	**success.nitanandi@gmail.com**
City/ Country	:	**Hyderabad, India**

Binita Nandi is a Life Coach, Parenting Coach, Career strategist, DMIT (Dermatoglyphics Multiple Intelligence Test) analyst, certified Numerologist and NLP master practitioner. She has done her Master Degree in Science. She has started her career in 2008 as a Counselor in the Dept. of Health and Family Welfare in State Govt. of West Bengal. As a parenting coach, she has helped many parents on positive parenting to gain a better understanding of their parental journey.

Binita Nandi is the founder and CEO of Happy Life Society. It is the one stop solution for life's four major parameters as Health, Relationship, Career and Spirituality. Mission of Happy Life Society is to help people to become an emotionally content, economically fulfilling and physically healthy and their best version in terms of developing happy and thriving societies.

Keywords : Bonding, Commitment, Love, Understanding, Respect

Marriage is not a bond of birth; it is a social bonding between two people above all two families and society. Therefore, it is possible to nurture carefully, but it is also impossible to maintain carelessly.

Our lives are dynamic, volatile, and uncertain too. But we spend a huge portion of our life journey riding on this marriage chariot. And on the four wheels of this marriage chariot are faith, love, respect for each other and above all self-respect. Even if one of them is damaged, the chariot wobbles. And then the responsibility of protecting this relationship rests on both of the spouse.

Self-sacrifices, the ability to accept and adapt, the patience to love and understand others, all these qualities of both husband and wife combined their happy conjugal life. It has no exact quantity or quality; the chemistry of every marriage is tremendously new and alive.

Here I am going to narrate the tale of a King (Husband) and Queen (Wife) duo from their own conjugal kingdom. The queen sent an open letter to her king.

Hello My dearest Hubby,

Today after a long time I am writing something to you again. I want to ask you a small question that if I want to give you half of my entire sky, would you able to find your existence in it?

You can say that being together for a long time is a habit or a bad habit. Sometimes such things happen like if there is a disagreement, I will stab you with unbridled words, you also don't go any less then, your words also hurt me a lot in the same way, At the end of the fight, when both of us are in two poles, it seems that everything is over and we don't need each-other anymore. But immediately I remember that the gems of all qualities as love, compassion, kindness, loyalty, adaptability, respect and those pearls of my mind that I sometimes lose when I quarrel with anger but I want to find them again and again and carefully stored them in the closet of my heart.

This is how the sun rises and sets and how the day passes, but anger, sadness is like stars at night sky, even though they stay up all night but fall asleep at dawn after being tired at last. But as soon as the sun rises of the next day, this marriage of ours became excited with the new enthusiasm of life. It is not less amazing than magic. That is the power of the bonding of a conjugal relationship. It's like sour, salt and sweet memories combined two persons in a single thread.

After all war, perhaps peace is the only thing, desired. Let it be our promise in the future that no matter how turbulent the family and social situation may be, but we walk the same way throughout our lives as each other's companions. One last thing I would like to say is that I really like losing myself to you.

From

Your Indispensable Habit (Wife)

Sipping a cup of a tea on a sunny morning, I wondered whether my marriage is a blessing or a curse. Whatever we get in our life depends on how we accept it.

The marriage is a journey. There is no perfect destination and perfect relationship. But we always try to accept and enjoy each and every shade of our life. For me the RAINBOW colors of my marriage life :

R- Respect each other's thoughts

A- Accept each other as we are

I- Intense trust on our relationship

N- No question about love for each other

B- Breathing space between us

O- Obvious support to one another

W-Wonderful understanding between two people.

In conclusion, I want to say one thing while writing this article, I realized that getting and not getting in life is very relative. Forgetting all the give-and-takes of life, the husband and wife are united in the blessings of God, these two beings on the stage of this short-lived life and by accepting and adapting themselves to the role of the Hero and Heroine of the play and they are able to create heavenly feeling in the theatre of the world.

|| ॐ ||

A Tight Rope Walk

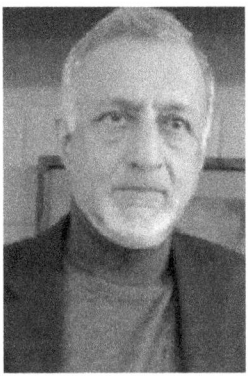

Author's Name	:	C. P. Belliappa
Qualification	:	M.E. (Chem. Eng)
Current Profession	:	Agriculture
Age	:	78 years
E-mail ID	:	bellicp@yahoo.com
City/ Country	:	Karnataka, India

C. P. Belliappa is a chemical engineer. After working for companies such as Indian Oil Corporation, Rallis India, and Humphreys & Glasgow Consultants, he returned to his hometown in Kodagu, in Karnataka where he manages his coffee plantation.

Belliappa is an educationist, a pragmatist, a rationalist, and a Darwinian evolutionist. Writing is his hobby. He has written numerous articles and essays in leading newspapers, magazines, and websites. Rupa Publications has published 5 books authored by Belliappa.

Keywords: Marriage, Bliss, Curse, Soul-mate, Joy

Bliss and Curse are at the two ends of the marriage fulcrum. My wife and I have been, by and large, blissfully married for over half a century. So, I consider myself reasonably well-qualified to write on the subject based on my own experience and that of my friends and relatives.

For many, marriage represents an unmatched companionship. Sharing life with another person (in the modern world, sometimes of the same gender), offers emotional support, financial stability and mental well-being. The everyday companionship that a like-minded spouse provides can be a source of immense joy and strength. Through gains, losses and mundane routines, having a committed partner can lighten burdens and multiply joys.

A stable and steady marriage often provides a nurturing environment for raising children. From celebrating birthdays and anniversaries to facing adversities together, shared family experiences enrich a couple's life. These collective memories of agonies and ecstasies strengthen the bond between partners, offering a treasure trove of memories to cherish.

Conflicts are an inevitable part of any close relationship. However, unresolved disputes and persistent misunderstandings can lead to resentment, emotional distress and a feeling of entrapment. Financial issues are a common source of tension in marriages. Differences in spending habits, financial goals or unexpected economic hardships can create stress, leading to conflicts and even erosion of trust within the relationship.

Effective communication is indispensable in a healthy marriage. Couples who communicate well are more likely to resolve conflicts amicably and sustain their bond. My wife believes that couples who fight and argue and later make up are more likely to have stable marriages.

Respecting each other's individuality and supporting personal growth is crucial. Recognizing and appreciating differences rather than trying to change each other can enhance mutual respect and love. When two individuals, united in marriage, become soulmates, it's pure bliss.

While the simplistic view of marriage as either bliss or curse oversimplifies ground reality, it captures the extremes of common experiences. It is natural for people to find their marriage oscillate between joy and challenge. Recognizing that marriage is a dynamic relationship involving continuous effort can lead to a more nuanced perspective.

Younger generations tend to view marriage differently. GenX and GenZ as they are known, seek bliss by remaining single or having live-in relationships with minimum commitments. It is fashionable for GenX and GenZ couples to be DINKs – Double Income No Kids. In fact, in the West, the very idea of marriage is under threat. Whether they ultimately achieve happiness by living a bohemian life is debatable.

It is not uncommon for a marriage to completely fall apart, become an unmitigated curse, and end in divorce. When this fracture takes place, and if there are children involved, the break will be hardest for the children and will remain a lifelong pain for them. Melinda Gates had this to say about her divorce from Bill Gates:

"Getting a divorce is a horrible thing. It is just painful. It is awful when you realise you need one."

Whether a marriage is blissful or becomes a curse depends on personal experiences, compatibility between partners, and the ability to navigate the complexities of life together to keep the marriage boat from rocking. By fostering communication, respect, and shared values, couples can tilt the balance towards bliss. Acknowledging and addressing challenges honestly can prevent potential curses.

In the final analysis, marriage is a tightrope walk, a delicate equilibrium swaying on a fulcrum. It is about finding harmony between bliss and curse.

॥ ॐ ॥

Grief to Gratitude

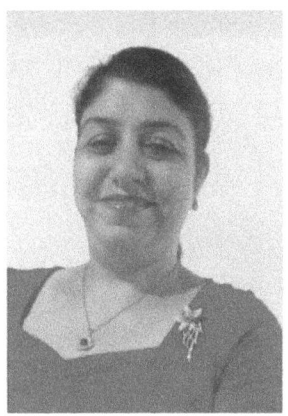

Author's Name	:	CA Meenaz Cyrus Surty
Qualification	:	B.Com., C.A.
Current Profession	:	Service in Government Sector
		Consultant and Counselor in Occult Science
Age	:	51 years
E-mail ID	:	**meenaz.surty@gmail.com**
City/ Country	:	**Surat, India**

Meenaz is a Chartered Accountant by profession. She was a ranker throughout her school days and had a bright academic career. She has completed her silver jubilee (25 years) in her profession with wide range of experience in private and government sector. At present she is serving as an officer in a semi government organisation.

In the field of occult science, she has acquired knowledge in Automatic Writing, Angel Card Reading, Access Consciousness Bars Practitioner, Numerology, Handwriting Analysis, Crystal, Healing through frequency and artificial intelligence and many more modalities like Spirit Animals, Dream Analysis, etc. She specialises in Talk Therapy and is eager to learn Mediumship. She considers herself as life-long learner. She is the founder of "MYSTICAL MEENAZ- Follow your Heart", a brand where she practises all her healing, spiritual and occult modalities.

Keywords : Communication, Dream, Evolve Together, Transform Together, Understanding

Marriage is supposedly the oldest known social system for the set up of a "civilized" society. It is a sacred institution that brings two souls together in love and commitment. For some, it's a blissful journey of growth and happiness while for others it is nothing short of a curse. For some it is a partner to share life's joys and sorrows and to laugh and cry together. But for others, it can become a curse, a constant struggle and source of unbearable pain. The once deep love turns into bitter resentment and suffocating chains. The journey that began in dreams and hopes ends in disappointment and despair. The bliss of marriage requires effort and dedication but the curse of a bad marriage can be devastating. 'Communication and Understanding' are the keys to avoiding the pitfalls and nurturing a life-long bond. Unfortunately, whether marriage is a bliss or a curse depends on the couples' willingness to work together and cherish their love. With 'commitment and love', marriage can be a beautiful journey but without it, it can become a life-long regret.

For a marriage to work, one requires these important qualities, which are hidden in the spelling itself-

M - Motivation

A - Affection

R - Resilience

R - Rapport

I - Intimacy

A - Appreciation

G - Grateful

E - Empathy

"Marriage", every single teenage girl, especially in India, has a fantasy, a dream that some handsome prince will come on a white horse and take her to her dream destination. But when the actual event (Marriage) happens, the dream of almost 90% of the girls is shattered, that too in such small pieces that sometimes it becomes difficult even to gather those pieces. Today I am narrating about one such girl. She too had dreams and aspirations about the life after her marriage and about the husband and his family. But as it happens in most of the cases, none of her dreams took the shape of reality. In the eyes of the world, the marriage was a perfect one. But only she knew how she adjusted in the new environment, where none of her desires were fulfilled about the life after marriage. Days and years passed with adjustments in personal and professional life. In between she was blessed with two beautiful children, a girl and a boy, which made here family 'complete'. But there was always a dissatisfaction deep within her which made her irritable, full of anger, frustration and broken from within.

As if all this was not enough for her, the health of her kids did not keep well. She ran from pole to post of hospitals, doctors and even religious places in the hope that some miracle will happen. The positive attitude then turned negative when one day her daughter did not wake up from her sleep. She lost the battle of life. She was completely broken and shattered to pieces. However, she gathered some strength so that she could at least save her son. But few days later she lost her son also. Losing both the children was a blow that no mother can withstand. She was totally into depression and had thoughts of suicide as she felt that there was no purpose for her life now. The struggles which she faced to be in the marriage had now converted into the struggle to just simply 'live'.

However, it is said that there are many turning points in life and this was one among the many, in her life. After about three years of struggling to just 'live', she managed to survive and restart living her life. Though being dissatisfied with her married life, she was now left just with her husband. Now both of them were having a common battle where she was displaying her emotions while her husband was silently dealing with it. Both of them tried to live coping with the grief and sorrow.

However, as every cloud has a silver lining, the grief and pain got them closer. It brought more compassion and empathy in them towards life and humanity. The purpose of life was found by both of them in serving others and working for humanity The pain brought about a 360 degree transformation in the marriage. Now both knew that they had to be the pillar of strength for each other.

She had tried hard to come out of the grief of her children and become busy with her office life, devoting more time and energy there to distract her from the pain of loss. But as destiny wanted to take her to other path, some unprecedented things took shape in the office whereby she was forced to isolate herself. But a lioness she is, not ready to quit, she took this as an opportunity in disguise and that started her spiritual career. She utilised her time for learning new things and did many courses and upgraded her knowledge. The by-product of these learning opened up new perspectives in her and that even improved her relationship issues. Not that the issues disappeared, but now she was well equipped with various tools and techniques to combat these low feelings in relationships.

We are often taught to understand and adjust in any relationship. But the actual fact is that understanding and adjusting by a single person only creates grudges and bitterness deep down in the person which at a point of time is reflected in the personality. So, instead of understanding and adjusting, 'effective communication' is the key from the start of the relationship. Marriage is a journey of 'growth and transformation', where two individuals evolve together and shaping each other's lives. Effective communication, empathy and trust are essential catalysts for transformation in marriage, helping couples navigate life's challenges so that they emerge stronger. Transformation in marriage requires embracing change, letting go of ego and adapting to new roles and responsibilities of 'working as one'. Marriage transformation involves moving from 'me' to 'we', surrendering individual desires for the greater good of the relationship. Transformation in marriage is not a one-time event but a continuous process, requiring effort, patience and dedication from both partners. As couples transform together, they develop resilience, learn to forgive and create a more profound, lasting connection. Upgrading oneself with knowledge develops the correct understanding towards life and also helps to understand and deal any relationship in a more better way. Find common activities of interest, give surprises, going out for drives, enjoying common passion and spending quality time together are some tools which helps to keep the relationship fresh. "The most important decision of life is to choose the correct life partner" and therefore this decision should be taken after deep thought so that it turns out to be 'Bliss'.

|| ॐ ||

Psalm of Life

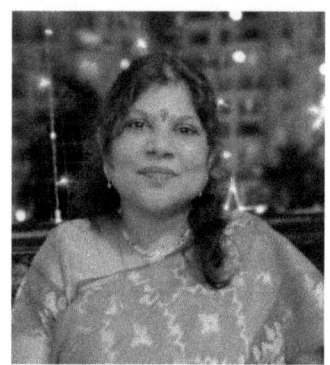

Author's Name	:	Deepa Jain
Qualification	:	B. Com., Course in Public Speaking
Current Profession	:	Home Maker, Helping Hand of Husband
Age	:	52 years
E-mail ID	:	**deepasuren1995@gmail.com**
City/ Country	:	**Mumbai, India**

Deepa Jain is skilled in house management and helping hand of her life partner, sharing his responsibilities as an entrepreneur in the field of banking and correspondence. She always had a keen interest in penning down her deep thoughts in form of poems and stories. She also takes interest in dance, music, meditation etc. She is good counsellor too.

Keywords : Challenges, Expressions, Struggle, Support, Mental Peace

Today I was stuck in morning chores I received a phone call from my hubby. I said good day and he replied I took your spectacles for the meeting by mistake along with mine. So, this is what mostly marriage is about where you share each moment of your life, where you want somebody to grow old with. It takes a lot of compromise, work, understanding and acceptance. It is choosing the right battles and let love and peace win.

It is about moving ahead and always forgiving spouse's mistake. So, every marriage is different. Bliss or curse you have to decide. Are you ready to embrace your spouse with acceptance the most important factor?

Gestures, expressions, body language are key factors. Also, they are silent signals. A gentle touch, a reassuring smile or sitting close can convey support and love without a single word being spoken.

For many, marriage represents a deep emotional bond, companionship and the joy of sharing life with a partner. The love, support and shared goals can create a fulfilling partnership that enhances personal growth and happiness. Marriage can be seen as both bliss and curse, depending on individual experiences and perspectives.

Conversely, marriage can also present challenges that may feel burdensome. Issues such as communication problems, financial stress and differing life goals can lead to conflicts. In some cases, these struggles can overshadow the positive aspects, making the relationship feel more like a burden than a blessing.

Ultimately, the experience of marriage varies greatly from one couple to other based on the long-bred ideas, values and beliefs inculcated in them through their living environment and experiences.

Two people joining each other in a holy union, "a marriage". Marriage is a union of not only two individuals but two families, two cultures and myriad beliefs. Life is a mosaic of many pictures of which marriage happens to be the most abstract one; nobody has actually been able to say if it is a bliss or sheer curse. In today's fast paced world, marriage is losing its charm among youngsters. Marriage brings responsibility and compromise on one hand but on the other hand it brings stability and utmost joy.

Marriage differentiates a human from animals, otherwise animals also satisfy their carnal desires. Marriage brings stability, companionship, emotional support. It gives a friend for life; a person definitely has to put efforts to make marriage happy but when these efforts lead to the formation of a lovely family, nothing can be more beautiful. When you have your next generation to pass on your values and what you have learnt would be the betterment of whole human race,

When you see through the ups and downs of life you have somebody to share your joy and lend you shoulder to cry upon; Life becomes easier, Marriage comes with bumps, you will not agree with your partner at multiple times, you will have clashes but isn't that what happens with your parents and family too. At the sunset of life having someone to listen to your bickering will definitely be a bliss. A relationship without marriage can be convenient, but it can never bring peace and contentment. Someone who has been with you at your best as well as worst time will definitely be your best consort.

Marriage has its own pros and cons but undoubtedly the pros are a way more valuable and marriage definitely is a bliss.

Feeling blessed to get the opportunity of penning down my thoughts. Always wanted to be an author and my dream came true. Thank you, Mr. Abhishaik Chitraans, Mrs. Rainu Mangtani and Mrs. Kala Malpani, for believing in me and given me a chance for the same.

In my article I have tried to share my view point about marriage a beautiful journey, a psalm of life. Marriage a golden dove gave me care, devotion, peace. It carried a divine message of the beginning of a new era, symbolic connection to hope.

'A relationship without marriage can be convenient, but it can never bring peace and contentment.'

|| ॐ ||

From Wife to Wonder Woman
How Marriage Transformed My Life 0^0 to 360^0

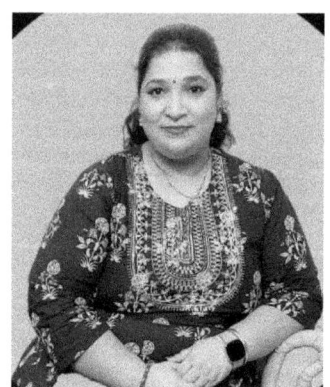

Author's Name	:	Deepti Sood
Qualification	:	Graduate
Current Profession	:	Certified Life Coach & Healer
Age	:	40 years
E-mail ID	:	**ndmmsblogs@gmail.com**
City/ Country	:	**Mumbai, India**

Deepti sood is a certified life coach, healer, tarot card reader & an influencer. She is passionate about life. Her mission is to help women to discover their life purpose & possibilities to fulfil all their dreams. She served as big sister in a reputed organization and helped more than 100 women's to transform their life journey. She had accomplished her excellence in being Reiki Healer, ho'oponopono healer, crystal healer, aura healer, angel card reader, tarot card reader, A youtuber and an influencer. She is a very loving person who is creative and compassionate about life and is a true fighter. Today she is most grateful for the gift of happiness and gift of gratitude.

Keywords : Adjustment, Anxiety, Challenges, Dream, Fingerprint

A successful marriage requires falling in love many times, always with the same person. Marriages are like fingerprints; each one is different and each one is beautiful.

"Being a woman in this world is not easy"

Every woman has her own dreams and goals so as I, when I married with Nitin, I imagined a life of shared dreams and quiet domestic bliss. Little did I know that my journey from wife to wonder woman was just beginning, and marriage would transform my life in ways I never anticipated. Before marriage, I had successfully cleared an interview, but due to personal reasons, I was unable to join. That was my first dream, and it remained unfulfilled.

Then I got married and became busy with family life, especially after the children were born. Taking care of them and managing the household became my priority. The initial months were filled with adjustments, learning to cohabit, merging our finances, and balancing our jobs of being a housewife and him with his work with personal time. These experiences taught me resilience and the importance of compromise. I began to see that partnership was not just about romantic dinners and shared laughter but also about tackling life's obstacles together. Slowly and steadily, our lives began to fall into place.

Then, a devastating blow hit our stable life when my husband lost his job. Our world changed dramatically during those difficult times. We both tried our best to stabilize our daily lives, sometimes ending in conflicts and tears. During that period, I realized I needed to do something to secure our future. I began to lose my self-respect and felt neglected within my family. I started experiencing depression, anxiety and self-blame.

However, as every dark cloud has a silver lining, another job opportunity came for my husband, and he was transferred to another state. Our financial situation began to improve, but I remained in the same condition. I was alone with all the responsibilities on my shoulders, which triggered more pressure and anxiety, resulting in loneliness, negativity and sadness. Then, one day, I had an anxiety attack. After that, my whole life changed, and I decided to push my restart button.

My sister introduced me to a meditation course, which brought significant changes and increased my confidence. Then one day, a major change occurred and my husband called us to join him. From there, my life began to take a new turn. One day, while browsing Instagram, I saw a video about life skills. When I told my husband about this, he listened and supported me in joining it. He supported me emotionally and financially both. I joined my mentor's course, and my life began to change from 0 to 360 degrees. I understood myself, gave myself time, value, and respect, and noticed that my family also started to respect me. My children and husband supported me in moving forward. Today, I have transformed from a devoted housewife into Deepti 2.0 Life Design Coach and Healer.

In conclusion, marriage is a continuous journey of growth and adaptation between two imperfect people. It involves embracing each other's strengths and weaknesses, learning from experiences and supporting one another through life's challenges. This journey fosters a deep connection and helps build a meaningful, enduring partnership.

|| ॐ ||

Wedded Bliss or Near Miss
A Poetic Marriage Journey

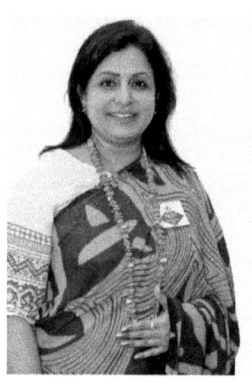

Author's Name	:	Divvya A Singh
Qualification	:	B Sc and B Ed
Current Profession	:	Consultant and Child Coach
Age	:	48 years
E-mail ID	:	**divvyasingh555@gmail.com**
City/ Country	:	**Gurgaon, India**

Divvya A Singh is a Co-founder of Selfwrite Institute of Holistic Development. She is an Educationist and Professional handwriting Analyst, Signature Analyst, Drawing Analyst, Date of Birth Analyst, Hypnotherapist and a Certified Published Author. She has more than 19 years of experience in the teaching sector and 3+ years as a Handwriting Consultant. She is a member of International Council of Graphologist. She is on a mission to empower children and adults and help them nurture their dreams through Graphotherapy, Hypnotherapy and other healing modalities.

Keywords: Marriage Celebration, Marriage, Counselling Marriage Journey, Wedded Bliss, Chemical Locha

Wedded Bliss or Near Miss: A Poetic Marriage Journey

In this journey of marriage, here's the lock and key –

Love, respect, and laugh, and you'll both be happy as you can be!

Remember, in laughter and tears,

Marriage is a journey of love through the years!

Keep the romance alive, with flowers and wine,

Don't hog the bed covers, it's a civic crime.

Cherish the moments-the good and bad,

Don't leave wet towels on the floor- it's really quite sad!

Embrace each other's quirks and routines,

Don't leave the cap of the toothpaste; if you know what that means!

Encourage each other to grow and improve,

Don't nag for small things; let some matters move.

Communicate openly about what bothers you,

Don't let frustrations build up and stew.

Form healthy routines that bring you both joy,

Don't forget to give each other enough space to deploy.

Laugh off the little annoyances that come your way,

Don't let petty grievances ruin your day.

Forgive mistakes with grace and understanding,

Don't hold onto resentment, it's too demanding.

In the tapestry of marriage, with habits woven tight,

Do choose love and kindness, every day and every night!

Welcome each other's families with open arms,

Don't let differences in traditions cause alarms.

Respect boundaries and communicate clear,

Don't gossip or complain, let love persevere.

Find common ground and build bonds strong,

Don't let misunderstandings linger for long.

Show appreciation for their love and care,

Don't let small disagreements lead to despair.

Communicate openly, with patience and respect,

Don't hesitate to compromise, always reconnect.

Give each other space when bad moods appear,

Don't take it personally, sometimes it's unclear.

Do offer support and a listening ear,

Don't escalate tensions, let calmness steer.

In the journey of marriage, through ups and through downs,

Do remember love conquers all with its gentle bounds!

Handle conflicts privately, with care and grace,

Don't involve others unless it's a serious case.

Seek advice from trusted confidants when in doubt,

Don't let external influences cause unnecessary clout.

In the journey of marriage, with unity as your guide,

Do cherish your bond and let it securely abide!

Stock up on patience, it's a precious supply,

Don't forget to replenish, when tensions run high.

Trust your partner's words and actions sincere,

Don't let suspicion cloud what you hold dear.

In the journey of marriage, where trust is the key,

Let love dispel suspicion and set your hearts free.

Honor theirs and yours dreams and passions with pride,

Don't diminish either spirit or push it aside.

Cherish individuality, strong and true,

Don't impose your expectations, let them pursue.

In the journey of marriage, where souls intertwine,

Respect identity, and let love shine!

Share the load, both the joy and the weight,

Don't leave it all to one, balance is great.

Communicate openly, about tasks big and small,

Don't let resentment build, hear each other's call.

Support each other through thick and through thin,

Don't forget teamwork is how victories begin.

In the journey of marriage, with responsibilities in sight,

Together you thrive, with love as your light!

Support each other's aspirations and dreams,

Don't let financial insecurities tear at the seams.

In the journey of marriage, with trust as your guide,

Face financial challenges side by side.

Cherish the commitment, strong and true,

In every moment, let your love renew.

Don't let distractions pull you apart,

Stay connected, heart to heart.

Embrace each other through highs and lows,

In each other's arms, let comfort flow.

Don't take each other for granted,

Keep gratitude always planted.

In the journey of marriage, where love is the song,

Find belonging together, where you both belong.

|| ॐ ||

Marriage is a Part of Human Journey

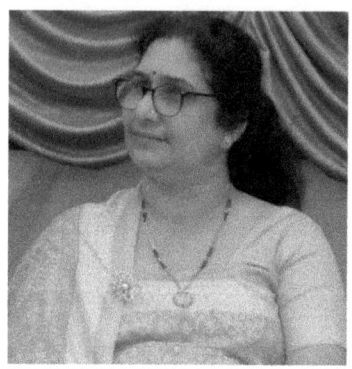

Author's Name	:	Dr. A S Poovamma
Qualification	:	B.AEd. M.A. M.Phil. Ph.D.
Current Profession	:	Rtd. Associate Professor, Former Principal and Vice Principal
Age	:	60 years
E-mail ID	:	…
City/ Country	:	**Gonikoppal, Karnataka, India**

Dr A.S Poovamma now retired from service as an Associate Professor in English in Cauvery College Gonikoppal. She has put in 37 years of service and served as a Lecturer in English, Associate Professor, Head of the Department, Principal and Vice-Principal.

She was the Co-coordinator of IQAC (Internal Quality Assurance Cell) of Cauvery College Gonikoppal in 2010-11 and got Grade 'A' to the institution. She was invited as the Chief-Guest speaker by several institutions and organizations during her long tenure of service. She is a life member of several Literary Associations like MLA, IACLALS, ISPELL. She was the past President of Rotary International organization; Gonikoppal.

She published Poems, Articles, and organized National and International seminars. She also presented papers in National and International Seminars in Hyderabad and in Innsbruck, Austria. She won several Awards like Karnataka Excellence Award in 2021 as the Best Lecturer in English.

Keywords : Journey, Ceremony, Contribution, Happiness, Understanding

Marriage is a part of human journey on this planet earth. As far as I understand human journey begins in the womb of a Mother. Sometimes when one is born end up there itself and one cannot know why one is born. Nobody knows why we are born and how long we continue our journey. If we observe human life; it takes us towards that world of confusion where we can never arrive at an understanding of why we are born and where are we heading towards.

First we dwell in our childhood stage and move up towards teenage and adolescence,; then begins our thought towards building our future wherein the institution of Marriage plays a major role. In India if we observe our culture, marriage is a holy ceremony wherein two Hearts come together with the blessings of our ancestors, seniors and divine grace. However, in my understanding Marriage is not just between two souls, it should be between two families. It has a larger space because, if the husband and wife love each other, understand each other and live together; they have to cherish their love and continue only if the two families understand each other and contribute to the couples wellbeing. As far as I can understand; I feel no human being is perfect; everybody will have some weakness or the other. Nobody is perfect. So if two families come together and understand each other they can in a clever way let one of the couple know what their weakness is, so that they can rectify it and develop into a fine human being to settle the differences. So, over a period of time the husband and Wife can gel with each other and move along to contribute to the progress of the society as well.

When the husband and wife understand each other and continue to live together with joy and understanding; children born to them will lead a very happy life. Then, Marriage is a bliss.

But Man proposes one thing and God disposes and then life becomes a curse. In my case, I had a blissful marriage of love and understanding for more than twenty five years and we were a happy couple but in 2022, I suddenly lost my husband and it was a time of sorrow and helplessness. I lost a wonderful partner and realized now Marriage can usher in curse. Till 2022 my marriage was bliss to me but after 2022 it suddenly rained a heap of curse on to my life.

To say that Marriage was a bliss in its early journey for me as God blessed me with Two lovely children: a son and a daughter, who take care of me in my husband's absence. This is my experience but if we generally observe, sometimes we see the couple opt for a divorce and live asunder. This separation I feel happens when the two families do not involve in understanding each other. That is why marriage is not just between two souls; it is also between two families. If there is common understanding between all the members of the two families the idea of divorce can be easily wiped out and the couple can live together in total understanding and happiness.

As human life operates through binary opposites, I think Marriage has also become a journey of Bliss vs Curse.

॥ ॐ ॥

Navigating the Peaks and Valleys of Wedded Life

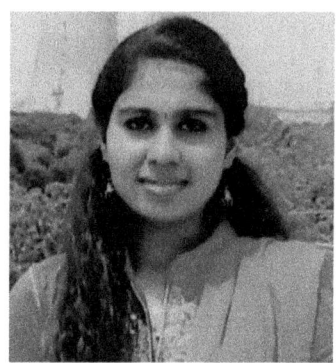

Author's Name	:	Dr. Agalya VT Raj
Qualification	:	M.A., Ph.D. (English)
Current Profession	:	Assistant Professor
Age	:	29 years
E-mail ID	:	**dragalyavtraj@gmail.com**
City/ Country	:	**Chennai, India**

Dr. Agalya VT Raj is an adventurous educator with a passion for communication and teaching. With a Ph.D. in English and a background in teaching and training, she excels in various teaching techniques. Her career spans roles as an Assistant Professor at SRM Institute of Science and Technology. She completed her Doctorate in English at Annamalai University, Chidambaram. Her research is in American Literature. She has published her articles in various Scopus, WOS, UGC Care listed journals and Peer reviewed journals. She has an impeccable writing and editing skills, public speaking, training program management, leadership, curriculum development, project management, and more. Multiple certificates of appreciation and participation in academic and professional development activities, including for NPTEL STAR certifications, NPTEL Translator certifications and international conferences.

Keywords: Commitment, Love, Partnership, Happiness and Harmony

Marriage, a cornerstone of societal structures, often oscillates between two extreme perspectives: bliss and curse. This anthology, "My Marriage: Bliss vs. Curse," encapsulates the myriad experiences of individuals as they navigate the intricate dynamics of marital life. It seeks to explore the joy, fulfillment, and companionship that a harmonious marriage can offer, while also acknowledging the pain, conflict, and disillusionment that can accompany a tumultuous union. By presenting a balanced view, this anthology aims to provide a comprehensive understanding of marriage's dual nature, encouraging readers to reflect on their own experiences and perceptions of this age-old institution.

In the delicate balance of life, marriage often stands as a pinnacle of human connection, capable of bringing both unparalleled joy and profound sorrow. For some, marriage is the embodiment of bliss a journey filled with shared dreams, mutual support, and a deep, abiding love. These individuals speak of waking up every day with a sense of gratitude, finding in their partner a best friend, a confidant, and a lover. Their stories are filled with moments of laughter, the comfort of companionship and the growth that comes from facing life's challenges together. For them, marriage is a sacred bond that enriches their lives, fostering a sense of belonging and stability.

However, not all marriages are tales of unending happiness. For others, marriage can feel like a curse, fraught with conflict, disappointment and unmet expectations. These narratives reveal the darker side of marital life, where love gives way to resentment, and harmony is replaced by discord. They tell of partners growing apart, communication breaking down, and the painful reality of living with someone who no longer feels like a soulmate. The sense of entrapment and the loss of individuality are recurring themes, highlighting how a once-promising relationship can deteriorate into a source of constant strife.

Yet, between these extremes, there are also stories of resilience and redemption. Some marriages weather the storm, emerging stronger and more united after periods of hardship. These accounts emphasize the importance of communication, compromise and the willingness to grow and adapt together. They demonstrate that even when marriage feels like a curse, it can sometimes be transformed into a blessing through effort, understanding, and unconditional love.

In my opinion, the most profound lesson from "My Marriage: Bliss vs. Curse" is the importance of maintaining open communication and mutual respect. Marriage, at its best, is a partnership, where both individuals feel valued and supported. However, when these elements are lacking, it can quickly become a source of distress. By acknowledging the potential for both bliss and curse, this anthology encourages couples to strive for balance and to approach their relationships with empathy and commitment. It reminds us that while marriage can indeed be challenging, it also holds the potential for immense joy and fulfillment.

"My Marriage: Bliss vs Curse" is a compelling collection that captures the essence of marital experiences. It reminds us that marriage is a complex, evolving partnership that requires effort, understanding and resilience. While some may find bliss and fulfillment, others may encounter challenges that test their limits. This anthology encourages readers to reflect on their own relationships and find strength in the shared human experience of love, struggle and growth within marriage.

॥ ॐ ॥

Fate's Chains

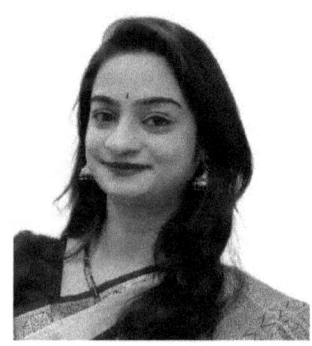

Author's Name	:	Dr. Anisha Mahendrakar
Qualification	:	M.Sc. Counseling Psychology PGDM – Clinical Hypnotherapy, PGDM – Sex Education and Intimacy, 19 Credit Courses – Techniques of Counselling, Methods of Psychological Diagnosis, Asian Healing techniques, PhD
Current Profession	:	Therapist & Healer
Age	:	32 years
E-mail ID	:	**anishamahendrakar@gmail.com**
City/ Country	:	**Bengaluru, India**

Dr. Anisha Mahendrakar is an internationally acclaimed Trainer and Therapist in the field of Psycho-Spiritual wellness. She is renowned for blending traditional values with contemporary techniques and diagnostic tools in psychological counseling. A UNO awardee, Dr. Mahendrakar has been recognized for her outstanding contributions to applied psychology, particularly in managing relationships and intimacy. A child prodigy with a natural talent for tarot card reading and healing, she is also the founder of the Healing modality Rapid Reiki-Quantum Healing. As the founder-director of 'The NewAge Therapist,' a psychological consultancy firm based in Bengaluru, India, Dr. Mahendrakar is dedicated to empowering individuals to blossom into their most authentic selves. She is currently pursuing her second doctorate.

Keywords : Arranged Marriage, Depression, Fate, Forced Union

Marriage is one of life's most significant decisions, yet it is often taken lightly. We spend more time deciding what to wear, and less time to decide, who we make our life and bed with. Often, as young adults we are not allowed to make these decisions, by yourself and the family helps. It is unfortunate, when the help comes as bulldozing and in turn destroys a lively person's life. This story is one of my landmark cases as a therapist.

I was in an elevator of a mall one day, when I saw a older women staring at me as if she knew me. She recognized me from one of my talks on psycho-spiritual healings. She asked me if I can please talk to her daughter Leela, who was married recently, and was now diagnosed with clinical depression. The family was distraught and really worried.

Leela was 21 when her life was irreversibly altered. In this society, a girl's value was often measured by the milestone of marriage, rather than her education or capabilities. Her parents insisted, coerced and convinced her, that nothing was more important than Marriage at this age. Soon, the groom was chosen, the wedding arranged, and Leela, like so many before her, had no choice but to comply.

Her new husband, Vikram, was a distant figure from the start. A young man with ambitions far removed from the life laid out before him, Vikram had been in love with another—a secret girlfriend from his college days. His parents, however, had discovered the relationship and forced him to break it off. They believed Leela, with her docile nature and good family background, would be the perfect wife to shape into their idea of an obedient daughter-in-law.

Both families had taken center stage in deciding the lives of their beloved children, Leela was clueless about what her life had in store for her. Vikram was forced to let go of a dear person and comply to his parents' wishes for the sake of family honor. Family honor was deciding the fates of many people here, rather than any feelings or emotions.

From the moment Leela entered her new home, she was met with cold indifference. Vikram barely spoke to her, his eyes hollow with resentment. His parents, on the other hand, expected her to immediately fall in line with their rigid expectations. Every mistake she made, every moment of hesitation, was met with harsh words and disapproving glances.

Days turned into weeks, and nothing seemed better. Vikram's mother would criticize Leela for everything—from the way she dressed to the way she cooked. His father was no better, constantly reminding her that she was lucky to have been chosen for their son. Vikram, still heartbroken over his lost love, took out his frustration on Leela, refusing to even share a conversation with her, let alone any semblance of affection. He would leave the house early and return late, avoiding her presence as much as possible.

Leela's spirit began to crumble under the weight of the unspoken misery that filled the house. The loneliness became unbearable, the constant criticism piercing through whatever remained of her self-esteem. She tried to reach out to her parents, but they dismissed her concerns, telling her that all marriages were difficult in the beginning. "This is your fate," they said, as if that could ease her pain.

The months that followed saw Leela's once bright eyes grow dull, her laughter disappear entirely. Eventually, her condition worsened, and she started to turn pale. Her body failing her. She was then diagnosed with severe depression. She had begun her journey with strong psychiatric pharmaceuticals, and therapy. With her spirit broken, and a sad questioning look on her face, as if to ask what did she do to deserve this, she remained unresponsive. Everyone spoke about her terrible fate and "poor girl" they would say, shaking their heads, "what a terrible fate." But the truth was, Leela's fate had been written by the hands of those who should have protected her. And now, all that was left was a hollow shell of the girl who once dreamed of a life filled with possibility.

The true essence of marriage—a partnership based on mutual love, respect and choice—is lost when it is forced upon individuals. Calling it "fate" is merely a way to absolve responsibility for the consequences of these decisions. When people are denied the right to choose their own partner, the concept of "fate" is often used to justify this control. But is it truly fate when the decision is forced? Such marriages, lacking mutual consent, often result in unhappiness, questioning the very foundation on which they are built. When personal choice is stripped away, the resulting unhappiness is not fate, but the outcome of coercion and control. True fate lies in allowing individuals the freedom to choose their own paths. Parents, with their extensive experience of people and life should be a guiding light to help them decide, not add on the young mind's anxiety and push their personal egoistical agenda. Only then can marriages thrive, rooted in genuine connection rather than obligation. It's time to reconsider how lightly we take such a profound decision.

Embracing Individuality in Togetherness
My Marriage is a Bliss

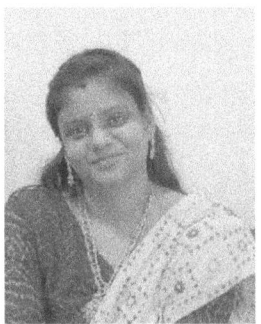

Author's Name	:	Dr. Ellakkiyaa Sankar
Qualification	:	M.A., Ph.D. (English)
Current Profession	:	Assistant Professor in English
Age	:	29 years
E-mail ID	:	**ellakiyashivasankar@gmail.com**
City/ Country	:	**Tamil Nadu, India**

Dr. Ellakkiyaa S is working as Assistant Professor in Erode College of Law, Tamil Nadu. She completed her Doctorate in English in University of Madras. She is a certified Phonic trainer and Handwriting Coach. Her research is on Indian Mythological Fiction. She has published her articles in various UGC Care listed journals, international journals and Peer reviewed journals. She attended 10 seminars, 13 conferences and presented paper in 15 various institutions. She has a better proficiency in English with good grammatical knowledge.

> **Keywords:** Love, Respect, Quality Time, Support, Encouragement

Marriage is often described as a journey, filled with peaks and valleys, moments of intense joy, and inevitable challenges. For me, this journey has been overwhelmingly positive and I am grateful to say that my marriage is a bliss. From the beginning, our relationship has been built on a foundation of deep love and mutual respect. We have always prioritized understanding and valuing each other's opinions, feelings and dreams. This mutual respect has fostered a sense of safety and trust that is crucial for any strong relationship. One of the cornerstones of our blissful marriage is open and honest communication. We have made it a point to share our thoughts and feelings with each other regularly. This transparency has helped us navigate conflicts smoothly, as we address issues head-on rather than allowing them to fester. We listen actively, ensuring that both of us feel heard and understood. Spending quality time together has been instrumental in maintaining the joy in our marriage. We make it a priority to have regular date nights, even if it's just a cozy evening at home with a movie and homemade dinner. These moments allow us to reconnect and keep the romance alive. Additionally, we enjoy shared hobbies, like hiking and cooking, which strengthen our bond and create lasting memories. A significant aspect of our marital bliss is the unwavering support and encouragement we provide each other. Whether it's pursuing career goals, personal interests, or tackling life's challenges, we stand by each other's side. This support system has been a source of strength, helping us grow individually and as a couple. Having shared values and goals has given our marriage a sense of direction and purpose. We regularly discuss our aspirations and make plans for our future together. This alignment keeps us focused and united, working towards common objectives that enrich our lives and relationship. Maintaining intimacy is crucial in any marriage. For us, physical affection and emotional closeness go hand in hand. We make an effort to express our love daily, whether through simple gestures like holding hands or more significant acts of kindness and appreciation. This continuous expression of affection keeps our connection strong and vibrant. While we cherish our togetherness, we also respect each other's individuality. We encourage each other to pursue personal interests and spend time apart when needed. This balance allows us to grow as individuals, which in turn enhances the quality of our relationship. Celebrating each other's achievements, no matter how big or small, has added joy to our marriage. We take pride in each other's successes and make it a point to acknowledge and celebrate them. This practice reinforces our bond and creates a positive and supportive environment. No marriage is without its challenges, but it's how we handle them that make the difference. We approach difficulties as a team, facing them with grace and a problem-solving mind set. This collaborative approach has helped us overcome obstacles and emerge stronger together.

My marriage is bliss not because it's perfect, but because we have cultivated an environment of love, respect and continuous effort. By prioritizing open communication, quality time, support, shared values and mutual respect, we have built a relationship that brings immense joy and fulfilment. It's a journey that requires dedication and care, but the rewards are immeasurable. For anyone seeking marital bliss, remember that it's the everyday acts of love and respect that build the foundation of a happy and lasting marriage.

Finding Strength in Adversity

Author's Name	:	Dr. Heena P
Qualification	:	AICC, Holistic Healing
Current Profession	:	Consultant and Practitioner
Age	:	50 years
E-mail ID	:	...
City/ Country	:	**New Delhi, India**

Dr. Heena P holds an AICC Certification, demonstrating expertise in holistic health practices. She specializes in: Detoxification and Personalized Weight Loss/ Gain Programs, offering tailored approaches to achieve health goals. Diabetes Reversal Management, providing strategies to manage and potentially reverse diabetes. Support for Lactating Mothers and Pregnancy Nutrition, offering specialized diets to support maternal health and mental health counselling. Sports Nutrition, advising athletes on nutrition to optimize performance. Meditation and Holistic Wellness, certified in AOL Happiness, VTP, DSN and Advance Meditation, Integrating holistic approaches for mental and emotional well-being. Yoga and Meditation Practices, with expertise in BR's Raj Yoga and Holistic Swar Yoga.

Dr. Heena's diverse skills contribute to promoting comprehensive health and well-being through personalized and holistic methodologies.

Keywords : Courage, Strength, Positive, Suffering, Healing

Today, after 25 years of marriage, I realize how swiftly time has passed and how unforeseen events have reshaped my life. Allow me to share the journey of a young, emotional and naive 24-year-old me – Dr Heena P.

From college to our family home, surrounded by loved ones and a few close friends, my world was comfortably small. Coming from a typical Indian middle-class family, my parents upheld traditional values. I had an elder brother, a sister younger by two years, and myself - carefree and always cheerful. We celebrated small joys with customs, special food, and surprises of gifts that brought smiles to everyone.

Then, tragedy struck nine months after my elder brother's marriage. On a chilly evening, my brother's pregnant wife was enjoying tea with us when suddenly, police arrived with devastating news - my brother had died in an accident. It shattered our family, leaving us numb. My mother lost consciousness, and our once lively home echoed with cries instead of laughter and chatter.

Despite the overwhelming sorrow, we clung together, ensuring the unborn child would not be affected. Days later, he was born - a ray of hope amidst our grief, a reminder of my brother. We poured our love and care into him, our lives now revolving around this precious baby with tiny hands and feet.

Three years passed. It was 1999 when my parents arranged my marriage. The groom, senior to me, had a good reputation, yet I worried. My father, eager for my happiness and seeing the groom as a pediatrician from a respected family, saw him as caring, smart, and the perfect husband material. Reluctantly, I agreed...

After a few days, I began adjusting to my new surroundings with unfamiliar people. But soon, they started demanding money and jewelry from me. Meanwhile, I found out I was pregnant. I felt trapped. I tried to smile for my family, but inside, I was struggling.

Then the abuse started. Slaps, punches, kicks became normal. I hid it all from my family, hoping it would stop. But it didn't. I gave birth to a girl, but the abuse only got worse. I even thought about ending my life.

In 2003, my son was born. He changed everything for me. Those two children became my whole world. But my husband's behavior didn't change. In 2004, I lost my father. It shattered me and my mother. I tried to cope, but the abuse, demands, and accusations grew.

After ten years, I couldn't take it anymore. I took my children and went to my mother's house. I was broken, losing my confidence. Then they took my son away without my consent. I felt trapped again, with no way out.

But then something changed. Through meditation and yoga, I found strength. I realized I wasn't to blame. I focused on myself and my kids. Then, my sister-in-law passed away suddenly, shocking us all. It made me rethink life. We handled our sorrow, and soon there were marriage proposals for my husband's younger brother. I wondered, "Is it that easy to replace someone like their life doesn't matter?"

When my kids became adults and got into a good college, something terrible happened to me. My in-laws accused me of theft and shamed me in front of everyone in our community. After a month, they realized they were wrong, but instead of admitting it, they tried to ignore what they had done and act like everything was normal.

After much thought, I decided to move forward with a divorce. It took a lot of courage to endure all the injustice and suffering. Looking back, I realize I made a mistake. Why didn't I speak up the first time my in-laws and husband mistreated me? Why didn't I defend myself against the abuse, despite being educated and capable? Why did I agree to endure it all?

Now, through meditation and self-reflection, I'm diving deep into positive energy and finding my way back with the support and guidance of loved ones. It's not easy and the wounds from that time won't heal quickly, I'm committed to becoming the best version of myself, no matter how tough it gets. Life isn't always easy—it's like handling a basket of flowers carefully and consciously, knowing that reality can be tough. Yet, I believe in the saying, "Every cloud has a silver lining."

Despite tough times, a person should remain committed to becoming their best self, believing every cloud has a silver lining.

|| ॐ ||

A Bond of Mutual Respect

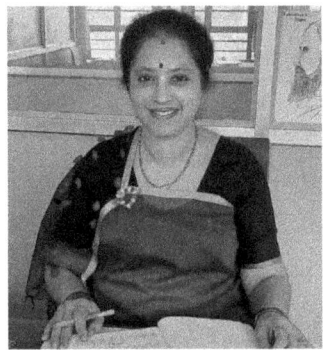

Author's Name	:	Dr. K G Veena
Qualification	:	M.A., M.Phil. LL.B., Ph.D.
Current Profession	:	HOD of English, Cauvery College
Age	:	48 years
E-mail ID	:	**veenaravindrak@gmail.com**
City/ Country	:	Virajpet, Kodagu, India

Dr. K.G.Veena is an academician and a lawyer. She was awarded the doctoral degree from the University of Mysore for her thesis "The Lotus and the Maple: A Comparative Study of the select Novels of Kavery Nambisan and Margaret Atwood. She is presently working as the HOD of English, Cauvery College, Virajpet. She has presented papers in various District, State, National and International Seminars. She has written a few poems and has also translated poems of Kannada and Kodava languages to English. Three of her poems are published. She has edited two books 'Women in Tiger Hills' and 'Inclusion of Kodava Language in the 8th Schedule of Indian Constitution' under the aegis of Karnataka Kodava Sahithiya Academy. She has been a resource person to various talks on 'English Language, Women Rights, Human Rights and in various Legal Awareness programs'.

Keywords : Trust, Understanding, Respect, Affinity, Love

Marriages are made in Heaven, is an ever recurring sentence spoken by the elders when an alliance is brought into the household for the most eligible bachelor or spinster in the family. If marriages are already made in Heaven then why should there by chaos in the married life? Why there are so many divorce cases in the courts? It must be believed that Heaven is created by us. There is nothing called Heaven out of our universe; it is we who create heaven or hell for us through our words and actions. This concept is very beautifully expressed by Kuvempu, a famous Kannada poet, in his poem 'Heaven if you are not here on earth'. To make our life worth living in this world we need to create heaven here on earth. So, heaven can be created in the married life through trust, understanding, respect, affinity and of course lots of Love.

Mutual Respect in the marriage, according to me, is the foundation upon which all the other feelings such as trust, understanding, affinity and love rely upon. A relationship is fulfilling only when the spouses show respect to each other's likes and dislikes. When the spouses respect each other, all the other relations follow the same. The partners must recognize and appreciate the qualities, strengths, beliefs and perspectives of each other to strengthen their relationship and promote equal status in them. Their effective communication would help them to face the challenges and problems of life with maturity and constructively. Respect for each other would bring emotional intimacy creating a sublime atmosphere for the partners to appreciate their feelings and opinions. Most often the partners would learn to respect each other when their acts of compassion, gratitude, support and forgiveness lead towards a strong foundation in their married life.

When the partners respect each other's feelings, there would be very less friction in their married life. During the days of my legal practice I came across a few divorce cases. I found it really absurd to see couples divorcing for silly reasons.

I remember one such case wherein a man seeks divorce just a week after his wedding. I was indeed shocked to hear that the couple was seeking divorce as the lady being an engineer with a scientific mindset didn't want to light the God's lamp (diya) in their ancestral house. She failed to respect her husband's dignity in the family. She should have understood that just a day's showcase of respect to her husband's belief and desire, could have saved their marriage.

Marriage is not just between two individuals but it is the bond that two families share. Every marriage sees its ups and downs. Mutual respect can make the couple understand each other's mood better before reacting to anger. Couple should never allow another person to express his/ her views on their marriage. Most of the marriages fail because every other individual in the house have a say in the life of a married couple. Most marriages fail when the husband does not stand for his wife and let relatives backlash his wife.

On another instance a possessive mother-in-law used to shout and ridicule her daughter-in-law in front of relatives and the husband becomes a mute spectator and does not stop his mother nor tries to convince his mother on her insignificant behavior. This created a gap between the couple and led to divorce.

To keep the marital bond strong each partner should feel safe and comfortable in each other's presence. My marriage is a blend of happy and sad events. But, I am lucky that I am able to voice my likes and dislikes. We respect each other personal space and never try to judge each other. As spice is the flavor of life, a few instances of discord has made our marriage more strong and reliable. Trust is inherently interweaved with respect. When partners showcase respect through their words and actions, trust naturally develops creating a stable relationship with shared goals and commitments.

To conclude, Respect is a fundamental requisition for a successful married life which can bring in love and affinity between the couple creating positive marital culture.

|| ॐ ||

Our Story from Chennai to Hubli

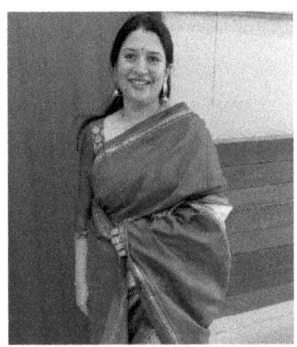

Author's Name	:	Dr. Mahima Mohit Dand
Qualification	:	M.D.S
Current Profession	:	Dentist
Age	:	48 years
E-mail ID	:	**mahima702002@yahoo.co.in**
City/ Country	:	**Hubli, India**

Dr. Mahima Mohit Dand is a Professor in Conservative Dentistry & Endodontics at SDM Dental College, Dharwad and owns Dr. Mahima's Dentistree in Hubli. A passionate educator, she co-authored a book and contributed to various topics in acclaimed text books, earning her the title of the Most Proactive Academician. She has several publications in national and international journals

An active humanitarian, Dr. Mahima has led impactful service projects as president of Rotary Club of Hubli - Vidyanagar, earning accolades such as Woman of Substance awards in 2021, Best President Award and 12 other honors.

Keywords : Marriage, Relationships, Adaptability, Cultural differences, Love

I always believed that love was the strongest force in the universe and my marriage seemed to prove it. It was a love marriage; the kind people often romanticize in movies. My husband and I met in a community organized trip. Our love story was quite like the movie Dil wale Dhulaniya le Jayenge, I fell head over heels and soon enough, we were planning a life together. But as blissful as our journey was, it came with its own set of challenges.

I hailed from a bustling metropolis in India, a city that never slept and offered a mélange of cultures, food and people. My upbringing was within a nuclear family, independent yet tightly knit. In contrast, my husband's roots were in a small town, a place where everyone knew everyone else and traditions ran deep. Marrying him meant not just merging our lives but also adapting to a new cultural landscape.

Initially, this shift was overwhelming. The small town seemed like a different world altogether. Though we were from the same community, the cultural nuances were starkly different. It was a cultural shock, but love made it all seem like an adventure.

The early days of our marriage were filled with laughter, long walks and endless conversations. We were like two pieces of a puzzle that fit perfectly. Yet, like any other couple, we had our share of disagreements and arguments. There were times when the house echoed with our raised voices, each of us trying to make our point heard. Sometimes, the arguments were about trivial matters like which movie to watch or what to cook for dinner. Other times, they were about more significant issues like finances or future plans.

One thing that stood out in our relationship was our ability to move past these arguments. No matter how heated our discussions got, the next morning always brought a sense of normalcy. We never let our fights fester. Instead, we picked up right where we left off, often forgetting what the argument was about in the first place. This ability to let go was, I believe, the cornerstone of our successful marriage.

Humans, by nature, tend to cling to the negatives and overlook the positives. But in a marriage, it's crucial to let go of grudges and move forward. This doesn't mean we never acknowledged our issues; we did. But once a problem was addressed, we didn't dwell on it. We learned, adapted, and continued to grow together.

Our adaptability was also crucial when it came to our daily lives. My father's teachings had always emphasized resilience, the ability to thrive in any environment, even the Sahara Desert if necessary. This lesson became a guiding principle in my marriage.

My mother's advice also resonated deeply with me. She often said that letting go and being a little submissive was not a sign of weakness but a strategy for greater harmony. This wisdom helped me navigate the ups and downs of our relationship. Despite our occasional clashes, the underlying love and respect remained intact.

Our professional lives also added a unique dynamic to our marriage. As a doctor, I had a demanding career that often kept me busy. My husband, on the other hand, was a businessman with his own set of challenges. People often questioned how our marriage would work given our different professions and social circles. But this diversity turned out to be a blessing. He had his friends, I had mine, and together we had a broad spectrum of perspectives enriching our lives.

What made our relationship truly special was the mutual respect and space we gave each other. Unlike the stereotypical Indian male chauvinist, my husband was incredibly supportive of my career. He celebrated my successes without any insecurity. His happiness in my achievements was one of his most endearing qualities.

"My Marriage: Bliss or Curse" offers a raw, exploration of marital bonds, intertwining intimate stories with universal truths. This captivating narrative invites readers to delve into the intricacies enduring partnerships. A must-read for those is seeking a deeper understanding of the multifaceted nature of lifelong commitments.

In essence, a successful marriage is about being simple, humble and occasionally submissive. It is about standing firm on significant issues but being flexible with the small ones. It is about looking for the good in your partner and cherishing the moments of happiness. For me, my husband is not just a partner but the best father my daughter could have. By compromising a little and letting go of minor grievances, we found true bliss in our marriage.

|| ॐ ||

The Life Journey of a Couple
Ammi and Abbu

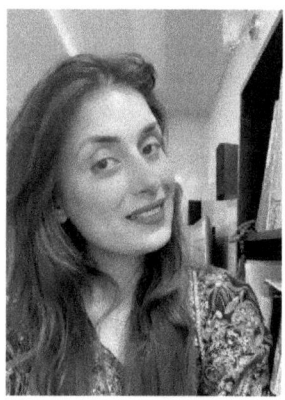

Author's Name	:	Dr. Mehjabeen
Qualification	:	MSc in Clinical Psychology, Doctorate in Psychology
Current Profession	:	Founder of Vision High Mental Wellness, Clinical Psychologist, Psychotherapist, Child Psychologist, Life Coach, Mental Health Ambassador @ Counsel India
Age	:	36 years
E-mail ID	:	**mehjabeen7778@gmail.com**
City/ Country	:	**Bangalore, India**

Dr Mehjabeen is an accomplished scholar and esteemed author known for her contributions to journal related to Mental Health and other helpful topics, which can make a huge difference in other lives. She has authored numerous publications that have significantly impacted relevant disciplines, where she has also been involved in ground breaking research. Her work is characterized by a commitment to specific themes, values or methodologies, making her a respected voice in her field. In addition to her academic pursuits, Dr Mehjabeen is actively engaged in such as community service contributions towards mental health public speaking, journaling further showcasing her dedication to advancing knowledge and fostering positive change.

Dr. Mehjabeen is a distinguished psychologist and the visionary founder of Vision High Mental Wellness. with an extensive background in psychology, she has dedicated her career to promoting mental health and well-being.

Keywords : Couple, Commitment, Determination, Nurture, Strength

Once upon a time, there was a couple known as Ammi and Abba, who were the epitome of a happy marriage. They lived in a cozy home with their four beloved children, fostering a loving and nurturing environment. Ammi and Abba were not just good parents but also best friends, partners who complemented each other perfectly. Their life, filled with laughter and love, was the embodiment of marital bliss.

Ammi was the heart of the home, with a nurturing spirit and endless patience. She ensured that their household was filled with warmth, traditions, and the sweet scent of home-cooked meals. Abba, with his gentle demeanor and wise counsel, was the guiding force, always ready with a story or a lesson from his own life experiences. Together, they created a sanctuary where their children thrived.

However, life has its way of throwing unexpected storms. One tragic day, their world was shattered. Ammi lost her beloved son and husband in a sudden, devastating accident. The once harmonious household was plunged into grief and sorrow. The pillars of Ammi's life, her sources of strength and joy, were abruptly taken from her, and the family was engulfed in a cloud of despair.

Yet, even in the face of such heart-wrenching loss, Ammi demonstrated extraordinary resilience. She knew that despite the overwhelming grief, life had to go on, especially for the sake of her remaining children. Drawing strength from her memories of Abba and her love for her children, she vowed to continue the legacy they had built together.

Ammi's journey through grief was arduous. She faced moments of intense sorrow and loneliness, yet she remained steadfast. She became both mother and father to her children, embodying strength and compassion. She encouraged her children to pursue their dreams, instilling in them the values and wisdom that she and Abba had cherished.

In time, the family began to heal. Though the pain of their loss never fully disappeared, it transformed into a source of motivation. The children, inspired by their mother's strength and resilience, grew into accomplished and compassionate individuals, always carrying the memory of their father and brother in their hearts.

Ammi's story is one of remarkable courage and determination. She turned the curse of her unimaginable loss into a testament to the enduring power of love and the human spirit's capacity to overcome even the most profound adversities. Her life became an inspiration to many, a beacon of hope for those navigating their own storms.

In the end, Ammi's tale is a poignant reminder that even amidst life's darkest moments, the light of love and resilience can guide us through. Her marriage, which once seemed a perfect blend of bliss and curse, ultimately highlighted the incredible strength that can arise from love and loss.

In conclusion Ammi's journey through the highs and lows of life—marked by the bliss of a loving marriage and the curse of profound loss—illuminates the extraordinary resilience of the human spirit. Despite facing unimaginable grief, she transformed her pain into strength, becoming a pillar of support and inspiration for her children and others around her. Her story is a powerful testament to the enduring power of love and the capacity to find hope and purpose even in the darkest times. Through Ammi's unwavering determination and courage, we learn that while life's storms may alter our path, they cannot diminish the light of our inner strength and the legacy of love we carry forward.

Compared to many present-day couples, Ammi and Abba's relationship stands as a powerful example of inspiration commitment and a great bonding, In a time when relationships often face the pressures of modern life, their story reminds us of the profound strength found in never giving up on each other. Despite enduring unimaginable tragedy, Ammi and Abba's enduring love and partnership showcased a timeless dedication that transcended life's challenges. Their legacy is a poignant reminder that true love and commitment can weather any storm, inspiring couples today to cherish and support one another through both joy and sorrow.

They were not a perfect couple and they made it stand by each other with their strong commitment.

A Testament of Unwavering Support and Motivation

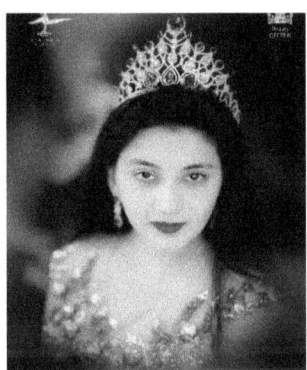

Author's Name	:	Dr. Navjot Kaur
Qualification	:	M.B.A., Ph.D. (Management)
Current Profession	:	Educationist
Age	:	31 years
E-mail ID	:	**drnavjotkaur29@gmail.com**
City/ Country	:	**Vancouver, Canada**

Dr. Navjot Kaur, is a young dynamic educationist. She is a Director of Administration of an eminent educational institution and an active member of the Advisory Board to schools. Adorning several crowns, she is a true beauty with purpose, an educationist by profession with the fundamental aim to enlighten several lives. She believes in imparting right knowledge and encouraging women to believe in their dreams and unleash one's true potential.

She received numerous international and national accolades and awards for exemplary leadership skills in the field of education. She is a woman with power and positive influence, who exudes unprecedented strength and valour with optimistic outlook to face all challenges of life tenaciously.

Dr Navjot Kaur is a truly epitome of beauty with brain as winning the national title of Mrs. India Planet 2022. She proved to be an inspiration and encouragement to ample of women to believe in themselves and vanquish greatness in life. With a vibrant blend of grace, intellect, and dedication, Dr. Navjot Kaur has made her mark, embodying the true spirit of an empowered and inspirational woman.

Keywords : Aspiration, Life Partner, Meaningful Exchange, Conversation, Commitment

Our story is a testament to the power of true love and understanding. My partner and I come from different parts of the world. Despite the miles and time zones that separate us, our bond is a living proof that true love transcends all boundaries. Though being in a traditional set-up of arranged marriage, love found its way.

Our story began in the most modern of ways, what started as casual conversations soon evolved into deep, meaningful exchanges. It was fascinating to discover how much we had in common despite our vastly different professions. Our daily experiences were different, but our values, ethos, dreams, and aspirations were remarkably aligned.

"Love happens like a wonderful cosmic accident, like a conspiracy of planets, like the alignment of the stars, by the will of fate."

From the outset, we were aware of the challenges that a long-distance relationship would entail. But instead of seeing this as a hindrance, we viewed it as an opportunity to strengthen our communication and commitment. Distance never sets us apart, the urge to be with each other has bound us even closer, proving that true love knows no bounds.

Living in two different continents and time zones, we are determined to build a strong communication, sharing little things and prioritizing each other, no matter how the day was. We enjoy each other's silence too. We have the power to make one another smile from far away, that's what truly matters.

Exploring the world together "Our Travel Tale"

Discovering the world together enriches our lives as we embark on adventures, weaving our experiences into a cherished travelogue. Every new destination has a story to tell, whether exploring the rich cultural heritage of India or the picturesque landscapes of Canada, discovering the breathtaking beauty of Southeast Asia, the mesmerizing cities of Middle East, adds a new chapter to our life story. Quite often we escape the real world, work pressures, various obligations and breathe the air, feel the warmth, energy and vibe of new places together.

Winning Together

Any accomplishment is not just a personal achievement, but a testament of the unwavering support and motivation we receive from each other. Our belief in one another is a constant source of our strength, propelling both of us to achieve new heights and vanquish greatness. Our journey is an exemplification of the pious bond our souls have with each other.

Our Fairytale

The beauty of our long-distance relationship lies in the ability to transform the ordinary into a magical fairytale. Our relationship has taught both of us to be resilient, to value each other's opinions, and hence building a strong foundation of understanding and love.

Distance never sets us apart, but the urge to be with each other has bind us even closer, proving that true love knows no bounds.

Our magical bond that can weather any storm is a strong foundation that can't be shaken by life ebbs and flows. Our unwavering trust and support for one another made us each other's confidants. We learned to navigate the ups and downs with grace and to focus on the positives. A successful marriage is learning, exploring and falling in love with all the imperfections and craziness every day.

Our relationship arching over different time zones and continents, is a celebration of love and understanding. Our story is a reminder that true love knows no boundaries and that with commitment, patience, and a deep sense of connection, anything is possible. Distance is temporary but the connection we build together is forever. Love is never easy but it's always worth it.

We hope our journey inspires others who find themselves in similar situations. Love, after all, is not about proximity but about the bond that two hearts share. No matter where we are in the world, we are together in spirit, bound by our eternal love, unwavering trust and understanding. In long-distance relationships or marriages, one has to be tenacious, committed and a magician. We have to make the real magic happen what seems unreal or impractical one has to believe in the divine grace.

|| ॐ ||

Wedding Day vs Married Life
Wheel of Life

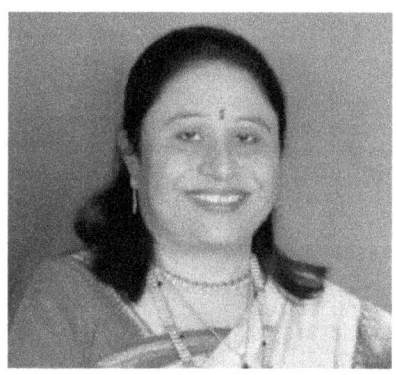

Author's Name	:	Dr. Noothan Rao
Qualification	:	B.Com, Doctorate.
Current Profession	:	Counselor, Astrologer & Graphologist
Age	:	52 years
E-mail ID	:	**noothan.wswrt@gmail.com**
City/ Country	:	**Bengaluru, India**

Dr. Noothan Rao- Counsellor, Graphologist. Formerly working for Canara Bank, currently involved in activities of integrated, holistic healing at ***"Write Strokes with Right Thoughts™"***, *Research Center, based in Bengaluru, India, offering services across globe.*

Professional qualifications: B.Com, ICWAI – Inter, Internationally Certified Handwriting analyst & Grapho-analytical Therapist, Certified Personal Counselor & Company Director, Doctorate & Professorship in Astrology, Honorary Doctorate in Advanced Graphology. Many more certificates in various Healing modalities. Presented papers at **National Women's Science Congress,** won best paper award & **Woman Scientist** award.

She trains people in personality development, goal setting, vision, Career guidance, Handwriting analysis, Grapho therapy and Art analysis to understand self/others. She is also working on various other interests of hers in the field of Counseling, Astrology, Tarot Reading, Dowsing Geopathic stress removal. She is giving integrated therapy to cure many medical problems. Her articles on all these areas are published in various websites, magazines, and Social Medias. Her interview has come in FM Rainbow (AIR India) under inspire program, California Radio etc. She has been called by TV for expert opinion on subjects.

Keywords : Belief System, Free Will. Perceived Expectation. Trauma Patterns. True Companion

All the creations of this world/ living beings are born with basic purpose of survive, reproduce and die. Human beings evolved beyond this basic instinct. They have additional brain functions which bring in curiosity, exploring, inventing, experiencing and expressing.

Humans are extremely social beings living in groups, community and society. Relationships bring a sense of belonging and purpose/motivation to live or do something. For example, a lady who experiences severe leg pain doing daily chores forgets all that pain when she has to do shopping or arrangements for her daughter's marriage.

The biggest epidemic in the future will be loneliness. It kills people more than any other diseases. We are born with so many relationships sans our choice. Parents, siblings, cousins, extended family members etc. We adjust, accept and live in those relationships.

Marriage is our first conscious decision of relationship in adulthood. Next is children. This brings in many more relationships without much choice. Whenever we have to decide/choose/face something, we will definitely have doubts, known/unknown fears etc.

When I got married, I had to take a tough call of giving up my Nationalized Bank job, because my husband got onsite program offer in Switzerland. I quit the job thinking that even if I work for my entire life, pooling money and going to dream destination of serene European countries and residing and exploring them will be near impossible. I had this confidence that if situation comes, I can pick up another job with all the skills I picked up all these years or I can curtail my desires and wisely manage money what my husband earns.

Later I took care of the child and family in such a way that I was available for everyone's needs and my own needs/desires were sacrificed. Sometimes I feel that people are ingrates, they come to me when they need something and never remember or do something to make me happy. I consoled myself that God has created me as giver and not as receiver and I should be proud of it. Also, if God has not created people to help me, then divine power directly helps me which made me more lucky and blessed.

My transformation happened through handwriting analysis, grapho therapy and counseling courses. From a mere housewife, I became woman scientist, writer, coach, trainer, therapist and successful in getting name, fame, money, opportunities, love, respect, blessings, happiness.

When we are prepared for any situations, exams, we don't fear. People prepare for wedding celebrations, not for married life. Understand yourself and express your needs and desires in a better way to avoid any undue perceived expectations and future complexities. A true companion is the one who likes, loves, cares, respects, protects, supports, and motivates unconditionally.

Now people expect everything to be there as served in platter. House, car, luxuries, believe me it is a beautiful experience to decide, calculate the possibilities of buying & go together to buy something with great care and remember those moments in future.

A married couple having children can rest in peace, when their children are healthy, happy, independent, sober, virtuous, focused, achieved, successful and become a contributor to society. My unwavering faith in divine plan helped me to achieve this goal and to become content in life.

My tryst with various psychology subjects, past life regression, occult science, association with clairvoyants gave me lot more insights into relationships and choices. Here are few such wisdom:

Our soul wants to go through all the experiences in its various life journey. Imagine, it will be so boring if all the life is very goody good, uneventful, sober. In one life it wants to experience the robber's life, another of police, another of beggar, another being king and so on. But, when we are born on this Earth, we don't remember that it was our choice. We keep cursing our fate, fear to take decision or give up on our life.

Our belief system originated from our childhood experiences affects our freewill /choice. For example, a soul which decided to have daughter in law life experiences has 3 free wills to exercise. One to become meek/submissive, another to become strong/rebellion, another as indifferent. Relatives may preach the child to be very obedient, respectful of elders or mother may encourage daughter to become very assertive, firm so that daughter won't suffer like her. After marriage when all the efforts to please others had not worked, lady may become indifferent to people and situations.

Sometimes souls choose similar (not same) patterns of life, and it gets etched as trauma patterns and life journey becomes very heavy, unsatisfactory. In short it is our choice as soul or as human being which leads to our situations. When the choice is yours, make it wise either by observing other's life or surroundings. This book is one such attempt to collect the life experiences of many people so that future generations can take a cue from these real incidents.

Wish you all a very happy married life.

|| ॐ ||

Dual Opinion in One

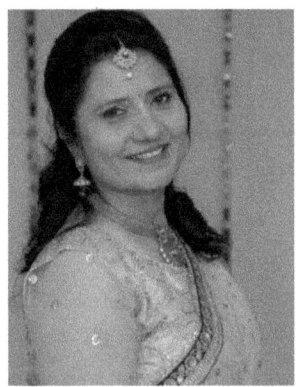

Author's Name	:	Dr. Priti Doshi
Qualification	:	Ph.D in Numerology
Current Profession	:	Healer and Professional Teacher of Occult Sciences
Age	:	49 years
Email ID	:	**pritidoshi809@gmail.com**
City/ Country	:	**Mumbai, India**

Dr. Priti Doshi is a certified numerologist, tarot card reader, astrologer and a diploma holder in graphology. She has various modalities to share and to recount a part of her personal life journey, how she was and motivated towards this profession. It is truly said that difficult times make you stronger. When she was 15, her father was retired, since he was an only medium of the financial securities. She took up an opportunity to support the family at the age of 15 years and sacrificed her dream to become a doctor since she wished her younger brother to study well.

Priti Doshi opted for B.Com. instead of pursuing her dream of becoming a Doctor. After working hard, She cleared B.Com, and got married and became a mother of two. Despite financial challenges, she began giving tuitions at 15, continuing for over 30 years, eventually becoming a proficient phonics and grammar teacher. Facing Vastu dosh in her new house, She started the journey in the occult sciences to heal her home and family members. For the past nine years, she has been constantly helping others as a professional tarot card reader, numerologist and astrologer.

Keywords : Family, Behavior, Compromise, Commitment, Communication

Marriage is often seen as both a blessing and a challenge, depending on various factors such as compatibility, communication and mutual respect. Ultimately whether marriage is a bliss or a curse depends on how both partners approach and nurture their relationship. It's a journey that requires effort patience & willingness to grow together.

There are dual opinions about marriage I would like to share my story I fell in love with a boy named Bhavesh from a different caste (Jain) we were deeply in love and despite families' disapproval, we decided to marry. We were in relationship for seven years my father, brother and however, my in-laws never accepted me due to their caste differences.

I faced immense emotional pain and struggled to adjust to our new family and since I had taken a step forward to get married I was firm that I will commit to these relationship. I tried my best to win over them , but their rejection and harsh words made me feel unwelcome. Bhavesh was caught between his love for me and his family's expectations, felt helpless.

One day, a turning point in my life was to be pregnant and I wasn't nursed well during my pregnancy but by the grace of God and divine blessings I delivered a healthy baby girl and I truly enjoyed being a mother as well as after few years I delivered my Son and this journey of motherhood was a bliss in my life I nurtured them with kindness and compassion and slowly my life began to change I got attracted towards Spirituality and even my family saw my goodness and realized that caste didn't define a person's character.

Over time, my in-laws came to accept and love me for who I was. The family finally united and I found happiness. The story highlights the power of love, acceptance and understanding in overcoming societal barriers.

One of my friend also faced several problems in her life due to lack of dowry any earning women from her family were treated well but just a simple home maker were taunted by her family members even though she worked throughout the day her life was under mercy. They never had any kind of entertainment or fun in their 20 years of marriage and due to lack of dowry the family members made her life hell.

Title of the book is very beautiful; there are several shifts we have seen in olden day's marriage and current day's marriage. Today's generation wish to live continue in relationship.

We can always transform our life with patience, but as a numerologist I have seen several problems in marriage today's situation instead of committing.

॥ ॐ ॥

Connect the Disconnect

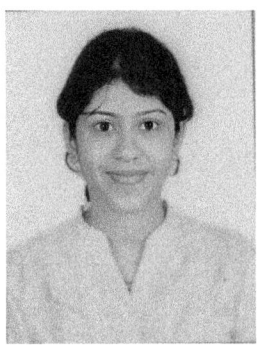

Author's Name	:	Dr. Priyadarshini MM
Qualification	:	MBBS, MD
Current Profession	:	Associate Professor Pathology
Age	:	39 years
E-mail ID	:	**log2piya@gmail.com**
City/ Country	:	**Kodagu India**

Kodavathi, Doctor by profession, Pathologist working as Associate Professor at the pristine Kodagu Institute of Medical Sciences nestled in a small Hill station, Kodagu, Karnataka. Took to poetry and writing after getting influenced by her Mother quoting William Wordsworth who said "Poetry is the spontaneous overflow of powerful feelings: it takes its origin from emotion recollected in tranquility". Writing and poetry came naturally during her moments of travel. Found solace in placing emotions on to words! Being a Doctor she has managed to create a perfect space to blend creativity and writing and has a Poetry book named 'Soul Baggage'- poetic captures of emotions.

Keywords : Marriage, Social Media, Digital, Chapter, Gen Z

Marriage!

Wondered life without it?

If All in the world felt the same!

How would one progress to another world?

Framed in the mirage of life,

Societal norms bind people

To the cycle of birth rebirth!

With changing times, meaning changed too,

Elusive today is married to social media!

"Connect the disconnect' is an article of the disconnected threads of marriage due to influence of social media.

Marriage has no definition. It isn't any logic to be explained or has no proven point. It's like a book which unfolds it's chapters to time.

We do visualize and conceptualize a perfect life, ultimately handle it in our own way as and when situations arise. Present day sees a threat to the Gen Z. They are digitalized!

In the present scenario social media playing it's game so perfect. How many posts on the fights and cries do we see? All we see is a perfect holiday on the banks of serene waters or a flight trip with day, date, time and a cuddly reel. World assumes and 'wows' the same! We start to introspect and find all possible negatives to entwine ourselves in an imaginary nonexistent world. All that which pleases our eyes, we wish the same in our lifestyle. Bound to the mercy of the social media handles parents, kids and emotions cry for some space. A space of their own which is not for the world to see. Who are we trying to please? The whims and fancies of an unrealistic world which has detached us from reality. We fail to communicate in real time instead its reel time fascination. Whilst the happy birthday and anniversary wish on Instagram let's not forget the person beside who deserved that wholesome care. A like on social media weighs more than what is actually expressed! Just contemplate-'Am I married to the social media?'

Its high time we take control of the situation. We need to set our boundaries, prioritize the time and limit comparisons as we thread the weaves of marriage. Today we have reached a stage where it takes effort to keep ourself away from a social handle but our life is the way we deal it. Proactive steps or handling mind with ease, whatsoever we need to understand the broad spectrum of the luring twines that lurks around us. Let's not fall to the trap of illusions instead unfold every chapter with understanding, content and peace.

A positive impact in any way is an imperative need in the world today. To bring a topic that will give it bigger perspective through shared thoughts will be a fulfilling task! A bountiful views will gather to bring about a constructive influence and a favorable outcome.

The Sacred Union of Shiva and Shakti
A Beautiful Balance of Devi and Devil Energies to Handle Life's Ups and Downs

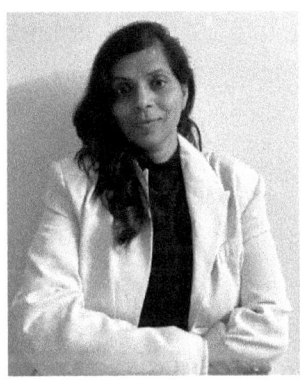

Author's Name	:	Dr. Shalini Garg
Qualification	:	Ph.D. in Psychology
Current Profession	:	Life Coach and Healer
Age	:	49 years
E-mail ID	:	**shalinigarg630@gmail.com**
City/ Country	:	**Alwar (Rajasthan), India**

Dr. Shalini Garg is a dedicated educator with a lifelong passion for teaching and learning. She completed her schooling at a convent in Delhi and graduated from Delhi University. She started her career as a computer teacher at a very young age of 19yrs.

After marriage, she had to take a long career break due to family expectations. However, she continued her academic journey, earning a Ph.D. in Psychoanalysis and later working as an English Professor.

Dr. Shalini Garg has authored two books that are soon to be published and she regularly writes blogs on Medium. Love writing poems that reflect her creativity.

She has also published research papers in UGC CARE-listed journals.

During the pandemic, she discovered life skills courses that provided essential tools for coping with the emotional challenges of the time. Inspired by the knowledge she learned from leading coaches and today she's a certified life coach, graphotherapist, Reiki healer and an inner child healer. She offers free online healing sessions as a part of her service to humanity. Her mission is to raise awareness and encourage people to take responsibility for everything happening in their lives, as all change begins within. She believes, change the perspective and the world around you will automatically change.

Keywords : Balance, Commitment, Existence, Harmony, Yin-Yang

Marriage is a profound and universal institution that almost 90 percent of people want to experience, regardless of their background and status, making it an unconscious goal to strive for.

It fulfills a deeper emotional need for companionship, beyond the bond of family and friends, as one seeks a lifelong buddy to sail through the journey of life sustaining the human race and legacy of shared existence.

The biblical story of Adam and Eve highlights the importance of marriage. Their act of eating the forbidden fruit—though a sin in paradise—became the origin of humanity on Earth, with the physical union of man and woman, the only means of creating life.

In today's modern world, where people have the liberty to stay in live-in relationships, marriage remains significant as it is not just a physical union of two bodies but a commitment, security, and a sacred space where two individuals evolve together, supporting each other through the trials and triumphs of life. Through this bond, they build families, raise children with and contribute to the society, creating a bond of love, values, and stability that is unique to marriage.

Marriage, once considered a sacred bond, is losing its significance in today's fast-paced world, where relationships are difficult to sustain. The Hindu belief in Shiva and Shakti or Yin and Yang, represents the union of masculine and feminine energies, Shiva being the masculine force of strength, decision-making, and authority, while Shakti symbolizes the feminine energy of patience, love, and nurturing.

Marriage is meant to strike this balance, with each partner complementing the other's strengths and weaknesses. But one must have the required skills to play the game of marriage that have never been taught in the traditional education system because of which people enter into marriage unprepared with unrealistic expectations assuming it will fulfill their unmet emotional needs.

Marriage is a medium projecting one's inner reality, where one partner acts as a mirror, reflecting the unresolved aspect of the other partner that needs attention.

The reason for disharmony in relationships nowadays is that both partners approach each other as emotional "beggars," asking for love, respect, and attention that neither of them has cultivated within themselves.

In this digital age, with technological advancements, life has become fast-paced and more connected on the surface, but ironically, the connection with our own self is lost. The root cause of this disconnection with self lies in disconnect with the source and origin of our existence, our parents who lay the foundation for all our future relations.

The key to healing and nurturing any relationship lies in resolving all complaints against the parents and filling ourselves with love. When we are fulfilled and content within, we will naturally radiate that love outward, attracting the same energy from our partner. We attract what we project, and creating a fulfilling marriage requires ongoing efforts from both the partners.

Marriage is not just a bed of roses or a fairy tale as depicted in movies or stories; The challenges, disagreements and hardships—are inevitable parts of the experience. The reason behind so many divorces and breakups today is that people only want to accept the good side of their partner; the love, attention, appreciation and which respect they experienced during the courtship period and avoid confronting the negatives and flaws which they get to know after marriage.

One must remember that life itself is a beautiful balance of contrasts—day and night, black and white, positive and negative, spring and autumn. Marriage is a means to balance this contrast between two genders, two attitudes and two energies. It's natural to have fights and conflicts between two people living together because of the other responsibilities that marriage brings in which is family, finances and social life. Even if circumstances prevent the continuation of a marriage, maintaining a workable relationship with the partner is essential to preserve the energy to attract fulfilling relations in the future.

To foster a healthy marriage, one must embrace all experiences, whether sweet, sour, or bitter. By accepting the full spectrum of marriage, couples can create their own paradise; otherwise, it risks becoming a continuous struggle, leading to dissatisfaction and disconnection.

In conclusion, I urge all those struggling in their marriages to take a step back and reflect deeply before making impulsive decisions that may lead to future regret. It's essential to understand that the root cause of marital issues often lies within, not outside provided one has the courage to confront and accept his reality.

True healing begins within. Once we embrace and resolve our inner struggles, external circumstances and relationships will naturally transform. Healthy relationships are the cornerstone of personal fulfillment. If one learns to manage the emotional intricacies that come with relationships, other aspects—such as health, career, and finances—naturally fall into place. This is because life is driven by emotions. If one feels emotionally content and balanced, that feeling radiates into every area of life, creating abundance and success. The emotions and feelings we experience are often deeply tied to our closest relationships, especially with the parents and the partner in marriage with whom we spend most of the years of our life. .

Seeking guidance from relationship experts or coaches can be invaluable in learning the skills needed to sustain healthy connections. Cultivating harmony within ourselves and our families not only leads to a more fulfilling life but also sets a powerful example of patience, tolerance and stability for future generations.

The anthology **'My Marriage : Bliss vs Curse'**, uniting 108 authors, is a remarkable initiative. By bringing together so many perspectives on the same crucial topic, it promises to offer guidance to countless individuals, who are struggling in their relationships and seeking clarity. The greatest challenge many people face today revolves around relationships—first with their parents and later with their spouse and children. These early familial bonds are the foundation that shapes our approach to all future relationships and yet, there is no formal education on how to deal with these complex dynamics that affect every other area of life.

This anthology, therefore, serves as an invaluable resource, offering diverse viewpoints and solutions. Readers will have the opportunity to find stories and advice that resonate with them, helping them find peace and direction in their relationships and ultimately creating a positive ripple effect in all areas of their lives.

|| ॐ ||

The Unique Journey of Marriage:
Life from Imperfect to Perfect One
Relationship Lessons from Self to the Next Generation

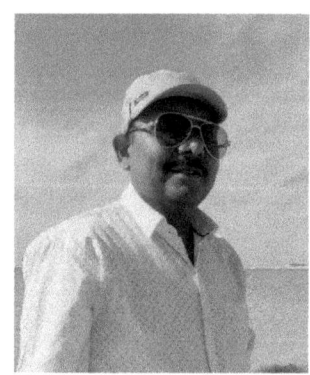

Author's Name	:	Giresh LD Chawda
Qualification	:	B.Com, Computer Hardware & Networking Engineer
Current Profession	:	Graphic Designer, Creative Artist
Age	:	42 years
E-mail ID	:	**gireshldchawda@gmail.com**
City/ Country	:	**Indore, India**

Giresh LD Chawda mainly belongs to the cleanest city of India, Indore MP. He has completed his graduation in Commerce and during his graduation, he completed his Diploma in Computer Hardware and Networking.

But as per his destiny, he is doing his ancestral printing work, which was being done by the previous generations as per the current new format and trend as the third generation, for this he has done Diploma in Graphic Designing along with printing and advertising as well. Having received training and certification, he has worked for many Corporate & reputed spiritual institutions, in Simhastha 2015 he worked for Namami Gange project in Ujjain, in 2018, done branding for IPL matches in Indore. He is providing advertising and printing services in his city as well as all over India as the director of Yash Enterprise,

Simultaneously, Giresh has a deep interest in the spiritual field, during pandemic period and lockdown, he studied Numerology and got certified training in Reiki and Marma Chikitsa for public welfare.

Keyword : Couple, Journey, Tradition, Relationship, Understanding

The journey of marriage begins with the union of two beautiful souls through nature or the universe. They both choose each other themselves in this present birth. If they have fallen in love with each other before marriage, otherwise as per our Hindu tradition, it is through search by family members to get met each other. This is the first step in the journey of both their lives.

Before marriage, this is a very romantic time for both the couples, getting to know each other's specialties, shortcomings and weaknesses, in which the talks of a few minutes do not end for many hours and this is the precious time, when love blossoms starts climbing for each other. And for those, who Love Marriage Couples, their love has already taken place and this is that special moment when this fast train of both of their lives, on two separate tracks, with the engine of the ecstasy of love, travels to the beautiful pubs of life filled with love. It begins to enjoy the valleys filled with love that come into her life with the moments and reaches the path of the second stage of her journey.

The train of life of both of them is going towards their next destination which is marriage. This Path becomes a complete blessing for most of them and the beginning of curse for some, let us see into this topic a little deeper to understand.

The curse applies to those couples, who have decided to get married going against their family and their religion, because in a marriage, the couple who gets married only both is on one side and everyone else is against them. Only 100% commitment towards each other can determine the success of a relationship in every situation. Otherwise, both relations dies in pain due to not being able to fulfil the responsibilities after marriage.

Ladies and gentlemen, I will not bore you all much now. When this relationship of marriage starts with the family in our India, then it is not just a marriage but it is a grand festival in which Both the couples get married as per our Hindu rituals on that special day with many family members present throughout their life with this relationship which includes parents, Brother-Sister, Bhai-Bhabhi, Bua-Phoopha, Mama-Mamai, Chacha-Chachi, Devrani-Jethani, A family rosary is formed by pearls in the form of family members., The bride and groom circumambulator a consecrated fire seven times (Saptapadi), reciting specific vows with each circuit. Vows made in the presence of the sacred fire are considered unbreakable, with Agnideva held as both witnessing and blessing the couple's union. now this train of marriage crosses the 3rd station with enthusiasm and joy, passing through many precious milestones of life.

The next stage of this journey opens the red carpet of the intensity of the relationship of both the couples, accepting each other's strengths and weaknesses and carrying on the love for each other while living with all the family members. In which one gets to live many beautiful moments of immense joy and fun. It suits those couples whose cards in life are in their favor and vice versa, whose cards are against their relationships, which often happens even after love marriage or arranged marriage, which is the lack of communication with your partner as well as all the people in your relationship and mutual shortcomings and weaknesses, respect and insults, your way of living your life, habits of unnecessary spending more than your family income. Even if a good married life is going on, it turns it into a mess and pushes it into a sea of Curse & Pain, which can be easily seen in the disintegrating relationships in today's current environment.

When two people enter into a marriage relationship, they have to complete this journey with blissful way, so both the couples have to know each other's strengths as well as overcome their shortcomings and weaknesses.

But instead of these shortcomings overpowering each other, one should enjoy the journey of life by making up for the shortcomings with good qualities. And if both of them are not able to figure it out then they can consult senior members of the family or through occult sciences expert like Astrology, Numerology, Spiritual Guidance, get information about yourself and your life partner, such as power ot the date of birth and destiny numbers, By Day of Birth it happened, the constellation in which it occurred, what was the zodiac sign of that time, Power of Both's Name for each other, by reviewing one's life with positive and negative aspects, one can live a natural life by solving the psychological & emotional problems arising in life, which turns the pain born with the unnatural understanding of those two couples into bliss because it is a very important part of life, because we did not learn these things even after spending crores of Rupees on our education. And the couple, who are still living in pain due to lack of spiritual knowledge, because they have not assimilated the medium of occult science and spirituality and especially it takes time and patience to understand these things and implement them in life - It is very important to have faith in the religion you follow. And all this can be the basis of innovation and peaceful life for the coming generations.

In the end, if the pain between the couple does not end even after doing all the above, then it is wise to end the relationship, because many times we meet each other by chance and get into a relationship, but in reality we feel suffocated between each other. If they are, then they are not made for each other.

A Pathway to Transform Yourself

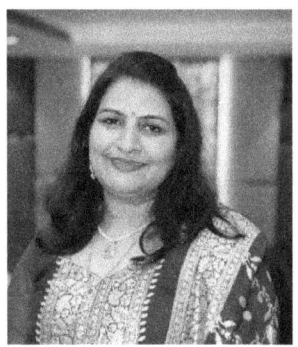

Author's Name	:	Harishita (Vicky Chauhan)
Qualification	:	B.P.Ed., M.A. in Yoga Diploma in Acupressure, Diploma in Neurotherapy
Current Profession	:	Life Coach, Counselor, Energy Healer
Age	:	41 years
E-mail ID	:	**harishita10@gmail.com**
City/ Country	:	**Noida, India**

Harishita, CEO and Founder of **Sacred Healing**, The Institute of Energy Healing, Occult Sciences and Research having global certification and recognition ie. ISO 9001:2015, She is a multifaceted healer and therapist with expertise in various modalities. Her specialties include Energy Healing: Focusing on balancing and restoring the body's energetic fields for improved physical, emotional and spiritual health. Mokshapatta Reading: Utilizing the ancient Indian board game for spiritual guidance and self-awareness. Tarot Card Reading: Providing insight and clarity through tarot, a tool for personal growth and decision-making. Neurotherapy: Addressing neurological issues by regulating the nervous system. Sound Healing: Using vibrational sound to promote deep relaxation and healing. Life Coaching: Guiding individuals toward achieving their personal and professional goals through holistic support.

Harishita's work integrates these practices to help clients achieve balance and well-being on multiple levels. She has experience of 15 Years in this field.

Keywords : Transformation, Family, Education, Emotion, Partnership

Marriage is often perceived as one of life's most transformative and defining experiences, a union that brings together two individuals in a bond of love, partnership, and mutual support. For some, it's a source of immense happiness and fulfillment—a bliss—where partners grow together, overcome challenges, and finds deep emotional connection. For others, however, marriage can turn into a complex web of unmet expectations, misunderstandings, and emotional strain—a curse—that weighs heavily on their well-being. For me, my marriage converted from curse to bliss. It is a union of two families. I belong to a Gujjar Community. I got married to a person, who belonged to a village, which is very backward for women. From childhood, I lived in Delhi city. My family and I had a very modern thinking. Everyone in my family was educated but my in-laws were uneducated. But now, there is good understanding and a great amount of love between us. Now, the relation between me and my mother in-law has changed to a mother daughter relation. I am very grateful that today I got a chance to write in Anthology book on the topic of Marriage, where we can read unheard realities about marriages of 108 wisdoms. I am heartiest thankful to Abhishaik Chitraans Sir for providing this opportunity to us.

I have heard from childhood that marriage is a relation, where you have to compromise, but I realised it today that marriage is a very beautiful and lovely relation from which I got my freedom, self confidence and a partner who understands me very well, supports me in every step of my life, believes and trust me with his whole heart. I got a family who supports me, understands me and love me a lot. My brother-in-law is like my brother, and my sister-in-law (Nanad) is like my sister. They treat me like their own sister. I have got these two relations, which are very priceless for me along with my husband's relation. When I got married, my life took a twist which was very unbelievable for me. I, a girl, who lived in a city and was a sports person, got shifted into a village where people's thinking was very backward. There was inequality between men and women. People there believe that only men have respect and women should not get any respect. They discriminate between a boy and a girl. They used to follow their old traditions. There was a saying that "Girls are a burden for a family. They shouldn't be born". I realised there that "A woman is an enemy of an another woman". I was from a total different background unlike my in-laws. So, I had faced totally different things unlike my previous life. I gradually started to understand their way of living. Then I thought that if my mother would be here so she would also tell me to do the things in this way only. So, I started believing that my mother-in-law is not my mother-in-law instead she is like my mother. With this intention I started to compromise in some things for good reason. I and my family realised that for a marriage to run not only husband and wife relation is important but also other relations are equally important. So, everyone in my family started to let go of minor mistakes of each other. My brother-in-law and husband supported me a lot to adjust in their surroundings. It's not like that only I compromised some things, but my family too. My mother-in-law gradually understood me and changed some things in her behaviour and rituals. Some things I changed for the sake of my healthy marriage relation. Not only me but also my family, we two gradually understood each other and changed some things according to each other benefits.

To conclude, I would say that we should FOCUS on what we want from our life. We should always remember one thing that what we give to others, the same we will get back from Universe. If we want happiness in our life, then we should think that we will get happiness by letting go or holding the grudges will give us happiness. For me, letting go of grudges will give us happiness. If we will give someone dissatisfaction, the same dissatisfaction we will receive. So, give happiness to others for receiving the same happiness back.

|| ॐ ||

Tips for Healthy Married Life

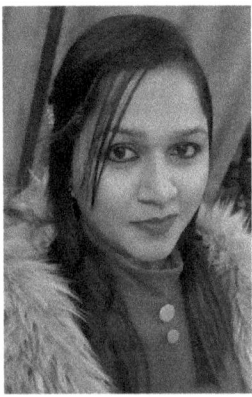

Author's Name	:	Harsatvir Kaur
Qualification	:	M.A. (History), B.Ed.
Current Profession	:	Teacher
Age	:	36 years
E-mail ID	:	…
City/ Country	:	**Mohali, India**

Harsatvir Kaur is a teacher, who has done her Bachelor Degree in Arts and Master Degree in History. After that she has done her Bachelor of Education Degree with Punjabi and SST subjects. She has also cleared the Teacher Eligibility Test. She has four years' experience in teaching. She has won many zonal and state level prices in co-curricular activates. Along with reading and teaching she also enjoys writing. And so, fourth slowly, she also works to put pearls of words in sentences. She is now budding author.

Keywords : Connection, Communication, Companionship, Differences, Lifestyle

It is said that marriage is a gamble or lottery, if you win in the lottery then its fine otherwise you will regret it rest of your life. "Marriage" whenever I listen this word many questions roam in my mind. What is marriage? Marriage is socially and legally recognised union between two people often a man and a woman that establishes rights and obligations for the couple and their children as well as their families. God designed Marriage for three primary purposes companionship, procreations and redemption. But why this union is important or we can say why it is necessary?

Marriage is a blessing. God has furnished us with present of this bond to add more colour to our life. A new person takes place in our life. We love him. Our life goes on. Our family getting large. We connect with society. In my opinion a person cannot be completely connected to the society. He/she gets to know its virtues and vices only in when he is in this relationship.

Now when this relationship has happened, a question rises if a marriage is Curse or Bliss? Is this question as easy as it seems? Can this relationship be understood in one day, one week, a month or a year? As per my opinion it's not, it takes long time to realize, whether marriage is curse and blessing is completely depended on our partner who have chosen by us or our family.

For many people marriage seems like a dream or hallucination. Exactly! the definition of Marriage is not just the union of two human beings rather it is union of two families also. A girl adopts herself in a new family sometimes this process can be complicated, it's totally depended on the new family observes or understand her. If the groom's family consider their daughter in law like their own daughter and correct her mistake like their own daughter, then it helps to adjust the new one to the family and also to live happy marriage life.

Simultaneously if the in laws consider her outsider or non-member from first day and reflect on her small mistake as crime and leave it on her that leads to reduce the chances of better relationship between them. I want to add one more thing here that if sometimes there is some misunderstanding between the families/ values and culture then one formula is always works that is the understanding between the husband and wife. That means if they understand each other value/ culture/ needs/ decision and also respects each other and their families will help them to live healthy and happy marriage life.

The marriage life can be converted into curse if we do not value our relationships. There are so many reasons behind it, one of them is poor communication between the partners like if we don't clear and communicate all the points with each other then it creates misunderstandings and gaps which convert the happy marriage life into curse. Second most important point is when the couples start follow the lifestyle of another one. Sometime we are influenced from others and we expect the same thing from our partner which will become the reason of day-to-day conflict that ruined our marriage life.

Finally, I can say marriage is bliss. Marriage is bliss of oneness. To be one with our spouse is one of the great rewards of marriage. This is the bliss of togetherness. Let's not take our marriage for granted. think about many women and men feel alone with no plus one. This is bliss of friendship and love. Marriage is bliss of family ties.

Marriage is union of two souls with the right partner. It may by far be the most fulfilling journey of life. Come! Let's be a comfortable couple and take care of each other. How glad we should be that we have somebody we are fond of always to talk to and sit with. "A great marriage is not when the perfect couple comes together, but it is when an imperfect couple learns to enjoy differences".

Dear Readers, I would like to share some words about this anthology book. First of all I would like to tell you that how I came to know about this book. Actually, my mother, who has been the student of Abhishaik Sir, told about his commendable work. After discussion with my husband, I contact Abhishaik Sir to become the part of this book. Dear Readers I am very glad to say that you can collect the knowledge of your important part of your life that is marriage. Now days the divorce/ separation are very common and no one guiding the upcoming generation.

In this book there are different opinion/ suggestion of multiple authors in a single book, which will help the new generation to handle the ups and downs in their marriage life. I hope you all would like the concept of this book and sincerely respect the sentiments of all the authors.

In the end I would like to Thanks the entire team, who consider me worthy of this. Hope you find this Anthology Book close to your heart and life as well.

|| ॐ ||

Colors of Life

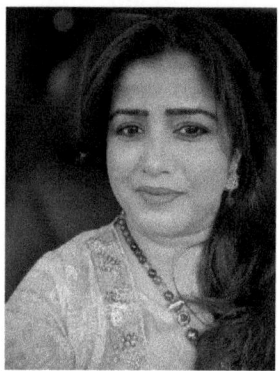

Author's Name:	:	Himani Bajaj
Qualification:	:	B.Tech. Computer Engineering, Harmonized Life License Qualification
Current Profession:	:	Entrepreneur, Financial Advisor, Occult Science Practitioner, AP with SKY Kundalini
Age:	:	47 years
E-mail ID:	:	**bajajhimani@gmail.com**
City/ Country:	:	**Toronto, Canada**

Himani Bajaj is an accomplished entrepreneur with over 15 years of experience in the financial industry. She is dedicated to empowering families through a deep understanding of financial concepts. Holding a B. Tech in Computer Engineering, she combines her technical expertise with financial insight to offer valuable guidance to her clients.

Himani emphasizes the importance of both financial and mental health, recognizing how much numbers can influence individuals and their decisions. She helps her clients make better choices in every aspect of their lives.

In addition to her work in finance, Himani is a Certified Numerologist and Vastu specialist/ consultant. She also serves as an assistant professor specializing in Simplified Kundalini Yoga (SKY) in Canada. SKY is an Integrated Wellness Program aimed at achieving health, happiness, and harmony in all areas of life, promoting holistic well-being and balance.

Keywords: Real-Life Journey, Unique, Challenges, Rainbow, Diversity

Everyone has heard stories about marriage; some are happy, some are painful. Some couples complete their journey with joy, while others break up along the way. But in the end, all these stories teach us lessons and show us different colors of life.

This is the real-life journey of Gauri, who lived in a town with her lovely family. She was the youngest, with an older brother and sister. One day, everything changed when her brother died in an accident, leaving behind his 8-months-pregnant wife. The family was devastated, but with time, they tried to overcome this tragedy.

Six years later, it was time for her sister to get married. There was hope for happiness, but it was also a challenge because her sister was unhappy in her marriage, facing abuse and blame. After seeing her sister's struggles, Gauri decided not to get married and wanted to stay with her family to take care of them.

"Life is like a canvas full of different colors, each representing a new chapter waiting to unfold. It's a play where everyone has a role, experiencing the rich variety of colors in life."

Gauri finished her studies, returned to her hometown, and started working in a multinational company. One guy named Shiv, who worked in a different department, always visited her department and tried to talk to her. They became very good friends, and Shiv started visiting Gauri's family. Shiv was new to the town and had a clear heart. We have all been through this stage when parents seek the best match for their kids. Gauri found out from a mutual friend that Shiv likes her and wants to propose. She knew exactly what to do. Although Shiv was getting other proposals, he decided to talk to Gauri about his feelings in a respectful manner. Gauri told him, "Shiv, you should talk to my parents. They have the right to make this decision." She did it the same way our Indian culture teaches us.

A couple of months passed. Shiv's parents chose a girl for him and he agreed, but he wasn't comfortable with the decision. So, he eventually said no and decided to talk to Gauri's father instead. They had a good conversation, and Gauri's father told Shiv to bring his parents to meet him..

Now it was Gauri's turn, but her father didn't ask her anything. When her sister came, the four of them sat down and had a conversation. It wasn't a good conversation. Gauri was blamed for some things, but she told her father, "I was not eager to marry him and never thought of it. I wanted to do everything with your consent. I will go with your decision. Her sister spoke to their father and said, "Whatever decision you make, do not rush like you did in my case." Shiv brought his parents, and both families agreed to the marriage. Gauri's father realized that Shiv's family was very humble and would take good care of his daughter.

A few days later, Shiv's sister also got engaged and her wedding was after couple of months. During this time, Shiv received his permanent residency in another country. This brought a new challenge. Shiv decided to go to that country first and then bring Gauri there so she wouldn't have any problems. However, Gauri's father insisted that Shiv take her with him because they were not comfortable with her going later. This dilemma continued until finally, they decided to get married before Shiv left.

After one year of marriage, they moved to other country. Starting their life from scratch was not easy, but they supported each other. A new bright colour came into their lives when they were blessed with a baby girl. However, many challenges followed. Gauri lost her father, Shiv lost his job, and Gauri had to leave her job because Shiv was not comfortable to take care of the baby, according to him mother can take care better. Leaving her job was a big sacrifice for her other pregnancy and career. She started helping Shiv with his business, and everything was going well until she lost her 8-month-old baby during pregnancy. It was heartbreaking for both of them. Shiv accepted this reality, but Gauri was in deep pain.

Over time, things changed and so did people. Shiv supported Gauri for a while, but later he told her she needed to overcome her grief on her own. He immersed himself in work, while Gauri focused on taking care of their first child. After few years, they were blessed with a second child. Gauri overcame her pain for her family's sake. She tried to join Shiv in his business, but they couldn't work well together. Whenever she tried to join him in the office, he felt the kids were a distraction and asked her to take them home, sacrificing her career for the children. It was hard for Gauri to accept this challenge, but she worked on herself. Gauri and Shiv had one good thing: they always kept business and family separate. Gauri started working on herself and become a life coach, helping others heal themselves. This helped her become a better person and play a better role in life.

Gauri and Shiv run their business together, each contributing in their own special ways while supporting each other. They've been happily married and live joyfully with their wonderful kids, enjoying a harmonious life together.

Challenges will come, but it's up to us how we see and react. Like the colors of a rainbow, marriages of different colors add to its beauty, each bringing its unique charm. Embracing diversity makes life more colorful and rich.

|| ॐ ||

Tradition Meets Modern Love
Bridging the Differences in Arranged Love

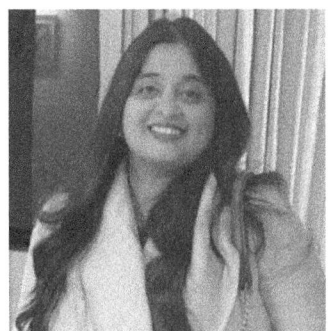

Author's Name	:	Himani Verma
Qualification	:	M.Sc. (Chemistry), B.Ed.
Current Profession	:	Educator
Age	:	29 years
E-mail ID	:	**himani221294@gmail.com**
City/ Country	:	**Punjab, India**

Himani Verma is an accomplished educator with a Master Degree in Chemistry. With a robust teaching career spanning over four years, she currently imparts her knowledge and passion for the subject at Quest International School. Known for her dedication and innovative teaching methods,

Himani has become a respected figure in the academic community, inspiring her students to excel in Chemistry and beyond.

Keywords : Belief, Contribute, Journey, Matchmaking, Support

Marriage is a journey filled with love and sorrows, challenges and triumphs, laughter and tears and often winning and losing. My own journey began in the city of lakes, Bathinda, I harbored dreams of finding love and companionship in marriage, but little did I know that my path would lead me to an arranged marriage, a journey that would shape me in ways I never imagined.

Growing up, I, like every other girl, had my fair share of fantasies about marriage. I dreamt of meeting someone who would sweep me off my feet, just like Cinderella, a prince will come someday and take me with him in his world, someone with whom I would share a deep connection and unwavering love. However, reality had different plans for me. In the backdrop of Bathinda's bustling streets and colorful festivals, my parents began the search for a suitable match for me. And I belong from a typical Rajput family, little did everyone know my Mumma hails from Himachal and my Dad is Punjabi, so I am a good mix of Punjab and Himachal.

And the search for a stereotypical "good boy" started in my family. The concept of arranged marriage is deeply ingrained in our culture, with families playing a pivotal role in matchmaking. It was no different for me.

Amidst the nervous anticipation and everything, I met Hitesh. He was a man of few words, with a gentle demeanor that put me at ease. He is actually calm to chaos. Our initial interactions were marked by awkwardness, as we went through the unfamiliar territory of arranged courtship. Yet, as we spent more time together, I discovered layers to his personality – his kindness, his sense of humor, and his commitment to his family. Growing up with two sisters, my husband was immersed in an environment, where the dynamics of female strength, resilience, and compassion were omnipresent. This upbringing ingrained in him a profound respect for women, shaping his interactions and outlook on life.

At least once in our life we all may have come across a fact saying "opposites attract", it became true when I actually met him. We are two different ends of a sky, which were never meant to be together. But one fine day we decided on "Forever".

He has always supported me to be the better version of myself. It is his support and perseverance that each passing day is a memory to hold on forever. His belief in me and my dreams is just another level. He`s the one person whom I will always find in darkness. He adds life to my monotonous days. Words will never be enough to describe what he means to me, but he`s my eternity and beyond.

I would rather say that a marriage is a transformative experience, shaping an individual into the person we never thought to be. Marriage is union of two people who come from different upbringings, but still finds peace in each other. This relationship of ours has made stronger in various ways. Love, friendship, trust are vital emotions that are the foundation of a strong marriage. Marriage is bliss in every possible way; it's how you perceive it. There is certain trade-off in the marriage, if we expect acclamation from the partner, we too should contribute towards his.

Embracing the Imperfect Beauty of Marriage
A Journey of Love, Growth and Transformation

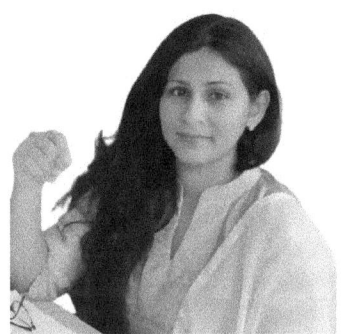

Author's Name	:	Isha Singh
Qualification	:	Pursuing MA Psychology, PG Diploma in Mass Communication
Current Profession	:	Graphologist, Drawing & Doodle Analyst, DOB Analyst, Parenting Coach and NLP Practitioner
Age	:	42 years
E-mail ID	:	**ishhasingh05@gmail.com**
City/ Country	:	**Gurugram, Haryana**

Isha Singh is a multidisciplinary expert in human behavior and development. With a Postgraduate Degree in Mass Communication and ongoing studies in Psychology, she has combined her knowledge with certifications in Graphology, DOB analysis, and NLP practice. As the founder of **Selfwrite Institute of Holistic Development**, Isha has spent over three years helping individuals understand themselves better through handwriting analysis, signature analysis and drawing analysis. Her expertise extends to parenting coaching, empowering parents to foster strong bonds with their children. Isha is dedicated to using her expertise to nurture the next generation's growth and well-being.

Keywords : Challenges, Growth, Imperfections, Love, Marriage

As I reflect on my marital journey, I am filled with a sense of awe and gratitude. This journey has been a transformative experience that has shaped me in ways I never thought possible. From the moment we said "I do," we embarked on a path filled with challenges, personal growth, and ultimately, a deep sense of fulfilment.

At the outset, I felt a mix of enthusiasm and apprehension, unsure of what lay ahead. But as we began our journey together, an underlying sense of joy and anticipation prevailed. We were two individuals with our own unique experiences, perspectives, and imperfections, and we were eager to build a life together.

As our journey unfolded, we encountered various obstacles and challenges. We discovered that our viewpoints and opinions sometimes collided, leading to intense discussions and disagreements. But through these experiences, we learned to communicate effectively, compromise, and understand each other's perspectives. We learned to embrace our imperfections and grow together.

There were moments when I questioned my decision to marry, but amidst the turmoil, moments of pure happiness and love reaffirmed my belief in our union. Our marital journey has been imperfect, marked by both triumphs and difficulties. We have faced challenges and moments of uncertainty, but through these experiences, we have emerged stronger as individuals and as a couple.

In retrospect, I understand that marriage is not a fairy tale or a perfect paradise. It is a journey filled with both high points and low points, successes and setbacks. But it is also a journey filled with love, companionship, and the unwavering belief that together, we can overcome any obstacle.

Ultimately, marriage is not solely about finding the ideal partner; **it is about being the best partner one can be** – imperfect, human, and committed to growth. I have learned that true love is not about perfection but about embracing imperfections and growing together. With effort, patience, and commitment, we will continue to navigate life's challenges and celebrate its joys.

For me, **marriage is a beautiful journey, not a destination.** It has the power to transform and enrich our lives and reminds us to approach it with an open heart, mind and spirit. As I reflect on our journey, I am grateful for the love, laughter, and lessons that have enriched my life. I look forward to many more years of deepening our love and flourishing together through life's ups and downs, surrounded by beauty, joy and the promise of a shared future. Our marital journey has been a beautiful adventure, and I'm excited to see what the future holds for us.

|| ॐ ||

The Blessings Instead of Curse

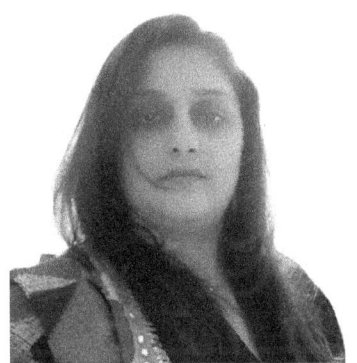

Author's Name	:	Jiggna B Bhatt
Qualification	:	Graduate in Commerce & Diploma in Software Engineering
Current Profession	:	Entrepreneur Deals in Rudraksh, Crystal and other Products used in Occult Science – Astrology, Numerology and Vastu etc.
Age	:	41 Years
E-mail ID	:	**jiggnabhattzee@gmail.com**
City/ Country	:	**Dubai, UAE**

Jiggna B Bhatt is a renowed Rudraksh and Vastu Specialist. She also specialises in Crystal remedies and Numerology. Jigggna B Bhatt has done her Graduation from Mumbai University and had been working as Banking Professional in UAE for almost 10 years. Presently she is a professional Occult Practitioner.

Being associated with many renowned senior Numerologists and Occult Practitioners like **Abhishaik Chitraans** of **M/s Ankakshr Miracless,** she has learnt many new methodologies in Numerology and has tried and helped many individual/ business houses in India and UAE as well.

Being a vastu and rudraksh specialist more than 1000+ clients have been advised and improved their lives and houses/ families across UAE, UK and India. Occult and Rudraksh products prescribed by her are really awesome.

Keywords : Understanding, Family, Community, Care, Couple

As we all know and understand about marriage. In India marriage means a blend of our ancient customs, which now evolved around modern practices, we all are strongly influenced by religion, family and community. Our marriages are now evolving since few years. We get a chance and approvals from society and family to choose our own partners and so now many couples today opt for love marriages, where they choose their own partner.

I also got a chance to do in my younger age, he came like a fresh breeze of love in life and we evolved together in marriage. As every normal couple we had many dreams to conquer the world and be the best. We have achieved quite a lot by now. But this journey had been a roller coaster ride at every stage for me and my spouse and me dealt with it and sailed the storms to make it a success. 20 years of togetherness and still counting. Like all others, for me also my marriage is blessings and I will refrain from using the word curse, because whatever I have learnt and achieved is all after my marriage. It was clearly a blessing, when I started to get the exposure of living freely as I wished, which I clearly always craved before my marriage.

My blessings :

1. Spiritual Growth : Joint spiritual development and self-realization with growing age have evolved us both to next level.

2. Emotional Fulfilment : Love, intimacy and emotional support is always there and with age priorities changed from intimacy to being loved and being validated.

3. Social Harmony : He has given me a Loving family, I have a good social as well as international status with respectful community to live in and strive for the best.

4. Progeny : My daughter is my biggest blessing in our marriage as we all agree that children bring joy and continuation of family lineage, I got to experience this while being happy just because I was married to a right person.

5. Material Comfort : My marriage bought me a financial stability and security which we jointly enjoy.

As I am mentioning about my blessings, I truly feel and believe my spouse also has the same respect and feeling about our marriage. Marriage can sometimes become a curse, if there is a mistreatment by siblings in the family. Especially if a female faces issues like disharmony, infidelity, financial constraints or childlessness, whenever any of the partners faces such issues, I will suggest one must take an expert help and talk to their trusted ones. This will help find a solution in a better way and we can hope for a marriage to become a blessing instead of a curse.

There are some keys to live happy married life :

1. Mutual Respect : Valuing each other's thoughts, feelings.

2. Trust : Unwavering commitment, loyalty.

3. Communication : Open, honest dialogue.

4. Compromise : Finding middle ground.

5. Spiritual Practices : Joint spiritual growth, worship.

We must keep these things in mind and work towards making the marriage, **Blessings instead of Curse,** and it is in our own hands.

|| ॐ ||

Balancing Dualities in Marriage

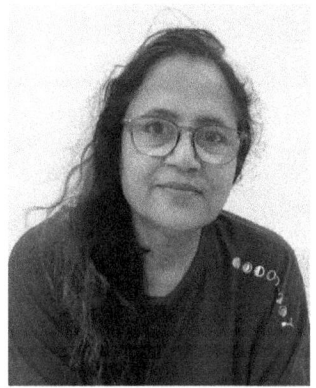

Author's Name	:	Kala Malpani
Qualification	:	HS, Certified Graphologist, Numerologist, Grapho-therapist, Logo Analyst & Designer
Current Profession	:	Graphologist, Numerologist
Age	:	64 years (45 years of Married Life)
E-mail ID	:	malpanikala1@gmail.com
City/ Country	:	Mumbai, India

Kala Malpani is a professional Graphologist, have been pursuing Graphology since 2011. She has a vast experience of teaching online and counselling in person. She has conducted more than 50 sessions in various collages n schools of cities like Mumbai-Bangalore, including medical institutions also. She has experience of doing corporate events in India as well as abroad. Her expertise is Grapho-therapy & Handwriting development. She is a numerologist and Logo analyst n designer too.

Besides all these she is socially active in her community organisations and have taken various posts there. She has performed responsibilities of different posts in organisations like Lions club also. Before coming in the field of Graphology, she was a renowned dress designer. There also she had a wide experience of 20 years. She was running a boutique successfully.

On top of all the above-mentioned fields, she is a homemaker, the area close to her heart.

Kala Malpani's rich background and diverse expertise make her a multifaceted professional, dedicated to her career, community and family.

Keywords : Harmony, Duality, Couples, Sacred Assignments, Shiva and Shakti

The concept of marriage embodies the principle of balancing dualities, where two individuals with different perspectives, strengths and weaknesses come together to bring coherence in life.

As per Hindu scriptures Shiva & Shakti symbolizes the union of dualities. In Vigyan Bhairava Tantra Lord Shiva explains Shakti (Parvati) about the extremities of universe, with 112 different examples – such as day & night/ Yin & Yang/ Purush & Prakriti/ Breathe-in & Breathe-out and so on and so forth. Finding a middle ground between these two extremes is the balancing factor of life. By understanding and integrating these opposites, one can achieve and harmony in their relationship.

In Graphology also, we call it 0 & 1 concept/ left brain and right brain/ emotional and logical.

Delving deeper one can understand that there are always two opposite energies at play, in the universe, which go hand in hand complementing each other. Only thing, one needs to balance them. We spend the whole life to balance these two energies. Whenever we succeed in creating balance at that exact point of time, we can call it bliss.

Life is not a linear equation, where 2+2= 4 will be the only equation. It's bundle of emotions and emotions don't have only two shades i.e.; black & white. It has all the colours of Rainbow.

In childhood, I read a story of a duck with 2 mouths. This story can be used as an analogy to bring out the intrinsic connection and interdependence in a marriage. Just like the duck with 2 mouths sharing one stomach, actions by one partner inevitably affect other. It underscores the importance of mutual care, consideration n the impact of individual actions on the relationship as a whole. This idea is a powerful metaphor for the shared fate and responsibility in a marital partnership. Both partners must be mindful of their actions and their impact on the other. Each decision & behaviour contributes to overall health of relationship.

Both concepts emphasize the need for mutual support.

1-In the story of duck, both the mouths must work together to avoid harm.

2-In the Bhairava Tantra, the teachings guide couples in balancing contradictory elements.

Marriage is not just a physical or emotional bond, but also a spiritual one. Incorporating these teachings can help create a more holistic and fulfilling marriage partnership, a strong and resilient, but deeply connected and spiritually enriched one.

There is no perfect couple who has only bliss in their marriage. It's the frame of mind at that particular point of time – couple feel blessed to get such a life partner or the opposite also.

I am also not any exception. I also have wasted lot of my bliss moments in creating harmony. Though it's not always in your hand, the other person has come on this planet with certain energies n qualities. It can be bliss if you consider the other person as human being, who can also make mistakes.

Spiritually speaking, our connections with others are sacred assignments, designed to teach us valuable life lessons. If we don't learn, we may need to reincarnate to master the same. Most of the time, the couples are opposite in nature n that's the greatest lesson they have to learn, to be with a person, who is opposite in nature & to share everything – again the concept of harmony in duality.

Different phases of life have different requirements –initially it's physical, then to create a replica of your selves as children is another bliss, which is possible only in marriage, in later age it is companionship. Here I remember the example of ring finger, which replicates our life partner. Rest all the relationships will depart from us, but our life partner remains there till the last breath.

It's the swing of time, which makes us swing from one extremity to another. Couples who understand it early can enjoy more bliss moments, otherwise they may have to suffer in the days to come.

It's like the song—"Maano tho Ganga maa hai, naa maano tho bahta paani". If you take it as a bliss, it's bliss or else curse.

"My Marriage : Bliss vs Curse" is a compelling title for an anthology that offers a balanced perspective on the realities of married life. It suggests a deep exploration of both, the joys and challenges that couples may face. The idea of this anthology will serve as a legacy for future couples.

|| ॐ ||

A Lifetime Companionship

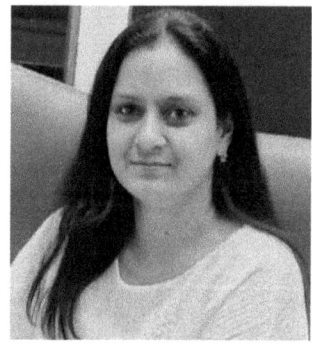

Author's Name	:	Kalpana Priyadarshi
Qualification	:	B.Sc., B.Ed., M.Sc.
Current Profession	:	Teacher
Age	:	42
E-mail ID	:	...
City/ Country	:	**Bengaluru, India**

Kalpana priyadarshi is a teacher and a writer. She has done her Master Degree in Biotechnology. She has graduated in life sciences.

She is also graduated in Education in physical science and life science.

Kalpana Priyadarshi, loves to write about society, life and feelings. Her writings have got special emphasis on the lives, conditions and feelings of females and the effects of society on their lives.

Keywords : Couple, Tradition, Family, Understanding, Imagination

According to Hindu mythology and scriptures, there is a story from the Mahabharata. Draupadi, the princess of Panchal region, was well-known for her beauty, audacity, and polyandrous marriage. The Pandavas, the five sons of King Pandu and Queen Kunti, were married to Draupadi. She, in her early birth, prayed to Lord Shiva for a boon that she could find a husband who would be noble, strong, skilled, handsome, and wise. Since it was impossible to have all five qualities in a single man, she got married to five men at the same time in her next birth, in order to get her wishes fulfilled. Out of her five husbands, Yudhishthir was noble, Bhim was strong, Arjun was skilled, Nakul was handsome and Sahdev was wise. As our ancient stories hint, it is never possible to expect for a multi-talented partner in a marriage.

Marriage is a companionship for a lifetime. Two people come together to stay and share everything in life. It should be a purpose to go home. It is a feeling of not being alone. It is a tranquillity, as everything has to be fixed by two partners.

A marriage, whether its love or arranged, becomes just a marriage, once done. While meeting an individual for an ephemeral, we can be splendid in the presentation and civility. But when we stay with someone forever, both have to be in realism. How that reality affects each other, the certificate of bliss and curse arrives from there. Before marriage, it's only the two of us, who are meeting and discussing their own personal things. Once married, thousands of other things have to be considered. If the onus of all the knots to be opened are left on either partner, the marriage becomes a curse and if both of them unite to cross each hurdle coming through their journey, it seems like a bliss.

Any marriage cannot run mere on the base of love and infatuation. It depends on what definition of love we have known. And the clear difference between infatuation and marriage is very coherent among the partners.

The notion of a blissful marriage arrives from two facts, either you are fortunate enough to get the best person as your soulmate, or you are wise enough to have the best understanding of the partner. The latter being the most uncertain part I believe.

My marriage was self-same. I met my husband, when we were higher secondary schoolmates and at that age, one does not have a conception of marriage. During those days, in our society, a boy and a girl being attracted towards each other, were believed to be in love and this bond was meant to result in marriage. At that tender age, the meaning of love for me was nothing more than this.

In the traditional families like mine, there was no display of both sides of married life. All we were told was, the life after marriage was nothing less than milk and honey. Forget about the unfortunate case studies related discussions. I guess these efforts were made by the families to make sure the girls do not have any negative imaginations about their upcoming journey. The terms like mutual understanding, respect, knowledge of a person, were not more than definitions.

We grew up listening that the husband was the only one we were supposed to look up on, once married. He was the one in this world, we belonged to. His wellbeing, his happiness, his achievements are ours and with all that, I got married at an age of Twenty-four.

I had countless glorious dreams in my eyes and boundless beautiful desires in my heart, just like any other girl at this age would have and of course, one delightful phantom was that, I had a complete understanding of my would-be husband, which I must say, was my greatest illusion, since it's out of the question to know even half of a person, if you have not stayed with him.

And after that, the life had been just a journey, trust me, which kept on teaching something or the other every day. Yes, I learnt and discovered many good things about me and realities of life during this adventure. And I was now completely out of the world of fantasy and waiting ahead was a very new and normal married life with its own possible challenges and a completely new person. He was a completely new personality, with whom I was never familiar with and since then, have known him little more day after day.

The lessons I have learnt gradually are, if you always had the back of your partner, if he has respected your self-respect and you are an identity for him like any other human being in his life, if you remain the same what you were earlier, and your heart is full of satisfaction, then cherish your marriage, as you are probably the luckiest.

But on the other side, things may always not fall in place. Maybe extra sour memories have been created than the candied ones, maybe the certitude of acceptance and warmth is still missing from the relationship, maybe the soul lacks some sort of contentment being in the alliance, but at least there is someone on whom you can count on, during the lowest chapters of life. There is a reason, for whom you want to make and be home. Certain duties of life and family get shared which otherwise were meant to be on the either one.

Perhaps, these are the criteria, for adjustments during a marriage, out of which, both the participants maybe evolving constantly and learning to live with each other in this institution, called marriage.

|| ॐ ||

Bliss If You Notice

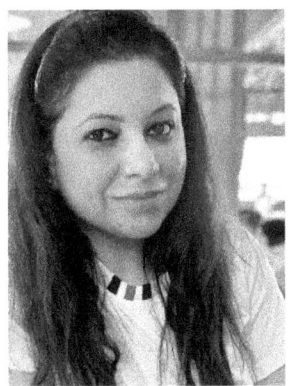

Author's Name	:	Kanan Jolly
Qualification	:	Graduate in Computer Science, Software Engineer
Current Profession	:	Working with MNC as Assistant Vice President
Age	:	43 Years
E-mail ID	:	**lifecoachkananj@gmail.com**
City/ Country	:	**Mumbai, India**

Kanan Jolly is a working professional and a happy single parent to a 13-year-old son. She is also playing a role of Certified Life Coach, Numerologist, Tarot and Angel Card Reader, also practicing NLP & Access Consciousness. She is a Motivational Speaker & Author. She is passionate about empowering Women to unlock their potential and have meaningful results in their lives. She is a Single Parent to a loving Son. She is a manifestor of the beautiful life, she is living.

Keywords : Abuse, Divorce, Love Marriage, Happy Single Parent, Blissful Life

Marriage is like, working as a team, filling in for each other, bringing out the strengths covering up the weaknesses, and creating a safe space to speak and share. When two distinct personalities decide to get married, that is when the real-life exam starts. I was 25 years old, when I decided to get married. In my head, I was thinking that the person I was getting married to, I was in love with, however, it was a short fairy tale story I was living at that time. We met at the workplace and became friends, we started liking each other and wanted to get married and spend our whole life together. Our families agreed to our inter-caste marriage, we had a small family ceremony to make this marriage official.

After a couple of weeks, the real challenges started and things became ugly, I could always feel that there was something, which is not working out but I was too young to make the decision and didn't dare to tell my mom, who was a single parent to me and my siblings, that I want to break this relationship and not get married to this person. At that time my priority was my Mom's respect and my sibling's future life, being the eldest out of all, I thought my sacrifice by going ahead in this marriage would be a good decision. I was scared of society as if I broke the marriage then people would say, what not to my Mom. I lost my father when I was 20 years old and the real face of the people around me, I had experienced that time, which I didn't want to go through again. Also, somewhere I thought things between us would get better once we start living together after marriage. With all my thoughts, feelings and emotions, keeping everything in mind, I got married to this person who was still a mystery to me.

As I said earlier the real exam starts after the marriage, we started living in a small rented home all by ourselves. Just like every couple to make the marriage work even I made compromises and adjustments, however, nothing worked. After going through a lot, again I thought things would get better once we had our child, I started working towards my health as I wanted to conceive and after a couple of months I got pregnant, the hope of things getting better between us was still there, during my pregnancy I was happy, I was joyful as I could see the drastic change in my partner's behaviour, which I was desperately waiting for. It was indeed a beautiful phase of my life. Then the day came when my Son was born in 2011. Our relationship & parenthood were going well until my partner joined a company in the city where his parents lived.

My life changed 360 degrees, when we shifted with his parents. With some good and bad times, I thought I would live happily for my child, but my destiny had different plans for me, slowly things started getting worse for me, mental and emotional abuse, physical abuse and financial abuse were part of my life, then. I was destroyed to a level that I had no option but to run out of that house for my Son and his better life. After 7 years of court cases, in 2022 I got my divorce decree from hon'ble Court. Today my Son and I are living a happy life. This marriage has given me both good and bad, kind of experiences. I have learnt and evolved as a person and a mother as well.

My marriage is bliss and not a curse, as it has given me the most beautiful gift of my life and that is my Son, I have seen good times as well for which I am always grateful. Marriage is the most sacred relationship, keep it pure with your love and trust for your partner and ignore the small arguments and life challenges. Contribute in every way, work towards it each day, be present in your marriage, and make it the most beautiful friendship of your life, however, if things are getting ugly in your marriage then have the courage to choose what makes you happy.

Gratitude!

|| ॐ ||

Are All the Mothers-in-Law Devils?

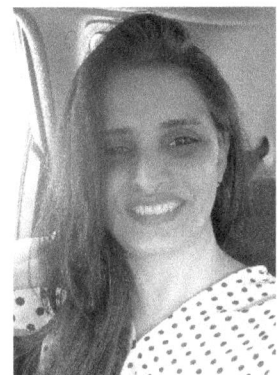

Author's Name	:	Kanchan Lakhwani
Qualification	:	B.A. in English (Lang. & Lit.)
Current Profession	:	Educationist (Student Tutor)
Age	:	44 years
E-mail ID	:	**harrshitagangwaanii@gmail.com**
City/ Country	:	**Mumbai, India**

Kanchan Lakhwani has completed her Bachelor's in English Language and Literature from Mumbai University. She is an Educationist and an Entrepreneur. She has been providing tuition services (for individual students and groups) to IGCSE, ICSE and CBSE wards for more than two decades now. She strongly feels that being around children has kept her grounded and sane; giving her all the more reason to continue with the profession that she is in. She also runs her small business of healthy roasted seeds like watermelon, muskmelon and hemp etc. – as recommended to patients by the doctor – She delivers on a pre-order basis. Her major clientele comprises corporates, who order healthy hampers during festivities, to give to their employees.

Kanchan has won 'Most Beautiful Hair' title, in the prestigious 'Mrs Maharashtra Iconic Diva 2020 – supporting Fight Against Domestic Violence' pageant, held in January 2020. Women across many walks of life came together to express their support to women who silently go through domestic violence inside the four walls of their cocoon.

Keywords : Marriage, Domestic Violence, Joint Family, Lessons Learnt, Perspective

Down the generations we have heard that mothers-in-law are devils, who love to create misunderstandings between the couple, leading to arguments and fights. It is also widely shared that they are dominating. But it's only when daughters-in-law step into the shoes of the mother-in-law do they realise the effort it has taken to get to where her mother-in-law is and why she does what she does. Sasha's story is a reflection of just this thought. The bond between Sasha and her mother-in-law shares another perspective (apart from the popular one) through my eyes. Despite limitations,

Sasha's mother-in-law does whatever she can in her capacity to empower Sasha with the knowledge and experience that she has gained in the five decades of her own marriage.

Are All the Mothers-in-Law Devils? / Everyone calls her a Demon

Sasha will be 45 years young in two days. It's a real blessing as she is in perfect health. She has been living a wonderful life and confesses to having learned some beautiful things from those around her. Living in a joint family may not be 'The Fad' in today's day and age but Sasha enjoys each and every moment with her in-laws and the extended family. You can raise your eyebrows at this thought but Sasha has learned the most crucial lessons of life from her mother-in-law. The latter has taught her how to live a sophisticated life, to respect non-living things, to live in a neat and clean environment, to cook with a wee bit more oil and a few more tomatoes, 'as little more oil brings a shine to your dish and a few more tomatoes add colour and taste to your veggies'. Sasha has become more disciplined under her mother-in-law's care and watchful eye and has learned to be more organised too.

Sasha learned how to budget the rations and to clean the fridge, and how things should not be strewn about carelessly all over the house but kept respectfully in their respective places; why the windows need to be cleaned till they are squeakily so and why cupboards need not be closed with a thud! Having married young, Sasha had come to her married home as a total novice and all these sudden changes in habits, did drive Sasha to the edge too but she also acquired patience over time with her mother-in-law's knowledge and understanding of the world. Sasha was also taught how to choose her battles. "Pick a few and leave the rest", her mother-in-law would calmly say after gauging the situation at hand. She was also careful about not pushing Sasha, when not required. However, where she knew Sasha could excel, she would leave no stone unturned. Such was her hidden love and belief in her daughter-in-law, who responded in kind.

Yet, all was not well in Sasha's world. Her mother-in-law was a silent spectator to her son's misdoings and she knew in her heart that tolerating his misdemeanors was very wrong. But because he was her son, she could not do much. Frail in health, she suffered too as she witnessed the domestic violence that her son rained on Sasha, for no real reason. The atrocities that Moksh committed on Sasha were way beyond imagination but his mother could do little or nothing as she had no finances or physical strength to battle it out with him. Worse, she knew that she would be at the receiving end of Moksh's wrath, if she came to Sasha's aid. Sasha, on her part, did not take the assaults quietly. She would retaliate with full force and even resort to calling the cops - if the need so arose.

There were times when Sasha resented her mother-in-law for not being able to take a stand. In retrospect, Sasha feels only gratitude and thanks her profusely for all of those lessons. Sasha confessed to being a brat when her mother-in-law had received the young girl in their gorgeous home, but she also patiently taught Sasha prudence. Sasha evolved gracefully to being a more mature person with all the behavioral ups and downs in the family. She became more accepting, understanding and tolerant. So, not all in-laws are evil. There are many in this world who are divine at heart and love their daughters-in-law more than they love their own off-springs.

Let's aim to eradicate this generational belief of mothers-in-law being the root cause of all problems and politics in one's married life. Sometimes it's not their fault at all. Let's forgive them, bless them and move ahead. It's just so that we can live more in peace rather than living with anger and hatred in our hearts and minds.

As there exist millions of people on this earth, there also exist an equal number of different mindsets. It's mind blowing how one particular topic can have such varied perspectives. Anthologies are a brilliant way to access these perspectives and a new viewpoint on subjects that we are conditioned to look at, in a particular way. They serve students and layman alike; to view the subject in a different light.

An anthologist has a purpose in mind and openly invites authors from various backgrounds to submit their works. The more authors, the more flavor in the book. It's as much fun for the anthologist to compile the collections as it is for the readers to witness a culmination of one idea from innumerable variations.

|| ॐ ||

A Dance Between Heaven and Hurdles

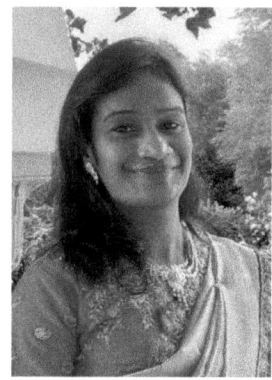

Author's Name	:	Kavitha Bhutada
Qualification	:	M.B.A., B.Ed.
Current Profession	:	Teacher
Age	:	38 years
E-mail ID	:	**sonikavitha111.ks@gmail.com**
City/ Country	:	**Mysore, India**

Kavitha Bhutada is an M.B.A. graduate and holds a B.Ed. degree pursued when she wanted to transform her passion of teaching into reality, currently working as a dedicated teacher. Alongside her professional career, she is a passionate artist with a talent for painting and a flair of creativity. She excels at various forms of craft, bringing her ideas to life with intricate designs and thoughtful details.

Kavitha is an accomplished homemaker. She is capable to balance her career and personal life, while nurturing her role as mother of two. As a mother, she is deeply committed in fostering her children's growth, providing them with love, guidance and the values needed to navigate life. She believes in nurturing their creativity and independence, always striving to be a source of encouragement and strength. Through her experiences, she brings a unique perspective on the journey of marriage, exploring the joys and challenges with authenticity and insight

Keywords : Relation, Celebration, Communication, Foundation, Memory

Marriage is a beautiful journey woven from so many moments of joy, laughter, and occasional struggles. After 12 years of shared experiences with my partner, I've learned that while challenges are an inevitable part of any relationship, the bliss we create together far outweighs those obstacles. From navigating the chaos of everyday life to celebrating significant milestones, each moment has deepened our bond and enriched our journey.

We've built a life filled with traditions and memories that serve as the foundation of our love. Through open communication and unwavering support, we've learned to face conflicts head-on, emerging stronger each time. The shared laughter over silly moments, the comfort of knowing someone always has your back,Resting peacefully in the warm embrace of a partner, feeling safe and cherished as dreams gently take over and the thrill of pursuing dreams together have transformed our marriage into a source of strength and happiness.

In this article, I'll reflect on the aspects of my marriage that bring me profound joy, the lessons we've learned along the way and how we continually nurture our love a midst life's ups and downs. I hope to inspire others to cherish the bliss in their own relationships while navigating the complexities that come with them.

Marriage is not a subject which can be described in an article or two, marriage is a relationship between two person, in which one is always right and the other one is husband !! jokes apart, according to me marriage is an **U** turn of life, which makes you and your partner's life upside down.

Not only for girls who leave there parents, siblings, friends, city, lanes and all the people who knew her from that fruit vendor who stands far away from the lane to that traffic police who caught her for license again and again from adjusting in a completely new family, new city and a new country in some cases. Exploring life with a partner where every moment whether smooth or challenging adds richness to the journey. Emerging as an individual having own preferences, choices, interest, likes and dislikes is challenging.

It's equally difficult for the boy too. A sudden drastic change in boys life, where a free minded bachelor suddenly starts being matured, started to work even harden trying to make more money so that he can take care of that person who just believed in him and came along with him, along with responsibilities there was always a huge pressure at home, everyone started judging that poor guy for every single move which was always the same, but now there were many 'microscopes' around on him, who always had their special report on the behaviour of both and then most importantly creating a special place of his partner in the family, striking a perfect balance between the family and the new person. It was equally challenging!!

The struggle was really hard, but the beauty of this relationship is that, almost instantly, you're welcomed into a web of new relationships and connections all new and yet so beautiful, I still remember one particular incident of mine when I was newlywed and the next day I was not well, when I opened my eyes after sleeping for a while, I saw whole family surrounded my bed with a doctor standing with a stethoscope, for a moment I was feeling like am I still in dream or what? I was so conscious. Then doctor diagnosed fever, because of the tiredness of so many marriage ceremonies and traveling. There were many such beautiful memories we shared together, where we both were made feel so special by both families. How can I forget challenges? It was not easy though, but for me I was having that particular person who stood always by my side in happiness and in sadness in health and sickness in fun and in pain!

And when we were exploring each other's perfections and flaws, then hits the best yet most difficult phase of marriage that is PARENTHOOD. The day when a child is born it changes everything from husband and wife to Papa and Mumma forever. Now we were not just two of us living carelessly now we have that bundle of joy with us who deserve all the best things in the world, but trust me it's not as easy as it sounds now, beautiful phase is the most challenging and tiring as well. But with my kids around now I feel life is so perfect and complete, my small world surrounded by the people whom I love the most, waking up with the person whose love will never change, pampered by kids the way I pamper them what else is needed in life! I don't expect anything more than this having love and trust in the family, care, concern and respect in each-other's eyes, unconditional support and that perfect soul mate who is always around u!

I feel marriage is like a train journey, we both boarded the train with excitement and anticipation, bags packed with dreams and hopes. The beginning of the journey is smooth, scenic and full of laughter. We make memories as we chug along through different landscapes. There are times when train hits few unexpected stops, or even a bit of turbulence. The journey can be long and tiring, but it's the company that makes it worthwhile. We learn to share the window seat, navigate through the crowded aisles, and find comfort in each other's presence, even when ride gets rough. And through it all, you hold on to the ticket you both chose to punch together, trusting that destination is worth every twist and turn, so relatable right…

This article is dedicated to my soul mate, who encouraged me to write and present my thoughts about marriage in front of the whole world through this book, Marriage is definitely a BLISS ! Life comes with challenges, miss understandings and troubles face them don't run away from them, face them together hold each other's hands and emerge as winners together! And finally I can say "In a great marriage, the love you receive is equal to the love you give." Cherish this phase and embrace the beauty of wedding lock.

Best Friends for Life

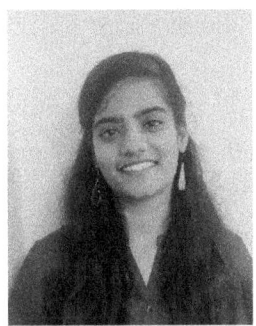

Author's Name	:	Keerthika
Qualification	:	B.E, (Bachelor of Electronics & Instrumentation Engg.)
Current Profession	:	Engineer
Age	:	26 years
E-mail ID	:	**keerthikab297@gmail.com**
City/ Country	:	**Bangalore, India**

Keerthika is the debut co-author of this book you are reading now and also a dedicated Engineer with a growing passion for writing. Alongside her budding literary career, she is deeply enthusiastic about cooking and is a nature lover who enjoys travelling.

She completed her Bachelors in Electronics and Instrumentation Engineering at Madras Institute of Technology Campus, Anna University and has been working for nearly five years as an Engineer in the Oil and Gas sector.

Rooted in a humble background, she constantly seeks opportunities that foster both professional and personal growth. She embraces new challenges with enthusiasm and is driven by a constant desire to explore and expand her horizons. Beyond her Engineering profession, she is dedicated to her culinary pursuits and writing, reflecting her diverse interests and talents.

This book is a testament to her passion for writing and she hereby shares her views on the title of the book as a co-author.

Keywords : Commitment, Friends, Journey, Meaningful, Understanding

In today's modern world, many people achieve success in their professional lives, but struggle in their personal relationships. This often stems from a lack of communication between partners or an inadequate understanding of how to live independently within a marriage.

Hence, this book will undoubtedly serve as an eye-opener on the institution of marriage, as it includes the perspectives of 108 individuals, making it more than just the view of a single person.

What's your take on Marriage?

Here it goes according to me ...

MARRIAGE is a **M**eaningful, **A**lluring, **R**esponsible journey of life filled with mutual **R**espect , an **I**nvestment in each other's dream, **A**ppreciation of efforts and a **G**enuine and **G**lorious **E**xperience to be **E**mbraced forever.

It is not a contract, nor is it simply a decision or a destination in life; rather, it is a beautiful journey. Coming to the topic of the book, to make it a bliss or curse totally depends on the people involved. Both partners should travel together on this journey of life as best friends. Marriage is a journey, where two individuals navigate all phases of life—Emotional, Physical and Mental—side by side. It is a commitment to hold hands through all of life's ups and downs.

Marriage is about understanding and it is a blessing to have someone with whom you can share anything and everything. God's purpose in creating the cycle of life—getting married, having children, and then seeing them marry—is rooted in the idea that throughout these 60 to 70 years of life, you need someone to journey with you. As your parents grow older and are no longer able to care for you, this person becomes the one who replaces them. Your siblings and friends may become busy with their own lives, so who will be there to support you forever?

This is likely why the concept of marriage was decided by God. It is a blessing to have someone with you forever as your best friend. If you ask someone who is alone, they will understand this even better.

You might wonder, why I haven't talked much about family. When two partners are clear about what they want and do, everything else tends to fall into place naturally. That's why I prefer to skip that part. Hence, in my view, it is ...

A lifelong commitment, a journey so fair,

Hand in hand, forever to share.

Built on trust, with understanding deep,

A beautiful bond, a promise to keep.

Not a better half, but wholly part of you,

Together it's a journey through life's every hue.

|| ॐ ||

The Journey

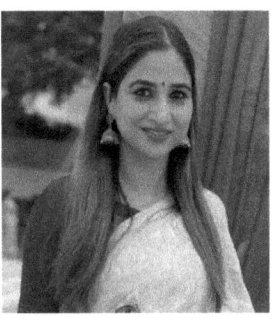

Author's Name	:	Kiran Yadav
Qualification	:	M.Com, M.B.A
Current Profession	:	Business woman
Age	:	36 years
E-mail ID	:	**kirany15487@gmail.com**
City/ Country	:	**Gurgaon, India**

Kiran Yadav is a Fantastic Educator. She has done her Master's Degrees in Commerce and Business Administration and holds a degree in Education. She has worked for more than 8 years as HR in reputed MNCs and the Hotel Industry. She has conducted many pieces of training for the fresher; later on, she was employed at various renowned International schools in Gurugram, India as a PRT Teacher.

She loves to enjoy nature strolls and listening to music.

She strongly believes if you love yourself, it's easy for you to spread love everywhere. It will help you to stay positive always.

Keywords: Trust, Respect, Forgiveness, Dedication, Affection

"do panno me kaise likh du mai, Teri-Meri ye kahani,

jise sirf mai janu or tu jane dilbar jani"

How can a marriage be good or bad? Two persons decide whether to make it simple or troublesome based on their expectations and ease. In today's Kaliyug, every woman wants a husband like Ram and a man wants a wife like Sita, however to tell the truth, neither today's husband will cross the seven oceans for Sita, nor is Sita ready to go into exile in her husband's terrible times.

As time went by, I have come to realize, that it's a continuous journey of self-discovery and mutual understanding. It is a melody of compromise and forgiveness of unconditional love and support.

I don't know what a husband looks for in his wife at the time of marriage. Still, I realize that when a girl comes from her father's house to her husband's house, she looks for all the relationships she has left behind in her husband; protection like a father, friend like a brother or sister, love like a mother. She needs everything from that one relationship.

It was not as if my fate was written with a golden pen, I have seen both paradise and damnation with him, I have also suffered a lot many times, the deeper the love the more the pain, however while falling we both managed to hold each other.

"Dard seene me tha kuch aisa,

Dard seene me tha kuch aisa,

Ki na ankho se bahaa aur na hothon se kaha"

Two people with totally different temperaments and personalities. While he had to remain connected to society and culture, my flight was very high. While he would get tired and look for shade, I had to spread my wings and fly.

Sometimes I laugh thinking about how we both managed to maintain this relationship through thick and thin.

The premise of every marriage is unique. Everyone has different desires, dreams and paths. The roots of my marriage is probably equality between both of us. Giving each other equal value and giving appreciation for one another's choices. When respect is mutual, clashes reduce, and the relationship thrives.

Even after knowing all this people forget to respect each other's opinions and one never knows when this relationship that starts with love and respect becomes a victim of circumstances and misunderstanding.

There were some such turns in our marriage too. Many times he might have overlooked my flaws and often I too might have overlooked his mood after seeing it. This is how a relationship is maintained.

"My love for him is such that I never let him leave me alone whether it be kitchen work, household chores or raising a child. I held his hand so tightly that I never let him go and always allowed him to support me".

It is not that we do not fight, fights are also necessary in marriage, otherwise, how will we know whether there is love or not?

Often people see fights as negative, but they can be transformative if handled constructively. It paves the way for growth, compromise, and a deeper understanding of each other's needs and boundaries. And the fun is that even after fighting, you cannot sleep at night without talking to each other.

And I feel that the key to a blissful marriage is to never sleep separately after a fight

"It is said that injuries to the body can be cured,

But there is no cure for injuries to the heart."

In marriage, you need to deal with the best of two lives. If you know each other's personalities, values and goals, it's simple for both to run on similar track.

All in all, my marriage is neither solely bliss nor curse; rather, it is a delicate balance of both. It is a testament to the resilience of the human spirit and the enduring power of companionship. As we continue to journey through life hand in hand, I am grateful for the highs and lows, the joys and challenges that have molded our common fate.

"Itni shiddat se hum ne tum ko sajaya,

Itni shiddat se hum ne tum ko sajaya,

Ki jalim khud sajna sawarna bhull gaye"

|| ॐ ||

Shaadi Ka Laddoo
Sweet or Sour

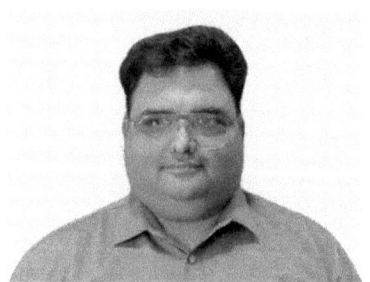

Author's Name	:	Lalit Sharma
Qualification	:	Under Graduate
		Certified Master Numerologist, Certified Vastu Advisor, Certified Palmist, Certified Astrologer, Certified Akashic Records Practitioner, Certified Meditation Practitioner, Psychic Healer
Current Profession	:	Occult Science Practitioner and Consultant
Age	:	48 years
E-mail ID	:	**anksatva@gmail.com**
City/ Country	:	**New Delhi, India**

Lalit Sharma is a distinguished occult practitioner with over three decades of experience in the fields of Numerology and Vastu Shastra. An internationally certified expert, Lalit has honed his skills through rigorous training at Bharatiya Vidya Bhawa, New Delhi and various prestigious institutes across India and Malaysia.

In 2015, he founded **Anksatva Academy**, a registered MSME and ISO Certified Institute dedicated to the study and practice of occult sciences. His academy offers a comprehensive curriculum that empowers students to explore and excel in their spiritual journeys.

Lalit is deeply committed to social causes and has actively participated in several initiatives aimed at environmental conservation and family welfare. He has volunteered with NGOs, contributing to projects like the CMS survey of the River Yamuna, as well as participating in movements such as Yamuna Satyagrah and Jal Sansad. Through his multifaceted expertise and community involvement, Lalit Sharma continues to inspire others on their spiritual paths while advocating for environmental and social change.

Keywords : Struggle, Success, Sweet, Sour, Life

This article is dedicated to those brave souls grappling with their 'Karmic Lessons' while uplifting their communities. Among them are lawyers, activists, bodybuilders, vloggers, and others who embody a positive outlook on life. Many of these generous individuals are married, while some are alienated fathers, facing the harsh realities of parental alienation. This societal issue takes a toll on fathers, leading to profound grief and complicated emotions.

Today, I share the poignant story of Manish Sharma and Risha Sharma, who wed in January 2015. Our paths crossed in March 2016 at India Gate during a Save Indian Family meeting. Their journey is a mix of heartbreak and resilience, aptly illustrated by the phrase **"Shaadi ka laddoo."** This popular Hindi expression captures the dual nature of marriage—both a delightful treat and a weighty responsibility.

Story begins, as Manish reflects on his wedding day, he recalls a celebration like no other—five rows of musicians, including a bagpiper band, dhol players and a grand procession featuring four magnificent horses. Fireworks illuminated the night sky as relatives danced joyfully, creating a magical atmosphere.

However, this euphoric beginning took a dark turn. After the celebrations, as rituals unfolded, the excitement of their first night quickly spiraled into shock. At 38 years old, Manish was filled with anticipation—only to be met with a revelation that shattered his dreams. When Risha switched off the lights, his heart raced with excitement, but the moment she turned them back on revealed unexpected scars—surgical marks that hinted at unshared struggles. This betrayal plunged him into despair, exacerbated by false allegations from her family that led to his arrest. The vibrant night morphed into a nightmare, leaving Manish reeling.

A Fight for Justice, Imprisoned briefly in Tihar Jail, Manish faced a devastating reality—false cases filed against him, even including the names of his beloved pets. Despite the overwhelming odds, a fire ignited within him. With the support of Men's Rights NGOs, he delved into legal texts, determined to fight back.

Four years of grueling legal battles ensued, fraught with frustration on both sides. Eventually, as the tide turned in his favor, Risha chose to settle the cases. In 2020, they mutually divorced, with no alimony or claims on his property—a bittersweet conclusion to a tumultuous journey.

Manish emerged victorious in the courts, receiving a ruling that criticized the Delhi Police for their mishandling of the case. This experience, while painful, transformed him into a resilient advocate for men facing similar battles.

Reflecting on these events, Manish learned invaluable lessons about communication and honesty in relationships. Had Risha been open about her past, their story might have unfolded differently. The five years spent navigating the legal system taught him about the complexities of Indian law and equipped him with the resolve to help others in similar situations.

When I, Lalit Sharma, asked Manish about his perspective on marriage, he shared, "It was a karmic lesson that I must clear. I must have done something to her in a past life." Regarding the prospect of a second marriage, he expressed a firm denial, stating, "I am happy with my learnings. I will never trust anyone solely based on gender."

In the end, Manish's journey exemplifies that while the "laddoo" of marriage may have been sour, the lessons learned along the way are undeniably sweet. His story serves as a reminder that even in the face of adversity, growth and resilience can emerge.

|| ॐ ||

A Beautiful Relationship

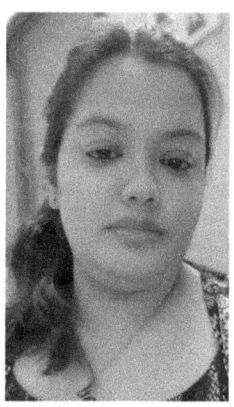

Author's Name	:	Leena Lalwani
Qualification	:	B.Com., Naturotherapist
Current Profession	:	Healer, Therapist, Numerologist Access Consciousness Bar Practitioner
Age	:	38 years
E-mail ID	:	**lalwanileena745@gmail.com**
City/ Country	:	**Mumbai, India**

Leena Lalwani is a Certified Therapist. She has done various therapies i.e Naturotherapy & Accutherapy. She is working in this profession morethan 10 years. She is also a Access Bars, Access Facelift & Body practitioner. She also practices as Numerologist and Tarot Card Reader. She has done Graduation in Commerce. She has changed lives of many people through her consultations and healing modelities.

She is also practices 8 modalities of healing and has successful results in Arthritis, Cancer, Depression, Parkinson, Dimentia, Asthma, Slip Disc, Cervical, Paralysis etc. She is also a Yoga Therapist and Yoga Trainer.

Keywords : Acceptance, Allowances, Adjustment, Relationship, Surrender

Marriage is all about acceptance and allowances...Acceptance and allowances for whatever is happening; it happens for our highest good. However, ensure that you do not immerse yourself so much in any relationship that you lose yourself.

- It's always good to serve.
- It's always good to give in.
- It's always good to compromise.

- **It's always good to make adjustments.**
- **All of these are requirements to live life.**

But if it breaks, you down and compromises your identity, learn to say no and stop there.

Hello,

To all beautiful souls reading this article;

Today, I feel blessed to be a single parent to my 13-years-old daughter. I have achieved my career without anyone's support and have changed many lives through my healing and therapy sessions. It was very tough being a housewife and standing up for my-self, especially in the early days of my marriage. I suffered from depression and even attempted suicide three times. Now, I understand that God has a different plan for me. **Surrender is a powerful tool**. I faced mental, physical, and sexual abuse in my married life, which shattered my confidence and made it hard for me to stand up for myself. However, with time, I realized that life was trying to teach me something. Instead of focusing on problems, I learned to focus on the **lessons in my journey.**

After disappointments in my life, I began to question God in my prayers: Why do I have to experience disappointments and setbacks? His reply was, "Because in disappointments, you learn to trust. In setbacks, your character grows." Why do I sometimes feel like life is filled with pain and helplessness? His response was, "In your weakest moments, I am by your side. Your pain builds your character."

Lessons Life Taught Me:

- **If you're rejected, accept it.**
- **If you're unloved, let go.**
- **If they choose someone or something over you, move on.**

Walk away not to teach them a lesson, but because you've learned your lesson from that.

How many more chances are you willing to give?

How many more times are you willing to be disrespected, unappreciated, manipulated, undervalued, and gas lighted by your partner?

He repeatedly undermined my worth and neglected my needs. I told him how much it hurt, but I still carried on. Walking away hurts, but it's an act of self-respect. Sometimes the lesson is known, when to put yourself first and safeguard your well-being. One day, God replied, "Don't think it wasn't seen by me, my child. One day you will not only recover but flourish. Remember, my plans for you are to prosper you and not to harm you. I am with you every step of this journey, mending every fracture, healing every wound, restoring every lost hope. Trust in me. I am your faithful protector, your healer, and your redeemer. You will see that my grace is sufficient for you." My last lesson was: Paying attention to a man doesn't keep him. Being beautiful. Being a good human being. Being honest. Being kind hearted No matter how good you are, it still doesn't keep a man, because the only way to keep a man is if he wants to be kept by you. So, don't hold on to a man or person who has already given up on you or the relationship.

Marriage is a beautiful relationship. Marriage itself is not bad, but our choices can be. It was my own choices that prevented me from attracting the right partner at the right time. The moment you decide to help yourself is the moment the universe will support you from all directions.

I Think 'ANTHOLOGY' is a great concept for many writers to come together & write their own experiences, thoughts & solutions on any topic. So, the person who chooses to read novels or other books can choose their own relatable topic with various tastes in one book.

"Be the best version of yourself."

|| ॐ ||

A Story of Endurance and Bliss

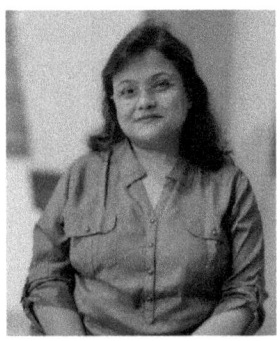

Author's Name	:	Lipiie Banerjjee
Qualification	:	B.Com., PGDBA
Current Profession	:	Consultant, Coach & Author
Age	:	54 years
E-mail ID	:	**banerjeelipi121@gmail.com**
City/ Country	:	**Mumbai, India**

Introducing a multifaceted and internationally renowned expert, **Lipiie Banerjjee** is an accomplished author whose works inspire and educate a global audience. As an NLP Trainer, she empowers individuals to unlock their potential through the power of language and mind. A Reiki Master, she provides healing and energy balancing, helping people achieve physical and emotional well-being. Her profound knowledge in Numerology and Astrology allows her to offer deep insights into life's patterns and cosmic influences.

She holds the prestigious titles of Gita Graduate and Advanced Vedantin reflecting her deep understanding of ancient spiritual wisdom and practices. Her journey from a successful corporate career to a dedicated spiritual catalyst is a testament to her commitment to personal growth and helping others. She combines her extensive expertise in various disciplines to guide individuals on their paths to self-discovery and transformation, making her a beacon of hope and change in the spiritual and personal development realms.

Keywords : Couple, Dream, Laughter, Melody, Wedding

Vivahadinamidam bhavatu harsadam

Mangalam tatha vam ca ksemadam

(Marriage – A Melody by Swami Tejomayananda)

May this wedding day bring to both of you happiness, auspiciousness and well-being.

Congratulations!!

Once upon a time, In a quaint village, lived a young couple, Arun and Meera. Their love story was the stuff of legends—filled with joy, laughter, and shared dreams. As they stood together on their wedding day, they promised each other a lifetime of love and companionship.

The Bliss

Pratidinam navam prema vardhatam,

Satagunam kulam sada hi modatam.

(Marriage – A Melody by Swami Tejomayananda)

Day by day, may you discover new love for each other. May it grow a hundredfold and may your family ever rejoice.

In the early days of their marriage, Arun and Meera found immense joy in each other's company. Every morning started with shared smiles and whispered secrets. They dreamt of building a home together, and as they painted the walls of their new house, their laughter echoed through the halls. Their emotional connection was strong, a sanctuary where they found comfort and peace.

Arun supported Meera's dreams of becoming a teacher, and she, in turn, encouraged his passion for gardening. Together, they grew not just as individuals but as a team, facing life's ups and downs with a united front. Their love was their strength, a beautiful bond that grew deeper with each passing day.

The Challenges

But like all fairy tales, their story had its share of challenges. Disagreements began to surface—small arguments about household chores, financial strains, and differing dreams. The conflicts sometimes felt overwhelming, casting shadows on their once-bright days. Arun struggled to maintain his sense of self, feeling lost in the daily grind of responsibilities. Meera, too, found herself yearning for the idealized version of marriage she had always imagined.

Personal Reflections

One evening, as they sat under the stars in their garden, Arun turned to Meera and said, "We need to talk." What followed was a heartfelt conversation about their fears, hopes, and frustrations. They spoke openly, sharing their feelings without judgment. This moment of vulnerability brought them closer, helping them understand each other better.

They decided to practice patience and empathy, reminding themselves that they were on this journey together. Arun began to find time for his gardening, while Meera dedicated time to her teaching aspirations. They celebrated small victories—Meera's first successful lesson plan, Arun's flourishing garden—and found joy in these everyday moments.

The term "vivaha" (marriage) originates from the Sanskrit verb root "vah," which signifies the act of carrying. That entails assuming the specific obligations associated with being married.

The primary obligation is to ensure the success of the marriage. The second duty entails providing assistance and ensuring the well-being of both the immediate and extended family, as well as fulfilling social obligations.

This phase of life is referred to as the grihasth ashrama, which literally signifies residing at home. The homeowner remains at home and assumes the duty of providing support to others, making them crucial for the continuation and upkeep of society.

In the end, Arun and Meera realized that marriage was neither purely bliss nor curse. It was a journey of love, patience, and growth. By nurturing their bond and embracing both the joys and challenges, they transformed potential hardships into opportunities for deeper connection.

Their story reminds us that marriage, with its ups and downs, is what we make of it. With love, respect and understanding, the potential for bliss far outweighs the challenges, turning a shared life into a beautiful tapestry of moments, both- bright and shadowed, woven together with care. Discover new love and respect for each other and let them grow each day.

In love they found both joy and strife,

Through bliss and trials, they forged their life.

With open hearts and hands entwined,

In marriage's dance, true strength they find.

॥ ॐ ॥

The Knot that Binds

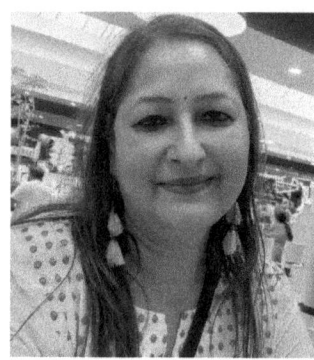

Author's Name	:	Madhu Soni
Qualification	:	Graduate
Current Profession	:	Graphologist, Grapho Therapist, Handwriting and Signature Consultant, Tarot Card Reader, Numerologist, Counselor, Coach and Mentor in moulding life.
Age	:	55 years
E-mail ID	:	sonimadhusatish@gmail.com
City/ Country	:	**Mumbai, India**

Madhu Soni is a multifaceted individual with a unique skill set that encompasses various fields such as graphology, drawing and signature analysis, doodle analysis, numerology, tarot card reading, handwriting analysis, grapho-therapy, and counseling for children. She possesses a deep understanding of human emotions and thought processes through which she provides valuable insights into analysing their personality sketch by underlying issues that may be affecting their personal and professional life.

Madhu Soni's unique blend of skills with her holistic approach reflects her unwavering commitment to empowering individuals of all ages to unlock their potential, overcome challenges and lead fulfilling lives guided by self-awareness and personal growth.

She has done various school projects about the awareness programme to improve handwriting for personality development. Apart from that she puts up stalls at exhibitions to encourage writing for self-improvement, focus and discipline.

She is the founder of **"miindgraphs"** wherein online/ offline consultations are done.

Keywords : Emotions, Experiment, Growth, Harmony, Mindset

Marriage is a sacred institution that has been around our culture throughout history. It is a union between two individuals who commit to sharing their lives, love, and support. However, the perception and experience vary greatly from person to person. Some view it as a blissful and fulfilling journey while others see it as a curse that brings more harm than good. In this article we will explore both views and try to understand whether marriage is a curse or bliss.

It's a universal truth that basic idea behind the concept is to cherish love union and create a beautiful environment of trust respect and security mutually. Partners play their unique role and grow together mentally and physically which makes them wiser and efficient for future together. They now become ready to face any setbacks and challenges by mere holding a partner's hand and upgrade their potentials. Now the question is that is the idea working smoothly as it has been since years. The answer is No with ample modifications and evolution. The reason lies in the changing value system desires and technical mindsets.

Today's world has been bombarded with technologies, machineries, computers home gadgets and facilities which has given us prosperity and finance comfort and luxury on one hand but taken away our peace harmony and emotions on another hand. Now our next generation born in this mechanical so called modern world are clueless and confused about emotions and connections. They are not to be blamed for this; we have given them this environment. Earlier human touch was everywhere to be seen but now we seldom see organic get together without any returns. Gen Z is learning diplomacy Independency financial security as priority and are far away from values like helping to care for family taking responsibility and be trustworthy and honest. These are hampering them to be committed and more intensive.

Relationships are superficial and based on benefits which are instrumental for divorces, live- ins, infidelity, breakdowns, and loneliness. We can see these very regularly and it's sad and scary. But again, nothing is impossible and with proper guidance and awareness we can prep the coming generation to trust the process. Coming to marriage it must be worked upon 24/7 for better and smooth functioning. We must go beyond curse to make it a bliss. It must be experienced to understand the feeling of a team and togetherness. It's a journey of 2 persons with different mindset beliefs and background coming together to live a happy life, upgrade each other, learn karmic lessons if I say so in spiritual terms. They unite to finish up their pending tasks which can be good or bad depending on the dealings.

And to top it all families of both are involved which enhances the process. I will not say it is so easy and smooth, but definitely vouch for its beauty and intricacies. One day u might feel it's all over but then some strange connection and conviction will make u go again head over heels in love. Its magic and power of the universal love language, which can surpass any endanger.

It's sad to see the beauty of marriage losing its grip over young adults. They are escaping the fact that no one is perfect, and Marriage is the combination of imperfect perfect where no one is perfect and imperfect either. That's where the catch is the trial and errors, fighting, loving having fun in smallest of things together actually keeps life energetic and interesting. It's also seen women mostly opting out of marriage may be due to newfound gender equality, job profiles, or losing out on their identities. They don't need a man to complete a life and vice versa and here is that they are losing the script. It would be wonderful to see modern smart yet rooted youngster tying the knots and enjoy their life.

I really advocate Marriage as a bliss from my experience of 33 years as it has made me a person. who I'm today who can handle almost everything and anything in this world by getting the support advice criticism and love of my husband and children, which has made me complete with my own baggage of sorrows dreams confusions and solutions.

This is a great opportunity for all of us as co-authors to share our experience and understanding of topic which we hope shall guide the future generation to believe in the system of marriage and to enjoy a blissful union of love and understanding.

|| ॐ ||

Marriage is a Learning, to Enjoy the Differences

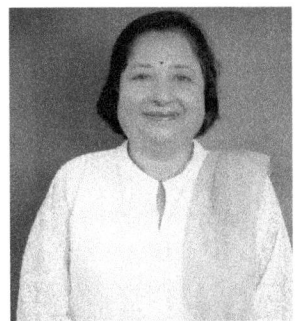

Author's Name	:	Manissha Shah
Qualification	:	B.Com., CA, CWA, DISA (ICA)
Current Profession	:	Counselor and Coach
Age	:	55 years
E-mail ID	:	**authormanissha@gmail.com**
City/ Country	:	**Ahmedabad, India**

Manissha Shah, academically is a Chartered Accountant as well as a Cost Accountant, with nearly 30 years of rich experience, focusing in the area of Information Systems Audit.

After many years of rich experience as a Chartered Accountant, she decided to go ahead with her burning desire and passion to create a positive change in the lives of people. She studied to be a Life Coach, a Relationship Coach, NLP Coach, Law of Attraction Coach, Master Practitioner of Graphology, Spiritual healer and many other peripheral courses. She not only has successfully transformed lives of hundreds of people in the areas of mental and emotional health and wellbeing, physical health challenges, relationship challenges, career challenges, financial challenges, but has also helped them create abundance in life.

Having very successfully, transformed cases of marital discord and those on the verge of a divorce into very beautiful marriage relationships, she decided to pen some of her thoughts, to inspire people to instill romance in their marriage.

Keywords : Courtship, Dating, Couple, Respect, Responsibility

Marriages are one of the most beautiful institutions of life, where both, husband and wife lovingly grow with each other. But today, marital discord, fights between the husband and wife finally leading to divorce, are increasing at an alarming rate. Therefore, here is an attempt to draw people's attention to 108 different perspectives to help create a beautiful marriage.

It is truly said, 'A great marriage is not when the 'perfect' couple come together. It is when the 'imperfect' couple learns to enjoy the differences. As human beings, none of us are perfect – we all have our own set of flaws. Let's accept that, for ourselves and others too.

Life seems so beautiful during the courtship or dating days for a couple – because, we tend to impress or woo each other with everything that the other would love, even if it meant, going out of our way, at times. Their eccentricities are taken as excessive caring, selfishness is loved, showering gifts are considered as an expression of love, carelessness is acceptable and many more. Life seems a total bliss.

If this bliss remains, Both of them would love to be with each other, enjoy life with each other, face challenges that come their way with double the courage and strength, both of them complete each other, love and trust growing leaps and bounds between them, even the biggest of challenges/hurdles in life are overcome easily, the kids grow up in an environment emphasizing peace and harmony and much more.

Post marriage, we start taking each other for granted. Our happiness depends totally on whether our spouse behaves, does things exactly the way we want them to do or not. When that doesn't happen, in majority of the cases, troubles start. Some of the trivial complaints that commonly came up during the course of my counseling sessions with couples:

(The first part is the complaint and the second part Is the response of the spouse)

- He doesn't ring me (from office) that often, or talk to me that frequently – I am busy in the office and she doesn't have anything new to tell me.
- She doesn't cook new things for me, or the food I like – This is the best that I can make, with the given constraints.
- He keeps finding faults with every little thing I do – If I tell her something once, she thinks I am always fault finding.
- She keeps on nagging – He doesn't understand if told once.
- He doesn't want to spend time with me once he comes home from office – Am tired, after slogging it out the whole day.
- Even though, both of us are working, he doesn't help me with the household chores or the kids – She doesn't notice everything I do

Every time we are confronted with complaints, can we :

- Avoid generalisations or exaggerations in our arguments?
- Remember all the good acts done by them before we raise our voice for something 'not right'?
- Avoid assuming things or taking out a different meaning for what our spouse has said or done?
- Have easy Rules to enjoy good things in life and difficult rules to be affected by the bad things in life?

For those who are looking out for a partner to get married to, prioritize :

- Inner beauty rather than Outer appearance: In today's times, if a boy is handsome or a girl is beautiful and charming, they are always preferred. It is preferred to select someone with rich inner beauty and values.

- Earning ability and responsibility rather than Earnings and Financial status : Rather than be awed by the cars, bungalows and foreign trips respect their responsibility, intelligence, capability to earn money.

- Matching 'values': If 'family' is of highest value to one and 'Money' is to the other, the match may not be proper.

- In India, a marriage is supposed to be between 2 families, rather than 2 people. So, a due diligence as to how much both of them respect each other's families also, is important.

- Last but not the least, please value your parents' and family opinions about each other also.

Let's take the onus of having a beautiful marriage on us. Let's take charge of the small differences and work on them. Let's apply the due diligences while choosing our life partner. Aptly said, 'Every successful marriage has 3 parties involved – the husband, wife and a coach (who guides them at every step)'

॥ ॐ ॥

The True Essence of Married Life

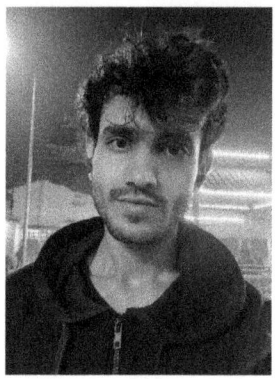

Author's Name	:	Mayur Ghate
Qualification	:	M.Sc.
Current Profession	:	Pursuing Ph.D.
Age	:	33 years
E-mail ID	:	**mayur.ghate3@gmail.com**
City/ Country	:	**Dombivli, India**

Mayur Ghate is currently pursuing his Ph.D in the field of Biotechnology at Indian Institute of Technology, Roorkee (IIT, Roorkee). He has done his Master Degrees in Biotechnology at Banaras Hindu University, Varanasi (BHU, Varanasi).

Apart from his PhD, he has enrolled in other certification courses like Neuro Linguistic Programming (NLP). Ho'Oponopono and EFT program, Handwriting analyst, Law of attraction coach.

Keywords : Acceptance, Astrology, Independence, Responsibilities, Values

I'm a boy belonging from middle class family, where we as kids are taught to study well, get good grades, find a job and if you get a good job, you will land up having a life-partner. After this you have to take responsibilities of the children and look after them as we did. Since I was a child, I have experienced a chaotic married life of my parents and my dad used to say, "Never be submissive or surrender in front of your wife, don't listen much what she says otherwise she will sit on your shoulders". After marriage your dad struggled a lot between his family and wife's family", I have screwed up my whole life! Now imagine after listening all this from my dad, what was the view of marriage in my mind?

Due to my chaotic situation, somewhere I got convinced that marriage is like a spell where we have to suffer a lot. I have grown up seeing how my parents, despite being together were completely separated emotionally. This was pricking me like a pin every day with lot of ego clashes, quarrels and blame game and what not and then I decided to be away from this quarrelsome atmosphere, pursue good education and become independent. Fortunately, I got the opportunity to move from my hometown and today its being 7 years, I am away from my home and I don't feel any homesickness, moreover I visit my home once in a year! Along with this, I literally lost all of my interest of thinking to marry someone and in my due-course, I was deeply involved in my growth and got habituated to independence. It was damn hard for me to even think of marriage, after which I have to sacrifice my independence, having to start the same lifecycle as my parents. Apart from my formal education, I loved astrology and I gained basic knowledge of reading charts, in our charts the ascendant and 7th house which is of our spouse are entirely opposite that reinforced my belief that marriage is hell. Well I did not understand the true meaning of this disparity until this time. I kept learning, because the formal education was satisfying my physical and materialistic needs, but at the end of the day I would feel alone and low, despite enjoying my solitude. To combat this loneliness, I started watching videos related to law of attraction, I got familiar with this law, but understood it truly only after 8 years. This awakening came after me enrolling into specific detailed courses of law of attraction and human values. In English, wife is called as better-half and in Sanskrit is called as ardhangini, in astrology we see opposite traits and true law of attraction talks about fulfilling each other's values. It was a great eye-opener for me, your life-partner is the reflection of the traits that are missing in you and the main purpose of the life partner is the acceptance of yourself as a whole and same for her. We are here to accept each other's values. If you truly accept the opposite side of you, you accept yourself which is the most blissful moment of your life.

To conclude, I would like to say we as humans have come to this earth to experience the true essence of life. In our whole lifespan, the life partner is the person who spends the longest duration of journey with us and the day we get married, our journey to self-acceptance begins which should be cherished. If you think it's a curse, just imagine that trait is in you and you have disowned it, simply accept it, the married life will be blissful. Just accept, accept and accept, life will automatically become blissful.

This anthology provides a great opportunity for the persons like me who wish to write and become an author. I know and comprehend the current scenario of the society and willing to convey my learning and make people familiar with the truth. Through anthology, it becomes possible to reach to thousands and thousands of people and change their lives for the betterment. As this platform is the amalgamation of precious thoughts and experiences of authors, people can easily relate with their own experiences that can add value in their lives. Finally, it bestows confidence among people and motivate them to become expressive.

The Double-Edged Sword

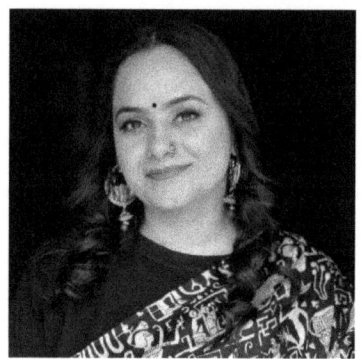

Author's Name	:	Mehul Gupta
Qualification	:	B.Com.
Current Profession	:	Smile Coach
Age	:	37 years
E-mail ID	:	**mehulgupta.8611@gmail.com**
City/ Country	:	**New Delhi, India**

Mehul Gupta is an independent woman and a dedicated smile coach, bringing joy and positivity into the lives of those she counsels. With a gentle heart and a nurturing spirit, she embodies the essence of an angel, healing people around her with compassion and kindness. Her mission is to inspire and uplift and guide others toward a happier, more fulfilled life through the power of smiles and positive energy. She believes in the transformative power of genuine connection and strives to create a ripple effect of happiness. Every smile she shares and every heart she heals is a step towards a brighter, more compassionate world. www.guptamehul.com

Keywords : Companionship, Connection, Communication, Couple, Commitment

Marriage, often described as an institution, serves as a foundational societal construct that encompasses various dimensions, including emotional, social, legal, and cultural aspects. It has evolved from a primarily economic and strategic alliance to a partnership based on love and mutual respect. Marriage offers companionship, emotional support and a sense of belonging. It can be a platform for personal growth and self-discovery, as partners navigate life's challenges together. Marriage often provides emotional and financial security, contributing to overall well-being.

From the outside, our marriage appeared idyllic—a perfect blend of love and companionship, laughter and shared dreams. Friends envied our connection, seeing only the blissful moments that peppered our lives like glittering stars in a clear night sky. But beneath this shimmering surface lay a tangled web of unspoken words, suppressed emotions, and unmet expectations. Our marriage was, paradoxically, a curse wrapped in the guise of bliss.

The Bliss

Our story began with an enchanting whirlwind of romance as Typical Indian family where the girl and the suited partner are met through relatives. The Indian girl always dreams of tall dark handsome man who will love her like the Bollywood shows. He was everything I had ever dreamed of—charming, ambitious, and attentive. Our wedding was a grand celebration of our love, filled with promises of eternal happiness.

Living together, we created a sanctuary of love and understanding. Our home was filled with joy, from lazy Sunday mornings spent in bed to evenings spent with family, movies, dinners etc. He used to be running errands to sooth and calm our lives .We shared dreams of a bright future—traveling the world, building a family, and growing old together.

The Curse

But as time passed, the cracks in our perfect façade began to show. The bliss we once reveled in became a mask, hiding the growing discord between us. Our love was genuine, but so were our flaws and the mounting pressures of life.

Our conversations dwindled to mundane exchanges about sleepless nights and schedules, devoid of the depth and intimacy we once shared. Miscommunication turned small disagreements into monumental battles. Our arguments, once rare, became frequent and fierce, leaving emotional scars that neither of us knew how to heal. We each clung stubbornly to our viewpoints, unable to bridge the growing chasm between us. The love that had brought us together now felt like a chain, binding us to a life of perpetual discontent.

The societal and familial expectations of an Indian tradition began to weigh heavily on us. Both sets of parents had their own views on what our marriage should look like, often leading to unsolicited advice and veiled criticisms.

The Duality

In the end, our marriage was a bittersweet blend of joy and sorrow, love and pain. It was a curse disguised as bliss, a relationship that taught us both the heights of happiness and the depths of despair. Our journey was a testament to the complexity of love—how it can uplift and destroy, heal and hurt, bind and break.

As I reflect on our time together, I realize that the bliss and the curse were intertwined, each giving meaning to the other. Our love was real, but so were our struggles. And in this duality, I found a deeper understanding of myself, of Him and of the intricate dance that is marriage.

Lessons Learned

- **Understanding the Importance of Communication**

One of the most critical lessons I learned from our marriage was the paramount importance of communication. However, as time went on, our conversations became superficial, avoiding the deeper issues that were causing rifts between us.

Partnership took back stage and we got enrolled in our own ways of the upbringing of our only child. The archetypal Indian house wife and a mother serving the family with herself at the back seat, giving unlimited care love to every person in the family without reciprocation.

- **Resilience in the Face of Adversity**

Our marriage taught us resilience. We faced numerous challenges that tested our commitment and love for each other. I learned that I could endure hardship, adapt to change, and emerge stronger. This resilience became a foundation upon which I added feathers to my career rebuilt myself, transforming struggles into opportunities for growth.

I started my venture of a cloud kitchen, and also was awarded with Women's Achiever Award for it and Women Change Maker of the Year. These recognitions brought courage , strength and smile to my confidence and later started adding more feathers to me, I became a smile coach treating and helping women to speak volumes of what was unsaid in their marriages and vouch on themselves to stand strong against all odds.

- **Embracing the Complexity of Love**

Now, with the clarity of hindsight, I see our marriage as a journey—a beautiful, tumultuous journey that shaped who we are. The bliss and the curse were two sides of the same coin, each essential in our story. Our love was a complex tapestry, woven with threads of joy and sorrow, laughter and tears. And in that complexity, I found a profound truth: that love, in all its forms, is where you can think its worth the journey.

- **Redefining Love and Partnership**

In this new perspective, I embrace the beauty of imperfection and the richness of shared experiences. I understand that a successful marriage is not one without challenges, but one where both partners are committed to navigating those challenges together with love, respect, and a shared vision for the future.

My Marriage – My Lifeline

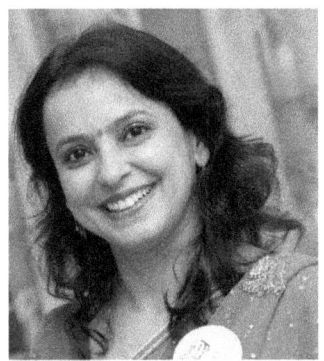

Author's Name	:	Mini Baijal
Qualification	:	B.Sc. B.Ed with PG Diploma in Management
Current Profession	:	Headmistress in a Private School
Age	:	52 Years
E-mail ID	:	**minikbaijal@gmail.com**
City/ Country	:	**Gurgaon, India**

Mini Baijal is the Headmistress of a renowned private school in Gurgaon. She is in the field of education for more than 22 years. She is a passionate educator who bagged **'School Spirit Award'** in 2018 and **'Best Teacher Award'** twice in 2019 and 2020. She was honored with **'District Performance Excellence Award'** 2019-20 by Science Olympiad Foundation. She was also conferred with **'Rotary District 3011 Excellence Award'** and a certificate of achievement for significant contribution at Sakshar. Her effort of imparting knowledge to the 21st Century Learners was appreciated and was felicitated at the Rotary Annual Award ceremony on 5 September 2023.

Keywords : Commitment, Mutual Trust, Respect, Understanding, Communication

Marriage is a beautiful relationship between two individuals. It is like a commitment between two partners. The partners must complement each other while respecting the differences they have as individuals. This commitment may be a lifelong commitment or it may end up in separation or divorce if the partners are not compatible. As the saying goes marriages are made in heaven but it is the couples who make it work on earth. In the initial years of marriage, everything seems to be like a dream or a rosy picture, but after facing rough times together the union becomes more beautiful. A Marriage may be bliss or curse depending upon how the two persons tied in a knot treat each other. They should have respect for each other. Most problems can be solved by sharing your feelings, listening and taking time out for your partners. No marriage is perfect. You learn each day and discover more about your partner. At times it is treated as a compromise but no one will be happy in such relation. There is no hard and fast rule or a tested method for a successful marriage.

Every couple has to create their own recipe and add ingredients of love, respect and trust to make it wonderful. The bond between the couple becomes stronger as they grow older together. Sooner or later they become the blessing for each other.

My marriage is certainly bliss. I can say that I am on the blessing side of the coin. It is not that we have not gone through rough phases but every time we have evolved with more understanding and stronger bonding. Mine was an arranged marriage. We had a courtship period of four months which I still cherish. Met a very simple person, with a heart of gold, 25 years back, but then I could not understand that God was blessing me with lifelong happiness. We did hit a rough patch. We also had fights, difference of opinion and long periods of silence but, then we decided to keep the channel of communication open to come to a solution.

The fear of losing someone is the biggest anxiety. I had gone through this four years back. That time I realised that he is my lifeline. Sometimes we take our partner for granted without knowing how deeply rooted he/ she is there in our breath, blood and heartbeats. He was suffering. I could not see him in so much pain but I had to be strong just for him. How could I lose hope? I had to make him believe that nothing bad would happen to us. By the grace of god he could be saved in time. Sometimes couples don't know how much they love each other. It cannot be measured but yes it can be felt. My marriage is the most fulfilling journey of my life.

I feel bad for those couples who separate. Many times it happens just due to the lack of patience, understanding or a respect for each other. Most of the problems faced by the couples can be solved by simply keeping the line of communication open. Respecting each other's opinions, dreams and differences is important. If the elderly members of the family intervene and counsel both partners, a marriage can be saved. Children are majorly affected by these broken marriages of their parents. They suffer a lot so one must try to save it as far as possible. If the relationships are bitter and on the verge of causing physical harm, then it is good to separate. A marriage is a bliss or a curse is different experience for different couples.

Marriage is a Blissful Curse

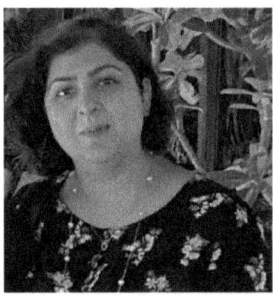

Author's Name	:	Neelam Khemani
Qualification	:	M.B.A
Current Profession	:	Consultant
Age	:	46 Years
E-mail ID	:	…
City/ Country	:	**Hyderabad, India**

Neelam Khemani has done her MBA in Finance. She has 18+ years' experience of Product Management and Operations in the areas of Business Research & Analysis in India and U.S. as well. She is a mother of a beautiful girl and a nurturer. She loves movies and music on long drive!

Keywords: Bliss, Brutal, Sincerity, Deceit, Love-hate

What is Marriage really ? … A Blissful Curse.

Marriage comes with a bundle of emotions – complete bliss, feeling wanted and accepted, a sense of belonging, feeling emotions that you never thought you were capable of feeling, selflessness. Well, this is all very rubicund… Then, why is it a curse?

While some understand and appreciate and value the commitment, the partnership is subject to a lot of internal/ external forces. And to be able to withstand such brutal forces and hard realities of life, it takes maturity, decency and sincerity to pull this through. While there are those few who can fit into that mould, there is a large set who cannot and make it the most terrifying institution ever where the borders of love and hate collide and cause so much damage that it can shake one up for lifetimes.

Twisha, a modern, feisty, independent, idealistic girl waited patiently for her Mr. Right to come into her life and day dreamed of having a large loving family which she craved after an empty long 30 years of her materialistic life. With love to give, the nurturer in her arose very naturally. But the people on the receiving end were not in for the same reason… little did she know she was falling prey to a narcissistic man and a flying monkey, who helped her husband with whatever he fancied and then devalue and discard.

Largely oblivious of narcissism and innate strong belief that she has found her home to love, nurture and to create a sense of belonging and permanency – she was welcomed by rude and a spiteful mother-in-law from day zero, only to question from here on – what kind of a son she must have raised? Someone who was so unhappy with her own life and her own circumstances that her son was her only crutch. Her reputation of being unkind and a manipulator preceded her. Number of the relatives had warned Twisha of her and the son. With the nuptials done, she felt it was too late. Nonetheless, she decided to move forward by giving her all and waiting for time/ fate to unfold what was in store for her.

As Twisha yearned to spend quality time with her husband on their honeymoon, she got a nasty shock when she was asked to shell out half the amount spent on it. She believed all the "hisaab kitab" had ended until the point of marriage where each family paid half of all the expenses. She was still determined to make a family for herself despite having the nagging feeling that this is not going to work out. She was soon made privy to how the previous alliance was broken and that had raised very logical questions from an educated and a logical girl. The partnership between son and the mother just never seemed right.

While on one side the honeymoon period was on, all stops were pulled by the mother-in-law to show immense dislike towards Twisha while she was doing her very best to help in the kitchen, pay for her food and grocery expenses, and fit into the family. Every bit of effort was put in to train Twisha to be the full time maid of the house. Everything was done not to make her not feel like a family member and where the mother continuously displayed her obsession and control over her son and his likes, dislikes, sleeping habits, etc. She was made to feel the third well in this equation.

Twisha's entire life was spiraling out of control with multiple events henceforth like moving into another house to restart their newly married life, bliss of movies and restaurants, second chances, intimate moments, building a friend circle and hoping to build a solid base to grow old with the man she believed was made for her as they did get each other at a lot of levels – emotionally and intellectually.

But as life stirred forward with a child, movement to the U.S, travelling on account of friend's coercion, conceiving the second child, losing it, taking care of home, child, and working at office and paying half for everything, never given any love or a gift or ever made to feel special/ needed in her husbands' life – until he found his way to exit the marriage and get rid of Twisha and their son. After the love bombing and devaluing phase, it was the discard phase which eventually saw the natural death of the marriage.

Once all the check boxes were ticked for him – of marriage, child, well settled job – he had to move to greener pastures devoid of any commitments, responsibilities to tie him down while Twisha was asked to go back to India with her son and raise the child on her own and never bother him again.

|| ॐ ||

Marriage Through My Eyes

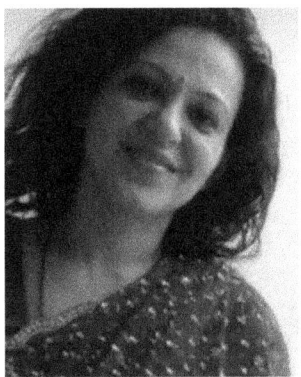

Author's Name	:	Neena Puri Nagpal
Qualification	:	MBA (Finance)
Current Profession	:	Director, Private Banking
Age	:	46 years
E-mail ID	:	**neenapuri@yahoo.com**
City/ Country	:	**Gurugram, India**

Neena Puri Nagpal is a BFSI professional with 17 years of Indian and Offshore market experience. Presently working as Director with India's leading bank. She is learner for life, always seeking new experiences and always embracing new opportunities. She is an incredible multi – tasker, someone who always strives for excellence in all domains, be it professional or personal. Most of all, she firmly believes in hard work – and that there's nothing in the world that cannot be achieved with hard work and patience. She is doting mother of two adorable kids, who loves a simple and wholesome living – a living that prioritizes self-care and mental health while balancing all other aspects of life

Keywords : Evolution of Marriage, Live-Love-Laugh, Non-judgmental, Self-awareness, Societal shifts

Marriage is what you make of it. Marriage is an institution in itself which was promulgated in olden societies for structuring of a family unit. It also was a monetary transaction, business or political agreement with concept of division of labor at the center stage, defining roles of man and woman. This provided a framework for meeting physical, financial, emotional needs of individuals involved. It evolved to an extent when apart from two individuals, two families ended up getting married! It has always been an important sign of commitment and transition into deeper and more serious relationship. With evolution of societies, various age-old traditions have assumed newer forms and colors and marriage has been no exception either.

Been married for good 20+ years myself that too into a large joint family system with three generations still coming together under one roof in good and bad times, there are a plethora of experiences that have played a definitive role in greatly shaping who I am today. The good ones stay as positive memories, the not so good ones need to be taken lightly for the show must go on. As they say, relationship between husband and wife is very psychological; one is Psycho and the other is Logical!! Husbands are the best people to share your secrets with. They'll never tell anyone because they aren't even listening.

The institution of marriage is breaking down and divorces no longer carry the stigma they used to. But that sad ending need not be. Its pivotal to understand oneself through self-awareness. Basically, an understanding of your triggers-what drives you and what drains you. Without self-awareness, it is almost impossible to know what we want from life, what we can give to our partner and expect from the togetherness of the relationship. Marrying early just because one has met the important milestones of "completing education, starting a job" can be safely replaced with later marriage when some maturity and expectation from marriage is clearer. Finding someone who patiently waits for you to calm down, who understand oneself and you, who knows that you know your own time and space are mature love is timeless.

Another piece of advice is to not love (read marry) on potential. Loving someone and having them love you back is the strongest emotion in the world. Marrying on potential will lead to a lifelong push and pull of changing your partner to fit into your image of your deserving companion. "I like the person this much and the rest I see as potential which I will work on, "this thought process is suicidal. The resistance in the relationship from forced push and pull can be detrimental leading to quiet quitting by either or both.

Worldwide societies are gravitating to the new concepts of grey divorce or bracing the new normal of never getting married. For marriage hinders your chances of moving forward from an ended relationship. The likelihood that a couple will get back together is generally minimal once a couple has separated. Not being married can make your future options more flexible should things not work out. Also in many parts of the world, marriage is socially considered to be the norm, but for the most part, the push for romantic relationships to have an end goal of marriage has become more casual.

Topic wants us to explore, decipher the intricacies of the institution of marriage. How the concept has evolved and is still evolving given tremendous societal shifts worldwide. Is coercing to think about marriage from one's own lens and perhaps can share few key lessons from one's own journey of married life. The pauses and reflections of one's one journey have helped experience myriad emotions and have been therapeutic in a way. For the articulation helped to become firmer in belief of being nonjudgmental and hold my ground assertively remaining kind and broad minded to others' journey

Whatever it is, I personally am averse to judging a marriage as everyone's journey is and remaining kind towards each other is the only ingredient for a happy society. A strong marriage is a union of two people, who choose to love each other even when they struggle to like each other. On a lighter note, when someone is murdered, the police tend to investigate the spouse first. Doesn't that tell you everything about marriage?!

|| ॐ ||

Tides of Togetherness Embracing Growth in Marriage

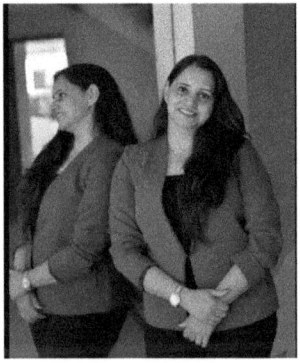

Author's Name	:	Neetu A Beel
Qualification	:	B.Com.
Current Profession	:	Numerologist, Graphologist
Age	:	42 Years
E-mail ID	:	**accessvibrations@gmail.com**
City/ Country	:	**Kolkata, India**

Neetu A Beel is a distinguished Numerologist and Graphologist with over 12 years of experience, dedicated to helping individuals transform their lives. As a certified Bach Flower therapist, she specializes in healing emotional wounds that often manifest as physical ailments.

Neetu's expertise extends to Past Life Regression therapy, guiding people to uncover the hidden roots of their present challenges. Her mission is to empower others with knowledge of the unseen forces that shape their lives, offering profound insights into the invisible but powerful energies that influence our existence. Neetu is passionate about educating and uplifting people, helping them unlock their full potential and lead a more balanced, harmonious life.

Keywords : Communication, Respect, Share Same Goals, Trust, Understanding

Marriage is a profound journey that weaves the fabric of our lives, teaching us invaluable lessons along the way. This sacred bond challenges us to grow, adapt, and become better versions of ourselves. When we embrace the karmic connection with our spouse, marriage becomes a blessing, a sanctuary where we learn to navigate the ebbs and flows of life with empathy, understanding, and a renewed sense of purpose. However, if we succumb to bitterness and constantly curse our relationship, it can turn into a curse, a heavy burden that drags us down. The true essence of marriage lies in our willingness to learn from each other, to celebrate our differences, and to nurture a deep, abiding love that transcends the inevitable ups and downs. It is in this journey of growth and self-discovery that we find the true meaning of a blessed union.

Our scriptures are rich with stories that beautifully illustrate the unique and sacred bond between husband and wife. The relationships of Ram and Sita, Vishnu and Lakshmi, are prime examples of this profound connection. These divine unions highlight the idea that marriage is more than a mere partnership—it's a karmic bond that transcends lifetimes. Every soul on this planet is intertwined with their life partner in a similar way, bound by fate to walk the path of life together. The true purpose of marriage is not just companionship, but the mutual upliftment of both partners. Together, they strive to fulfil a higher calling, supporting each other's spiritual growth and contributing to a greater purpose. Just as the divine couples did, every married pair has the potential to achieve something extraordinary by nurturing their bond and walking hand in hand on their shared journey.

A blissful marriage is built on several key elements, each as vital as the wheels of a car, ensuring the journey is smooth and fulfilling. The first of these is respect—the cornerstone of any relationship. Respect means truly valuing your partner for who they are and appreciating their presence in your life. Without respect, the foundation of the relationship can waver.

The second and perhaps the most crucial, is trust. Trust is the bedrock upon which love and partnership are built, allowing both individuals to feel secure and supported.

The third essential element is communication. Clear and open communication is the key to understanding and resolving differences, ensuring both partners feel heard and valued.

When both partners share the same goals and work toward them together, it creates a shared 'sense of purpose' that strengthens their bond.

Finally, a deep understanding of each other's needs and emotions—often without words—fosters a connection that transcends the ordinary.

Just as a car cannot run with a damaged wheel, a marriage cannot thrive without these five essential elements working in harmony.

Marriage is one of life's most beautiful experiences, offering the opportunity for deep connection and personal growth. While not everyone views their marriage in the same light—some finding joy, others encountering challenges—the underlying purpose of this union is to evolve as individuals and souls. The journey of marriage is not always easy; some may walk a path lined with roses, while others may face a road of thorns. However, regardless of the challenges or blessings, marriage serves as a catalyst for growth. It teaches resilience, empathy, and understanding, helping each partner reach a better place in life. Through both the highs and lows, couples evolve together, learning valuable lessons that shape their character and deepen their bond. Ultimately, marriage is not just about companionship, but about personal evolution and the shared journey of reaching new heights together.

Your life partner is like a boat that helps you navigate the river of life. However, becoming too attached to that boat and burdening it with endless expectations can lead to chaos. To truly find peace and fulfilment, it's essential to set yourself free by understanding your life's purpose beyond just one relationship. When you focus on your own growth and path, your connection with your partner becomes more harmonious and balanced. Remember, the journey is about more than just the boat; it's about where you're headed and who you become along the way.

|| ॐ ||

Bliss or Curse – Depends on In-Laws
Saat Phero ke Side Effects

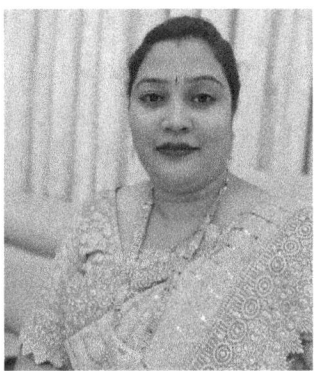

Author's Name	:	Neha Piyush Nashine
Qualification	:	Bachelor in Arts
Current Profession	:	Vastu Consultant, Numerologist, Tarot Card Reader, Author and Electrical Contractor
		• Proprietor - Shivansh Electrical and Infra Works
		• Director - Kulamama Resorts Pvt. Ltd.
Age	:	35 Years
E-mail ID	:	npnashine@gmail.com
City/ Country	:	Nagpur, India

Mrs. Neha Piyush Nashine is an Entrepreneur, Vastu Expert, Numerologist and Tarot Card Reader. She is also in Hospitality Business Director at Kulamama Resorts Pvt. Ltd. and A Proprietor at Shivansh Electrical & Infra Works. makes her an independent woman. She strongly believes in hard work and is an optimistic person. always ready to learn with a positive attitude. spirituality is her strength.

Keywords : Spiritual, Marriage, In-Laws, Effects, Housewife, Entrepreneur

Marriage, My Marriage is a blessing or a curse : Don't Know, they say that it is like a laddu, the one who does not eat regrets, and the one who eats it also regrets. I Neha, the one who was crazy to get married. When I was growing up, since childhood, some people asked me what will I become. I used to say that I would become a housewife and get married. everyone was laughing. My childhood was spent happily, I grew up, I had no interest in studies at all my father forced me to study B.A. first but I wanted to get married and go to my in-laws' house.

And then there was that day too. When a boy came to see me for marriage, the first time, I still remember the day, the boy liked me and I liked the boy, the date of our engagement came close, and we got engaged on this day. Then we got married, after marriage I went to my in-laws' house. My husband had a complete family. And right from engagement to marriage, we understood each other very well and there was love between us. my dream of getting married was complete after marriage.

My husband is also a very simple person. And he also loves me a lot, but after marriage new relationship is not only with the husband but also with relationship with husband's family, but that family never accepted the girl who came from outside, and the daughter-in-law was given all the time to realize that she is from outside and stranger. her in-laws never accept her from their hearts. that thing happened to me also. My husband comes home at night. I was the only one with my in-laws like a stranger.

In my in-law's House, there was everyone grandfather in law, Grandmother-in-law, father-in-law, Mother in law, Big Sister-in-law was married, Small Sister-in-law was unmarried, Sister-in-law used to stay in their parents' house mostly, I alone doing housework and mother-in-law and Sister in laws was going to shopping. During the day, At night, my husband and my mother-in-law said to him not a single work was done properly by the daughter-in-law. When I complained to him he said let it go, then its limits, when my mother, father, and brother-sister, came to meet me at my house, my mother-in-law complained my father about me that You guys teach nothing to your daughter.

My father did not spend time to my home, poor my father returned after this. Time was running two years later I was about to become a mother after many prayers, everyone was very happy. My mother-in-law told me a new word that first there should be a son and not a daughter, how can she say this when she herself has two daughters. My husband said let her go, it's his mother. Then the matter came to pass and the entire 9 months and 12 days I spent days in tension, I could not enjoy my pregnancy, Lord Mother Queen had approved of a daughter, I gave birth to a daughter as lovely as an angel, I named her Pari, my mother-in-law got angry, there were a lot of dramas, I stayed with my mother house for three months. Then time caught up and my daughter's has become one year old. my health was very bad. suddenly my doctor detected a stone in my gallbladder due to which my gallbladder will have to be removed, I was in a lot of pain at that time also my in-laws not help me.

My husband was with me but not supporting me. people from my maternal side were always with me. My little daughter, who had just given birth to me in my hospital, stayed with her maternal uncle for the whole day due to lack of time.... because I am admitted in hospital. Three years Later I had a son. Time has moved on 8 years later I was a worthless daughter-in-law, i was the one who had snatched the son of my mother-in-law, from her point of view. daughter-in-law Who did not serve to her in-laws For a long time, they think time changed. My husband bought a new house for us my house has changed in front of my eyes, my husband children and I moved to a new house. everything will remain, but my service to my father-in-law is mine, today I am everyone's daughter-in-law, my husband has taken me, a new place, according to my mother-in-law, I had separated her from my husband. It may have been my wish that I should move away from my in-laws, my god wish that I move on from my in-laws house.

I have been married for 14 years. Today I am a writer, but I am still a worthless daughter-in-law. The hard time for a woman is when she becomes a mother.

When she has a baby, she needs love. A human being can understand and support, but my mother-in-law cannot feel the pain of her daughter-in-law and I know that in those rare moments of my life, I experienced the feeling of becoming a mother who was worried only because of my mother-in-law, being troubled by a mother-in-law. the time that i spent in fear. I lost those very precious moments of being a mother. - This is my saying for which I will never forgive my mother-in-law and my in-laws.

Marriage is good, if the mother-in-law becomes a mother, she meets a girl in the in-law's house, when the mother-in-law gives love to the daughter-in-law mother-in-law give love and the marriage will become a blessing, not a curse because marriage is not a relationship between a boy and girl, it's a complete family relationship. If the all relationships are good then we girls get heaven feeling, we just do not need to get a good Husband with a good mother-in-law and father-in-law too. Then marriage gets Bliss.

|| ॐ ||

The Dual Nature of Marriage

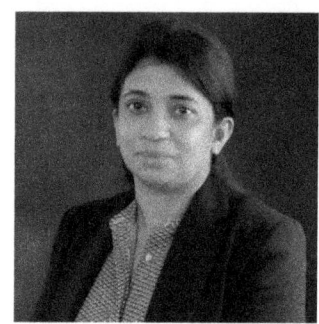

Author's Name	:	Nidhi Chugh
Qualification	:	B.A. English (Hons), Certified Graphologist
Current Profession	:	Consultant, Numerologist, Astro-Vastu Expert and Logo Designer
Age	:	49 years
E-mail ID	:	**numerologistnidhichugh@gmail.com**
City/ Country	:	**Gurgaon, India**

Nidhi Chugh is a self-motivated and hard-working individual who has made a significant mark in the fields of graphology, numerology and Vaastu. She is a Certified Graphologist specializing in handwriting and signature analysis. In 2011, she completed her advanced course in graphology from the International School of Handwriting Analysis (ISHA USA, California). Additionally, she undertook an advanced course from Power of Handwriting in India and currently serves as the Delhi NCR head of the organization.

Nidhi's extensive experience includes conducting workshops on personality development through handwriting in schools and corporate offices. She has also worked in the HR departments of several offices abroad, focusing on recruitment processes. Her knowledge in Vaastu, combined with her skills in numerology and graphology, allows her to assist individuals in overcoming a range of challenges, including delays in marriage, relationship issues, court cases, and financial difficulties.

For corporate clients, Nidhi acts as a solution provider, helping organizations recruit the right personnel through her expertise in numerology and graphology. She also works to balance the energies within corporate premises, contributing to a harmonious work environment. Nidhi offers consultations both online and offline, having successfully completed over 5,000 cases that include homes, factories, and commercial establishments.

Keywords : Emotion, Relationship, Companionship, Partnership, Support

Marriage means a lot to most people, making it a significant moment in life. But people often ask, "Does my marriage help or hurt me?" Now's the time to value how special this bond is. Sure, every marriage faces issues and challenging times, but many are peaceful, caring relationships that help both partners grow and feel happy.

Emotional Support and Companionship:

A happy marriage offers one of the most essential and lovely aspects: emotional support and companionship. Life can be tricky, so it's great to have a partner who stands by you through everything, helps you face challenges, and celebrates your successes. It's like having your cheerleader who experiences life's highs and lows alongside you.

In a happy marriage, partners listen to each other and heal each other's hearts. They feel at ease sharing everything from every day wins to deep concerns because their bond and shared feelings encourage this openness. This connection brings comfort, knowing someone always cares about your well-being and feels connected to you.

Growth Through Partnership:

Marriage helps people grow and impacts couples' development when they start living together. Once two people tie the knot, they begin to explore themselves, learn, and get better as a team. This sacred bond allows individuals to become contributors to society or reach their goals while also giving their partner the chance to chase their dreams.

A joyful family needs to respect each person's uniqueness, as this quality grows within the family unit. Partners push each other to keep pursuing their hobbies and personal growth. This support gives power and purpose making life's journey exciting. Nothing beats seeing your partner flourish when you know you've played a part in their success.

Establishing Confidence:

The foundation of every marriage is the trust between the spouses. In a happy relationship, you don't just stay faithful; you also know your partner will back you up no matter what. It's the certainty that both of you put equal effort into making each other happy.

Trust doesn't appear overnight, but it's key to a successful, lasting marriage. The idea is simple: when trust exists, you can turn to your partner, which helps ease stress and worry and allows your relationship to grow. This trusting environment leads to open communication, where each partner can share their concerns, desires, and appreciation.

Shared Joys and Memories:

Marriage holds a lifetime of shared experiences locked away in a treasure chest. Every relationship tells its own story brimming with amazing moments - joyful, hilarious, and affectionate by turns. It might be a cherished memory of the first date, a special anniversary celebration, or even the everyday moments spent together. All these add the perfect touch to a strong marriage, like frosting on a cake.

This is how feelings grow stronger - by remembering shared experiences together. These memories become part of their shared story, along with new events they experience as a couple. This happiness isn't fleeting; it forms the foundation of their bond and helps make it last.

At the heart of a happy marriage is love without conditions and total acceptance. As time passes, each partner gets to know the other's good points, flaws, odd habits, and shortcomings. Yet they still love each other, not in spite of these things but often because of them.

This kind of love doesn't rely on passing feelings. Instead, it grows from mutual respect, trust, and a real appreciation for who the other person is. In this way, marriage turns into a safe place where both people can be themselves without worrying about being judged. This acceptance creates a deep sense of emotional safety making the relationship feel truly happy.

Shared Responsibilities and Achievements:

Life can often seem too much with all its demands, from handling jobs to house chores and raising kids. But in a happy marriage, these loads are shared making them easier to carry. When both partners do their fair share in the relationship, the work becomes doable, and the feeling of being a team gets stronger.

Sharing responsibilities goes beyond household tasks. It includes emotional, financial, and intellectual aspects of the relationship. Both partners feel valued, respected, and understood. As a team, they face challenges, which makes their joint victories even more rewarding.

When you think about your marriage, focus on the love, support and happiness it provides. A happy marriage has its ups and downs, but it grows stronger through emotional bonds shared experiences, and mutual respect that partners build over time. Trust, unconditional love, and shared duties turn marriage into a beautiful journey—a source of joy, personal growth, and understanding.

|| ॐ ||

Learn from Mistakes

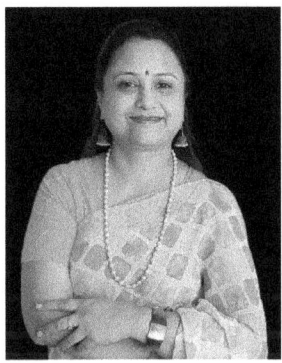

Author's Name	:	Nimishaa Mathur
Qualification	:	M.Sc. (Chemistry), B.Ed.
Current Profession	:	CXO @ Home
Age	:	42 years
E-mail ID	:	…
City/ Country	:	**New Delhi, India**

Ms. Nimisha Mathur is working as a full-time *Home Manager*. She is passionate for wandering, cooking, gardening and rhythmically tapping the floor. She is enthusiastic about social service and counselling. She is an empathetic listener and vocal on social issues. She is qualified as a Trained Teacher (B.Ed.) and M.Sc. in Chemistry with a long teaching experience.

Keywords : Believe, Communication, Interaction, Mistake, Responsible

Hey Reader! till now you have read experiences on marriage of my co-authors, I would like to say this anthology is kind of manual which will give you power packed sailing experience of high and low tides of marriage voyage.

Stand for yourself: Now I would like to share the essence of my marriage journey. Mine is a love marriage. So, it is quite obvious we both had to impress each other's family. When I disclosed this in my family there was literally a filmy scene and my parents tried hard to roll back my decision. But my mother was very firm, and her words really stuck with me. She said, "Alright, if you choose to marry him, don't come back to us for any kind of support.". At the time, it felt frightening and isolating, which made me become overly accommodating and submissive. My young mind was deeply affected, leading me to believe that once I left home, I had to adapt to my new family no matter what, or else I'd have no other place to go.

Now that I'm more mature, I realize that she was just trying to make me reconsider my decision out of her deep care and concern. Being the youngest, I was incredibly sheltered in my family. My husband also had a tough time getting everyone on board with our decision, especially since his mother wasn't at all ready to accept me. I tried all compromises by pushing my self-esteem to meet everyone's expectations. Most often I underrated myself and kept silent where I should have to take a stand. This empowered everyone to dominate and suppress my emotions. In fact, I was over committing, even changed my childhood habits, my tastes, and choices. This state was difficult to keep in the long run. And when it became intolerable and I was in phase of depression, I stood up for my rights. I decided to object the unfair treatment, I was immediately labelled as a rebel and uncompromising. My denial started bitterness in relationship with my hubby and in-laws, we had fights, disagreements with reluctant communication. The emotions which I suppressed for years erupted like tornado, caused me rude and loud.

This would not have been the situation if I had asserted myself from the beginning- gently, but firmly. The learning is never over power any relation.

Be Communicative: Another mistake in my marital journey was indirect communication. My husband was the go-between for me and my in-laws. Though, reason and intention were good, to avoid any chaos in family. The major loss due to this, I missed building strong relationship with my in-laws, based on personal rapport. Both the parties live departed and sharing complaints/opinions with the mediator and never came across to discuss and sort out with mutual agreement. So, be communicative and interactive with each one in the family.

I strongly believe, it is the moral responsibility of each one in partner's family to give the most adaptable environment and time to girl who came from different family, culture and social ground. At the same time the girl should also put forward her best efforts to understand the culture of the family, make bonding with each member in the family. Addition of a new member in the family brings lots of changes in routine life, old practices and existing cultural & social aspects, hence it is mandatory that both should give time to each other to adapt the changes.

My Bliss: Despite lots of odds, the prettiest and amazing bliss was that me and my hubby were truly willing to be together. We had a strong commitment of moving ahead together in our journey. With the time, we matured our relationship along with family progress and fought with all odds keeping dignity, respect and responsibility of a socially respected family.

The worse part of mismanaged marriages is dreadful impact on kids, they start hating marriage institution. And that I observed in my kids also, which changed our life and entire thought process. We realised this and started communicating with each other. It took time to make our kids realize that it was momentary and conditional.

It is a social responsibility of every individual to take forth the generation ahead legally and also to run the marriage institution in such a way that our coming generation feels excited about marriage. I trust, this anthology will serve the purpose of support and motivate to coming generations so that they believe in marriage, understand the sweet and bitter experiences of married life and learn to manage challenges with patience and intelligence.

Marriage is not always a bed of roses, but the roses with thorns. My tip for the Gen z is love and arguments are the two sides of a marriage coin. As intellectual individuals we have different mindset, opinion and different reactions to different situations. We should learn to understand, respect and deal with this opinion difference.

Time never remains the same, sometimes under certain unavoidable circumstances our feelings and emotions change for our partner, still try to keep some positivity by looking back to the happy moments of togetherness, turn the pages of photo album, remember the moments of intense love, situation where you were feeling sad and lonely and your partner hold your hand and said "don't worry everything will be fine, "main hoon na". These little things are very impactful and will always keep the spark of love and bond alive in your marriage.

I believe my journey and experience on marriage is helpful as you embark on your beautiful journey of togetherness to make lots of memories to cherish. My tips will bring you out of the foggy phase into the vibrant rainbow colours of marriage.

"Patience and willingness to be together is must for successful and everlasting marriage."

Dedicated to my love, my life partner

॥ ॐ ॥

A Journey of Support and Stability

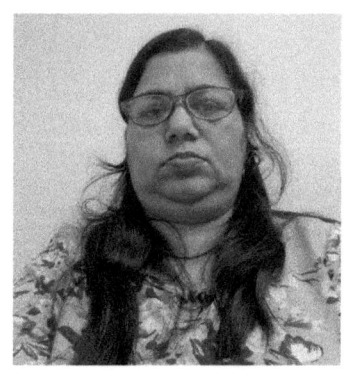

Author's Name	:	Nitender Mann
Qualification	:	B. Ed,, M.A.
Current Profession	:	Consultant and Counselor
Age	:	46 years
E-mail ID	:	**nitendermann@gmail.com**
City/ Country	:	**Toronto, Canada**

Nitender Mann is a budding Author and Certified Astro-Numerologist and Tarot Card Reader. She has done his Bachelor of Education in English and Economics. She has also done her Master Degree in Economics. She had worked more than 15 years as a teacher in reputed school in Punjab, India as well as in Canada. Now she is working in an accounting and insurance office as well as practicing in Occult Sciences.

Keywords : Marriage, Teamwork, Commitment, Couple, Support

Marriage is mostly a personal journey that people experience in different ways. It may differ greatly from person to person with respect to individual experiences, beliefs and value systems. It is imagined to be a lifelong undertaking of teamwork, shared goals, and mutual support. Marriage is about more than just sharing a home; it's about building a life together. It's making countless unforgettable moments, It's the everyday joy of growing alongside someone who is there for you through all ups and downs of the life. Marriage is not between two people, but between two families—their traditions and values,

Others view it is as a curse, especially when it brings more pain than joy. If they or those experiencing constant conflict, emotional strain, or a loss of personal freedom, then the marriage can seem like a heavy burden. In such situations, it might feel as if the relationship is more about enduring hardship than enjoying partnership.

Marriage is a blessing in terms of companionship, emotional support, stability and the chance to continue their life with someone they love. It is shared responsibilities between two is bond between two peoples as well as between families. As I said it depends on our personal experiences. If you got married and having a loving bond then the marriage is a blessing but if your experience is not good then it would be curse. And those who never get married they are not able to find it whether is a blessing or curse.

Everybody has different opinions but if I say what is my opinion then I would say it was a blessing given to me by God. Every marriage has ups and down but would never be a curse for anyone rather it teaches you to have patience, compromise, forgiveness, adaptability, selflessness, love and commitment.

Since I married to my husband my whole life had changed. He supported me in every part of life. After marriage, for every Indian girl it was hard to complete his further studies, but he supported me for further studies, Not only financially he also supported me physically. After my son birth I keep on studying and doing job. In this my in-laws also supported me. And when we moved to Canada from India he did not let me do the job as my son was quite small. He said I will earn and you take care of our son. I always felt like I a queen to the king, who always took care of my each requirement. In return I also always supported me in every part of the life. But every good story also had a bad part or phase of life. My bad part started very slowly, which I did not realized for making me queen he kept on ignoring his health issues and a time comes when we have come back to India for his treatments and after moving to India slowly his kidney stopped working and there comes COVID also which worsen our beautiful or blessed family. He went on dialysis and life become very hard, but we still both were together fighting between life and death. But could not fought more and he died in 2021. Now he is no more living but what he had given me are very good and nice memories or our marriage. After his death I moved with my son from India to Canada and achieved a lot but still felt that if he would see me as an independent woman, who takes care for everything he would be very much proud.

At the end, we can say that whether marriage will be a blessing or a curse would depend on the quality of the relationship, the level of commitment and communication attained by the two partners in the marriage. Every marriage is unique and lessons we learn also varies from individual to individual. And a successful marriage requires effort, love, commitments from both partners.

Ultimately, how marriage may be viewed as a blessing or curse depends on the particular circumstances and experiences of each couple.

|| ॐ ||

A Self Registered Bond of Trust

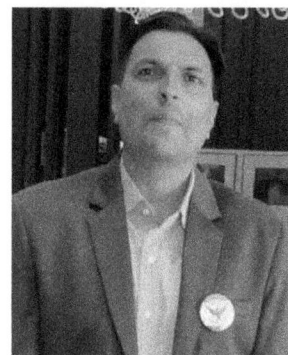

Author's Name	:	Om Prakash Priyadarshi
Qualification	:	M.A, LLB, PGDBM, PGDLL
Current Profession	:	Realtor, Film maker, Human Behavior : Expert, Inner Health Physician in handwriting, Professional Grapho Therapist Analyst & Coach
Age	:	38 years
E-mail ID	:	**Omprakashpriyadarshi612@gmail.com**
City/ Country	:	**Noida, India**

Om Prakash Priyadarshi is Real Estate Business Owner and also associated with an internationally renowned real estate company Exp Realty. He is Certified professional Handwriting Analyst, Inner Physician health in Handwriting & Professional Grapho-therapist Analyst from international council of Graphologist. He is also Certified in Occult Mastery program. He has done LLB, Master Degrees in politics, Post graduate diploma in business management in Human resources management and post graduate diploma in Labor Laws. He had worked more than 15 years in Central government in different locations of India.

He is also aspiring Film maker, Actor and Director working on different Assignments. As realtor and digital expert helping Businesses in team building and digital automation.

Om Prakash Priyadarshi is also Human behavior expert. He strongly believes that the parents and the teachers can become "Changemaker" of our current education system to make India proud to become land of education, along with he helps students of age group 11 years and above to solving their academic issues, emotional issues, financial challenges & different other challenges of study.

Keywords : Decision, Comfortable, Journey, Freedom, Human Behavior

Marriage is often seen as a blessing or a burden, but for me, it has been the biggest blessing of my life. When I look back, I realize that my wife has played a key role in every important decision I've made. She encouraged me to take bold steps, including leaving a secure government job to follow my dreams. With her support, I moved into the real estate business, something I had always wanted to do, but might never have had the courage to pursue on my own. Because of her, I was able to turn my passions into a reality and live a life full of purpose. My marriage has been a journey of growth, love, and shared success.

Leaving the Safety Net: A Life-Changing Decision :

My career started in the central government, a job that many would consider the perfect opportunity for a secure, comfortable life. The salary was stable, the work was predictable and there was a clear path to retirement. But deep down, I felt unfulfilled. I had a dream to start my own real estate business and a passion for teaching and personal development. The idea of leaving such a secure job was terrifying and I didn't know if I could actually go through with it.

This is where my wife stepped in. While others were hesitant about my decision, she was the one who believed in me completely. She saw my potential and encouraged me to take the leap of faith. Together, we decided to take the risk, and I left my job to pursue my dream of working in real estate. The road wasn't always easy, but her unwavering support kept me going through the tough times.

Now, I run a successful real estate business, helping buyers and sellers find their dream homes. I also help businesses streamline their businesses through team building & digital automation. Other side helping students of 11 years and above age group of different schools and colleges to solving their academic issues & different other challenges of study. He is helping them out in emotional challenges also. This wouldn't have been possible without my wife's belief in me. Her encouragement gave me the confidence to step out of my comfort zone and chase my goals.

Following My Passions :

Beyond real estate, I've always had a deep interest in human behavior, personal development, and teaching. I enjoy working with students and helping them develop the skills they need to succeed. Over time, I've also explored areas like Grapho-therapy, handwriting analysis, and the connection between handwriting and inner health. These passions have added even more meaning to my life.

Once again, my wife played a huge role in this journey. She never discouraged me from pursuing these interests, even when they were outside of my main career. In fact, she pushed me to explore everything I was passionate about, including my dream of becoming a filmmaker, actor, director. Her constant support has allowed me to balance multiple careers and interests without feeling overwhelmed.

Our marriage gave me the stability I needed to take on these challenges. I've been able to mentor others and help them grow, just as my wife helped me grow. Together, we've created a life that reflects both of our dreams and ambitions.

My Marriage is Bliss :

When I think about the idea of marriage being a "bliss or curse," I can confidently say mine has been pure bliss. A supportive and loving partner can make all the difference in life. My wife has always shared my vision and values, which has made our journey together easier and more enjoyable. We face challenges together and celebrate successes together. For me, marriage has been the foundation of all my achievements and I truly believe that without my wife's encouragement, I wouldn't be where I am today.

On the other hand, some marriages do become a curse when partners don't understand or support each other. But in my case, I've been lucky to have a marriage that has only lifted me higher. It's not just about love—it's about building a future together and supporting each other's dreams.

My marriage has been the greatest gift in my life. It gave me the courage to leave a secure job, start a successful real estate business, and pursue my passion for teaching and personal development. My wife's love, belief, and support have been at the heart of every success I've achieved. Our marriage is built on trust, shared goals, and a deep understanding of each other, and it has truly been the foundation for a life full of purpose and joy.

For me, marriage is not just a relationship—it's a partnership that has brought out the best in me and allowed me to live the life I've always dreamed of. Without a doubt, my marriage has been the ultimate blessing.

|| ॐ ||

Marriages are Made in Heaven

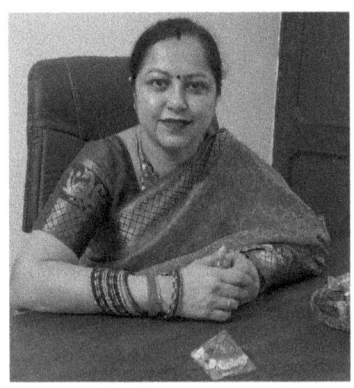

Author's Name	:	Pooja Gulati
Qualification	:	M.A., B.Ed.
Current Profession	:	Consultant, Numerologist, Vastu Expert, Crystal Healer, Switch Word Expert, Pendulum Dowser
Age	:	44 years
E-mail ID	:	**27poojagulati27@gmail.com**
City/ Country	:	**Meerut, India**

Pooja Gulati is a renowned and Certified Numerologist. She has done her B.Ed. and Master Degree in Arts and completed all her education from Pune University. She has worked as a teacher in a renowned school in Meerut for 10 years and is now working for the upliftment of people and helping them release their problems through numerology and other sciences of occult. She uses different techniques and remedies through switch words, crystals, healing numbers, pendulum dowsing, aromatherapy, color therapy, bachflowers to heal people.

Keywords : Adjustment, Challenges, Happiness, Social Arrangement, Trust

As with any relationship marriage can bring joy and challenges. Sharing a life with a partner can bring a sense of security, companionship and emotional support. The bond between two people can deepen over time and can lead to a life full of love. However on the flip side marriages can also bring challenges and difficulties. There can be frustration, unhappiness which changes joy into pain.

We all have heard the saying "Marriages are made in heaven" and we Indians believe that thoroughly. We believe that marriages are something divine and destined. It is a social arrangement for two persons to live together. Life after marriage can turn into heaven or hell depending on the understanding and attitude of the couples. Trust and love are the basics of married life and the main thing is adjustment. Men and women both have to do many adjustments in life. It is in our hands to make it a bliss or curse. My marriage, as I would say is a bliss for me. Mine was an arranged marriage and we never knew each other, but after marriage we came to know about each other's traditions, each other's way of living and many other things. There were adjustments made to cope up with each other which I think is necessary for a long lasting relationship. My husband has always supported me. He has always been like a pillar during my hardships. There are things which we do just for each other's happiness. There is no road map to make marriage successful. There had been many issues in life but we stood together. My husband says many times that he can't imagine his life without me, which I feel is a blessing for me to have such a loving and compassionate partner. I don't have any regrets in life. I have come so many miles and with his help I know I will surely reach to greater heights in life and I am thankful to God and blindly believe that marriages are made in heaven and everything is destined.

Marriage is a complex and multifaceted institution that can bring joy and challenges. By recognizing the dual nature of marriage we can approach with a realistic mindset by acknowledging that ups and downs are a part of long term partnership. Successful Marriages are built on a foundation of love, trust and mutual support where both partners actively work towards maintaining a harmonious and fulfilling relationship despite the challenges that may arise.

Balance of Personal Aspirations and Family Duties

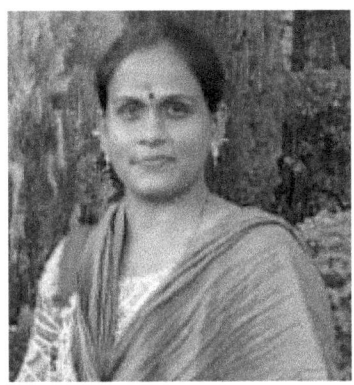

Author's Name	:	Pooja Saxena
Qualification	:	M.A.
Current Profession	:	Home Maker
Age	:	34 years
E-mail ID	:	…
City/ Country	:	**Bareilly (U.P), India**

Pooja Saxena is a dedicated individual lady, who has spent her total 10+ years of working along with shaping young minds as a teacher. After a successful career in education, she married into a joint family and she embraced the role of a homemaker, where her creativity and passion continue to thrive.

As a loving mother to a little angel, Pooja finds joy in nurturing her family, while exploring her talents in the kitchen as a passionate cook. In addition to her culinary skills, she has mastered the art of weaving and stitching, crafting various types of clothes with precision and care.

Pooja's journey reflects her commitment to both i.e. family and personal growth, blending her diverse skills with love, care and creativity.

Keywords : Commitment, Care, Creativity, Communication, Couple

My Marriage : Bliss Vs Curse is a personal reflection by Pooja Saxena, a former teacher, who has transitioned into the role of a daughter-in-law, homemaker in a joint family and a mother as well. In this article, Pooja delves into the dualities of marriage, exploring both the joys and challenges. She has encountered, as a passionate cook, mother to a little angel and a skilled seamstress, she finds fulfilment in caring for her family and creating a loving home. However, she also candidly addresses the sacrifices and identity shifts that come with leaving her career behind. Through her honest storytelling, Pooja questions whether marriage is a blissful partnership or a hidden burden or learning challenges, revealing the complexities of balancing personal aspirations with familial duties.

Before COVID-19 changed the world, Pooja Saxena was a teacher, enjoying the rhythm of her work and the satisfaction of shaping young minds, but when the pandemic struck, schools abruptly closed and Pooja found herself at home, her routine disrupted. As time passed, her mother grew anxious about her marriage prospects, fearing that uncertainty might delay this important milestone in Pooja's life. However, on November 30th, 2020, Pooja got married into a joint family of Parents with three brothers and one sister, stepping into a new chapter that was both exciting and challenging. She married with the second son of the family.

Life in her In-laws' home was a significant change. Adjusting to the dynamics of a large family wasn't always easy, but Pooja embraced the opportunity to learn and grow from these new experiences. Her husband's unwavering support became her strength, helping her navigate the complexities of her new roles. She wasn't just a daughter-in-law, but she also became a mother, when her little angel was born on January 31st, 2022, filling her life with immense joy and new responsibilities.

Over the past four years, Pooja has learned that marriage is a blend of highs and lows. While there are moments of bliss—such as the joy of raising her daughter and feeling the love and support from her husband as well as entire family. Balancing her identity as a former teacher, a homemaker and a mother often leaves her wondering where her individual aspirations fit in.

In Coming year 2025, her daughter will start going to school, a significant milestone that brings both pride and nostalgia. Drawing inspiration from her brother-in-law, Pooja has embarked on her journey with a sense of purpose, embracing each phase of life with resilience and hope. Though marriage has its complexities, for Pooja, it remains a journey worth taking—full of lessons, growth and love.

Marriage has been a journey of both bliss and challenges. On one hand, it has brought immense joy—a supportive husband, the love of a joint family and the blessing of a beautiful daughter. These moments of happiness make her feel fulfilled. Yet, the transition from a working woman to a homemaker, combined with the expectations of family life, sometimes feels overwhelming.

In conclusion, my marriage has been a mix of both bliss and struggle, but through it all, I've found my way. The joy of creating a family, the love from my husband, and the laughter of my daughter are the greatest blessings. Yet, the journey has come with its share of challenges—sacrifices, adjustments and moments of doubt. But marriage, I've learned, is not just about happiness; it's about growth, learning and resilience. As I continue this path, I embrace the blessings and face the challenges with strength, knowing that every experience shapes me into a stronger, more fulfilled person.

|| ॐ ||

Love, Laughter and a Merrily Ever After
And So, The Adventure Begins

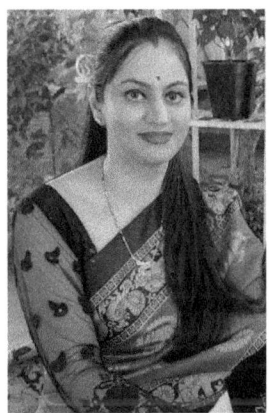

Author's Name	:	Pragya Sharma
Qualification	:	BJMC, MJMC, B.Ed., Certified Jolly Phonics Teacher
Current Profession	:	Homemaker
Age	:	32
Email id	:	sharma.pragya02@gmail.com
City/Country	:	Noida, India

Pragya Sharma has done her Master Degree in Mass Communication, Bachelor's Degree in Education and she is also a certified Jolly Phonics Teacher. She had worked with the entertainment section of one of the most renowned newspapers in India. She has also worked for more than 2 years as content writer for the magazine wherein she used to interview African Diplomats. Pragya had also worked as a primary teacher in the school.

Keywords : Adventure, Care, Cakewalk, Future, Responsibilities

I was a young girl from nuclear family living in Delhi and he was a boy living in joint family belonging from UP. It was a love at first sight for both of us. We both were 23 when we got married and far away from the reality as we never talked about our future. Every time, we used to meet, we would talk about honeymoon destination or the date night and the places we would like to visit together. It was an arranged marriage and we have been married for nine years now.

'9 years' seems good but let me acknowledge it was not a cakewalk. Few months, after marriage were smooth and everything was like a fairytale, but soon the reality hit me hard. It was getting really difficult to cop up with different mindset and there were so many responsibilities fell on my shoulder as daughter in law and as a wife which I think I have failed to some extent to fulfill and I have no shame in admitting this because every person learns from mistakes. Marriage is about learning from mistakes and to make sure you do not repeat those in future. Slowly and gradually, with the help of my new family members and little bit composure I got used to my new lifestyle and environment.

I would mention that my husband has also been my substantial supporter and has always helped me. I think a good marriage is something which allows evolvement in individuals.

Till date sometimes, I struggle to connect with my husband and at some level even not wanting to be near him when there is jolt of anger nonetheless there is nothing wrong in it considering I love him and he loves me. These are all emotions which you experience to evolve over a period of time. One thing I have learned through my journey is talk out, cry out and have heart to heart communication with your partner because parting and running away from problem is never a solution.

Taking 7 vows in the presence of your family members don't make your marriage last forever but what actually makes this institution last is when a couple stays whole heartedly dedicated to each other it.

Marriage is a blessing if both individuals love each other genuinely and are willing to never give up. Also, there should be a space, freedom and equality in marriage for it to work.

|| ॐ ||

A Union of Bliss and Challenges

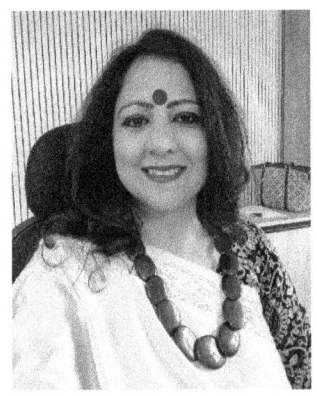

Author's Name	:	Priyaa Chauhan
Qualification	:	M.A. B.Ed.
Current Profession	:	Principal
Age	:	46 years
E-mail ID	:	…
City/ Country	:	**Gurgaon, India**

Mrs. Priyaa Chauhan, who is the Principal of G.D.Goenka Public School, is a distinguished figure in the field of education, boasting over two decades of experience. Her expertise stems from a robust academic background, holding postgraduate degrees in English & History, alongside a professional qualification in Education. Her illustrious career began at Amity International School, where she excelled as a teacher before ascending to various leadership positions in esteemed institutions across Gurgaon, including K.R.Mangalam, Lotus Valley, Shalom Hills, Laburnum School, The Pine Crest School and Mount Olympus School. Her dedication and talent have been evident throughout her journey, as she continuously strives to enhance the educational experience and nurture the minds of her students.

She has brought laurels to the schools she lead leading by winning various awards in the field of education, for an instance Award for best innovative school, Best Pre-school Award, Best school with happiness quotient and many more. Mrs Chauhan is leading the school with her vision, dedication, and passion for education. Her reputation for fostering a positive learning environment and commitment to academic excellence is truly inspiring.

Keywords : Decision, Harmony, Love, Marriage, Respect

Marriage is a word that rings bells in the ears of most of the girls and boys. Interestingly, I had always contemplated living with in-laws even before marriage and never gave a thought about the outline of the prospective husband…strange, isn't it?

Today, I have been married for 23 years. Initially there had been a struggle in adjusting with the new environment, full with people who had seemingly hijacked my life, making decisions about me without any consent. Though over the years I have come to understand that marriage is about compromises, adjustments, happiness, sorrow, boundaries, freedom, acceptance, and rejection. Since, we are social animals, it is imperative that we accept the fact of respecting each other and learn to cooperate.

Marriage has a beauty of its own if you have the patience to accept that the person standing opposite to you is just another human being like you, having an individual existence just like yours. When one begins to take the spouse for granted the same union can start seeming like a nightmare. Personally, it was a mixed bag of experiences at the beginning.

Being a young girl, it is difficult to manage all the emotions, especially when you have spent one part of your life with your parents who have a different set of aspirations, rules, bundle of emotions, different reactions to your problems, dreams or happiness. Another set of family suddenly intrudes in that comfortable zone and expects someone to immediately accept that change. I had had an arranged marriage. The girl who had never dated anyone and was even shy to talk to her husband got married. Later in life I started working and have no shame in saying that my husband has been a complete support to me, without whom I could have never got out of the house to work, which remains true even today.

An attribute that I lovingly and readily owe to my spouse is of patience. He is a soft hearted, pure person with no cunningness. He has loved me in all odds. We both have been patient with each other whenever the need arises. Though I have no animosity for love-marriage but as a person hold the view that such a vast institution of marriage should be taken with utmost care. While we are in love before marriage, we fail to acknowledge the faults of the partner even after dating for years. Marriage is not only the marriage of two human beings but of two families, their cultures, thoughts, expectations, experiences, and vices.

The perfect marriage- a word impossible to be seen or experience if not done with caution could easily destroy two families. Marriage as an institution is a sacred bond which should be carried on with proper understanding and respect. There might be difference of opinions, taste, likings but there should not be any place for disrespect. It is imperative that both souls be mindful of the dignity of each other.

In my own marriage, akin to others, there have been ebbs and flows, but we both have believed in it as an institution where we both are highly important for each other and the kids. Having both my sons is the greatest gift of God to me for which I cannot thank Him enough. We both have been instrumental in their brought up but what my husband has been doing for them should be big lesson for all fathers.

In my opinion all kinds of relationships involve disagreements and arguments. Marriage is no exception. So, for people who claim that marriage is of no use would find all people in their life repulsive. If someone is anxious about getting married, then I invite that person to think over the above lines.

|| ॐ ||

Every Heart Sings a Song

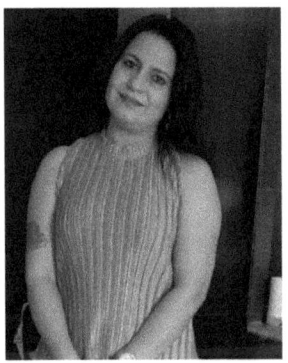

Author's Name	:	Priyanka Sapraa
Qualification	:	M.A. (Meditation & Yog) B.Ed., B.Lib., Diploma in Naturopathy
Current Profession	:	Occult Science Practitioner
Age	:	46 years
E-mail ID	:	**priyankaramansapra@yahoo.com**
City/ Country	:	**Gurugram, India**

Priyanka Sapra is working as a Vastu Consultant & Numerologist. She's started her journey into occult science 23 years back, when she's joined her Master in Meditation & Yog from Jain Vishwa Bhartiya University, Ladnun, Rajasthan and a diploma course in yoga from Vivekananda Yog Anusandhan Samsthan, Bangalore.

Later in life she's learned that Yog is not only a physical exercise, but it's a greatest path to move towards your inner journey.

Later she's learned about Vastu and got to know more how a place can make an impact of anyone's Life through land energy and the 45 devtas are present in under a roof.

Learning new skills like Reiki, Nakshatra Jyotish, Medical Numerology, Mobile Numerology are the helping tools of her to bring more peace & harmony in anyone's Life.

Keywords : Love, Dream, Humanity, Peace, Companionship

"A successful marriage requires falling in love many times, always with the same person." by Mignonette McLaughlin"

As I sat down to reflect and write about "My Marriage, Bliss Vs Curse", I had a train of thoughts about my own marriage and later of my nearer & dearer ones and their experiences. Most of these thoughts were hurtful stories that I can't forget till date. Finally, I decided to write about one of those stories, instead of my own beautiful journey of marriage. This story is about my childhood friend with whom I grew up. I still feel her pain and I am always there like a rock by her side. To maintain, confidentiality, I will refer her Megha.

The story dates to Megha's childhood which nurtured her belief system around marriage. Going down the memory lane, this day is when her dad brought home a color screen TV on which movies were shown every Saturday and Sunday. On one of those, Sundays, we watched the movie: "Satte Pe Satta," featuring Amitabh Bachchan, Hema Malini and Amitabh's six brothers. They lived together and had a deep love and respect for their sister-in-law. Watching it, she thought that one day her own home would be just as loving and filled with happiness. She dreamt of a husband who would love her like Amitabh and a family that would respect her. She could devote herself completely to such a family. Such are the dreams spun by the world of films.

Megha was enjoying a blessed life by the grace of God. This made her believe that she was always, destined to receive the best in all the spheres of life. Finally, her much awaited wedding day arrived. She married a handsome groom of her choice. She was still under the spell of the movie "Satte pe Satta" and was now looking for a similar environment. In her new avatar of the daughter-in-law, she found herself addressing her mother-in-law as "Mummy Ji," running around the chores following her mother-in-law's directions. Her parents had advised her, while leaving her home, to make her new house a paradise but missed guiding on the boundaries of giving respect and maintaining self-respect.

As the days passed, Megha's happiness bubble exploded. Her responsibilities kept increasing. Her special place vanished sooner than she expected. She felt as an ordinary outsider. Her job was only to care of them, regardless of their behaviour. Her husband's one-line statement summed it up: "You must take care of them whether they care for you or not."

Megha's husband's world revolved around his family and even their conversations were the same eg. "I fed mother on time and made sure she took her medicine. We also must arrange our younger brother's wedding. He was just waiting for our wedding to be over. It's been six months since you arrived. Now that you're pregnant, start looking for a match for him."

Despite request to delay the brother in law's ceremony, the engagement was fixed expecting Megha to take care of all the chain of events in her pregnancy. After the marriage her brother, so enamored with his wife would barely leave their room.

Both brothers had a joint business. While the elder brother managed everything, the younger brother had no obligations. All the responsibilities like looking after the parents, the younger brother, the business, the household and a new baby was on the elder brother and his wife, Megha. No one would even care about the baby. The new born baby would sleep in its cradle and Megha was expected to put him aside and continue working. The child started being cranky.

When she was taking care of the baby, her attention to the rest of the household chores got impacted. This did not go well with others. "Couldn't you have this baby six months after my wedding?" These words of her brother-in-law broke her heart. Even the mother-in-law heard this, but showed no reaction. No one took the responsibility to teach him manners. This behaviour was a common phenomenon.

That day she decided to rise and claim her life back. Her heart was broken. There was a mother, who did not in still values and in turn the younger son soon abandoned his mother. He took his share of the property and disconnected leaving all the responsibilities on the elder brother and Megha.

There were many questions in her mind. Is this what a family is? How do people live after abandoning their loved ones? How do they become so selfish, leaving their own behind?

My learning from marriage: "Every heart sings a song, incomplete, until another heart whispers back. Those who wish to sing always find a song. At the touch of a lover, everyone becomes a poet."
– Plato

॥ ॐ ॥

A Beautiful Married Life

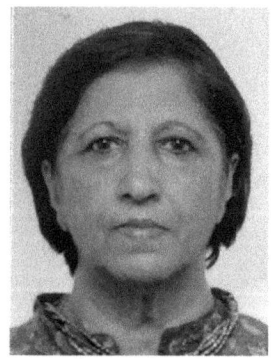

Author's Name	:	Prof. Sarojini Gupta Biddanda
Qualification	:	M.A. (English)
Current Profession	:	Retired Prof.
Age	:	71 Years
E-mail ID	:	**sarojgupta369@yahoo.com**
City/ Country	:	**Coorg, Karnataka, India**

Prof. Sarojini Biddanda (Retd.) is an educationist with a distinguished career as a Professor of English and Principal of Kavery College (Degree) affiliated to the University of Mangalore. Her creative endeavors include writing and directing plays, choreographing theme based dances and composing songs. Her published poems are about nature, joys and sorrows of life. As a member of Lions Club, she plays an active role in the environmental and rural development projects undertaken by the club. She is a globe trotter with a passion for learning foreign languages. As a member of the Karnataka Kodava Sahithya Academy, she was instrumental in organizing folk music and dances during her tenure. She is also involved with prestigious literary and cultural associations.

Keywords : Beautiful, Bliss, Life, Marriage, Vows

"Jivanam Sundaram Asti"

'*Life is beautiful*', This Sanskrit phrase encapsulates the inherent beauty of life. The divine presence within the hearts of all living beings guides the sacred journey of life. In this journey, we go through different phases… some dark and dreary, some bright and beautiful. There are roaring rapids and deceptive dips ere we reach green fields. When you share this journey with your spouse, who loves you unconditionally, life transforms into a vibrant, thrilling and deeply rewarding celebration.

Marriage has been a sacred institution from time immemorial. In our epics the marriages ordained by God, emphasize love, loyalty and spiritual connectedness. Marriage is a beautiful union of two hearts and souls provided it is founded on love, commitment, companionship, compatibility and respect. It can attain a transcendental aura.

Ability to adapt to changes plays an important role. Many moons ago, as a young bride, when I entered my new home, I had been assailed by the thought of navigating in uncharted waters. To my surprise, it wasn't a Herculean task. I was bubbling with youth and boundless energy. My positive mindset and the habit of applying myself to my tasks with éclat won my family's admiration. The freedom to pursue my career and passion was a boon.

One cannot enter into this phase thinking, married life is going to be a fairy tale or a summer romance. Changes come thick and fast. The transition can be peaceful provided the couples learn to look at things from a different perspective. Have a quiet moment of reflection to avoid gyrating in your own confusions. For a marriage to be successful, the couples require self-discipline and self-confidence. 'Yat bhavo tat bhavat' – You become what you believe. This belief will strengthen your emotional bonding with your spouse. This helps the couple cultivate a loving and thriving relationship, which goes on developing a vertical boost in the years to come.

Bertrand Russell, in one of his reflective essays, highlights the importance of an emotional balance and ability to handle life's twists and turns with resilience. A person who masters these qualities is always happy and makes for a happy marriage. Though marriage is a lifelong commitment, being imprisoned in a cocoon with too many taboos is suffocating. Impinging on each other's independence or personal space is not acceptable. But beware! Do not let the 'spacc' become a gaping hole, which can become a vast hiatus, never to be bridged. Whatever your preoccupations are, spending time together, dreaming together and contributing to each other's growth go a long way in cementing the married life.

On the other hand, if the couples are egotistical, it fosters traits such as arrogance and selfishness. It can undermine the marriage and turn life in to an inferno. Right kind of counseling and words of advice from senior members of the family, who give them living examples of love and harmony can help the couple save their marriage. Discussing a topic like "My Marriage : Bliss vs Curse" is a way of understanding the blessings and challenges of marriage. The ideas voiced by a galaxy of writers can provide inspiration to the couples to dispel their doubts and resolve their conflicts. It can gently prod them to get rid of excessive self-absorption and unrealistic expectations. It can remind the couples the significance of the marriage vows made by them.

In traditional church wedding ceremonies, the couples vow, "To love, to honor and to cherish till death do us part". How could they forget these words? The wedding ring symbolizes the eternal bond between the husband and wife. The "Vena amoris" or "Vein of love", is an ancient belief that a vein runs directly from the ring finger to the heart! Hindu wedding ceremony has a beautiful ritual celled, 'Sapthapadi' or Seven steps', the bride and the groom take seven steps together, each step symbolizing a vow they make to each other.

The sanctity of all these beautiful and meaningful rituals can never be ruined if the couples exile themselves from all negative thoughts and pessimistic views. Let them catapult themselves into a glorious stratosphere of joy and contentment. Let them humbly mumble these words from Rig-Veda - 'Let noble thoughts come to me from all directions'

'Aano bhadra krtavo yantu vishwatah'

|| ॐ ||

The Eternal Connection
A Soul Connection

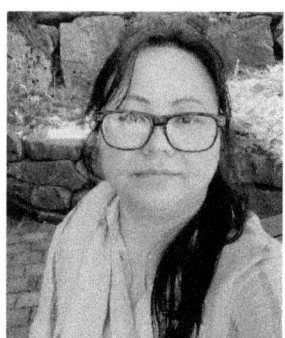

Author's Name	:	Promila Devi Sutharsan Huidrom
Qualification	:	Bachelor of Computer Science (B.C.S.), Diploma in Advanced Computing (C-DAC, Pune), MSc in Innovation and Entrepreneurship (Oslo, Norway)
Current Profession	:	Poet/ Author
Age	:	44 years
E-mail ID	:	**writerpromila@gmail.com**
City/ Country	:	**Jevnaker, Norway**

Promila Devi Sutharsan Huidrom/ Promila, being a modest Poetess, enjoys writing in Hindi and has been writing from a very young age. It has to be a path chosen formidably by her, quitting her Software and Business career. She has been residing in Norway for about 20 years now and settled and still write in Hindi and chose Hindi as the core language chosen for her writing, although her future books are coming in English and Norwegian too. She has won many Awards and accolades.

She is an active philanthropist and social reformer, who believe in giving the society back in the way, that which gave her an identity and life so beautiful.

Love life, live life and life is so beautiful.

Keywords : Boundary, Care, Compatibility, Eternal, Love

Marriage is said to be made in heaven. I believe it indeed is. Love is all for lovers, marriage is beyond that. A compassion, a care, a share, a team, a compromise, a compatibility- it's all about marriage.

When we grow, we become more rigid and it becomes difficult for us to adjust living with anyone or anybody. So, is to a man or a woman, who is married and decides to live together forever, must be something special and different. It indeed is a compromise in every step but compromise for good. Sometimes the wife does, and sometimes the husband. Adjustments is a crucial deal in a marriage.

How a ball and socket joint fixes a bone and together that arm works wonders, that is how a marriage is.

There are certain arguments and challenges sometimes in a marriage but the one who is more vulnerable should be given some space and vice versa. Life is a challenge so is marriage. If one decides to marry, then it must be a once in a lifetime project with lot of care and compatibilities.

Marriage fills the gap for one another. Husband in today's time contributes equally at home for chores which is a good thing. Definitely there are exceptional cases but since the wife works equally and contributes financially to the home, husband too must contribute in the chores of the home and take care of kid(s) equally.

Nowadays, women are equally the decision maker, so they should sit together and decide. The lady of the home has also have a word to say and it is happening in today's generation which is a good sign and the lady is independent with her thought and decisions.

Marriage is a mutual understanding with lots of mutual care and mutual support. It's a pure relationship. It's a soul connection as we know that husband and wife are not blood related, yet they create a blood relation, which is they kids and family and further on. So, it is special, we create a family tree. Two different souls from 2 different world create a family tree.

Marriage needs time and patience. There can be occasions where one is sulking and not talking then the other should give space and initiate the talk and further on, do efforts to keep it going. There come phases in time to time, one needs lot of patience and understanding to keep that relation going. It is really like planting a flower plant and nurturing it. It is like raising a baby, which needs love, care and efforts in every step of life. It is easy to break a marriage for one or another reason, but the real challenge is to keep going, unless there is a real serious reason to quit and move on.

Both husband and wife should have a boundary for some things like their computer, mobile and that space is personal, and nobody shares that with anybody. Trust should be there so much that it's not cheat. With right - comes the responsibility. So, it's very crucial that both have their space.

Marriage should not be done in the same gene pool, the farther the roots are the better the offspring(s). We all know that it's genetics and our offspring should be a better gene than us and not the other way. There is a right age to marry, one should follow that. Body doesn't wait for anybody.

We all know that marriage keeps the world going via the process of reproduction in a sacred space like marriage, unlike animals. Every age has a phase and like in "Sanatan" we say "Grihastha Ashram" that's the marriage life which is just for the couple and their kids, in-laws can stay nearby but not together. As they are always the key to disruptions in relationships, as too many balls rebound in a closed vessel.

Acceptance is very important in a relationship for one another.

Marriage is just once for me, and life moves on –

Live for today – Celebrate Everyday.

Together we stand – Together we raise.

|| ॐ ||

A Bond of Love

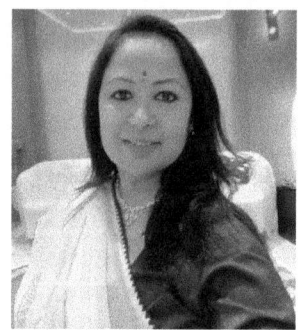

Author's Name	:	Punam Vishwkarma
Qualification	:	B.Sc., B.Ed., M.B.A. (HR)
Current Profession	:	Administration Head in School
Age	:	41 Years
E-mail ID	:	**punamvishwkarma055@gmail.com**
City/ Country	:	**Nagpur, India**

Punam Vishwkarma lives in tiger capital of India, Nagpur. She is a proud mother of two kids and wife of a handsome man. She is an Educationist, Guide and a Friend, these are her life blessings. She is a Tarot Card Reader and Numerologist. She helps people to decode the secrets of a successful life with numerology. She is a member of GLOAN, Global Alliance of Numerologists, which is a platform for Numerologist and Numerology seekers, all over the world to share quality information and conduct research in the field of Numerology.

Keywords : Marriage, Communication, Respect, Couple, Commitment

Marriage is a special bond between two people, who love each other and commit to share their lives together. It's a partnership built on love, respect and mutual support.

For me marriage is bliss, it's like having a teammate for life, someone who supports you through thick and thin. Plus there's all that love and companionship that comes with it!

My marriage is like blessings from heaven, a divine gift of love, joy and fulfillment in my life. Cherishing the blessings in our married is so important. It's about appreciating the love, happiness and all the wonderful moments we share with our partner. Take a time to be grateful for each other, for the journey you're on together and for the joy that marriage brings into your life. Embrace those blessings and hold them close to your heart.

There are ups and down in every marriage and relationships. It can be a roller coaster for many. It's all about navigating through those twists and turn together. In marriage, some common challenges can include communication issues, financial disagreements, and differences in values or priorities, lack of conflicts effectively. It's important to address these challenges together as a team.

In marriage, disagreements and conflicts are inevitable. It's normal for couples to have fights or arguments from time to time. However, it's essential to handle these conflicts constructively and with respect. Effective communication, active listening and willingness to compromise are key to resolving conflicts in a healthy way. Remember, conflicts can be opportunities for growth and understanding in a relationship. It's important to address issues openly, honestly and calmly to find solutions and strengthen the bond between partners.

According to me family plays a significant role in marriage. Family members can offer support, guidance and advice to the couple. They can help create a strong support system for the married couple, especially during challenging times. It's essential for family members to respect the privacy and decisions of the married couple while being there for them when needed. Communication and understanding between family members and the couple are the key to maintain a healthy and harmonious relationship within the family.

Additionally, family members can help create a positive environment for the couple by fostering open communication, respect, acceptance in the family. By being there for the couple during both good and challenging times, family members can play a crucial role in strengthening the marriage and promoting a sense of unity and togetherness.

Growing with your partner in married life is such a rewarding and fulfilling experience. It's about supporting each other, facing challenges together, and evolving as individuals and as a couple. As you navigate life's ups and downs side by side, you have the opportunity to learn, adapt and strengthen your bond. Embracing growth together can deepen your connection and create a strong foundation for a lasting and meaningful relationship.

I believe the key to a happy marriage is an open communication, trust and mutual respect, when both partners feel heard, understood and supported, it can create a strong foundation for a happy and fulfilling relationship. A happy marriage is like a never-ending conversation filled with love, understanding and support, keeping the conversation flowing in a relationship involves active listening, asking open ended questions, sharing experiences and thoughts and showing genuine interest in your partner's life. It's also important to be attentive, empathetic and supportive in your interaction.

A healthy marriage is indeed one that embraces change and supports growth. It's essential for both the partners to evolve individually and as a couple over time. Communication, understanding and mutual respect play crucial roles in fostering a relationship that allows for personal development and shared growth. Being open to change and willing to adapt together can strengthen the bond between partners and create a lasting, fulfilling marriage. It's all about growing together while respecting each other's individual journeys.

It is important to tell your spouse that you are thankful for having them in your life. Expressing gratitude and appreciation to your spouse make the bonding strong. Letting them know how thankful you are to have them in your life can make them feel loved and valued. It's always nice to take a moment to acknowledge and cherish the special bond you share with your partner. So go ahead and tell them how grateful you are for their presence in your life. It can truly brighten their day and strengthen your connection as a couple.

Showing gratitude in a relationship can be done in many simple yet meaningful ways. You can:-

1. Say "thank you" often for the little things your partner does.
2. Write a heartfelt note or letter expressing your appreciation.
3. Surprise them with a small gift or gesture to show you care.
4. Compliment them sincerely and acknowledge their efforts.
5. Spend quality time together and create happy memories.
6. Listen actively and be supportive when they need it.
7. Show physical affection through hugs, kisses or holding hands.
8. Share your feelings openly and honestly with each other.

These small acts of gratitude can go a long way in strengthening your relationship and creating a positive, loving atmosphere between you and your partner.

May the journey of marriage be filled with joy, growth and harmony, making each day a celebration of your bond and shared commitment, wishing all the lovely readers a lifetime of happiness and blessings in your married life.

|| ॐ ||

Composed of a Single Soul Inhabiting Two Bodies

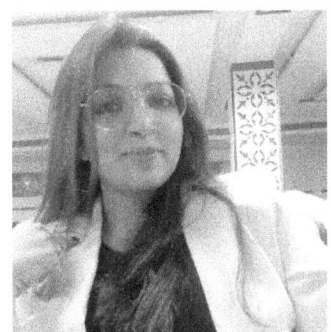

Author's Name	:	Radhika Devgan
Qualification	:	B.Sc. in Medical, M.C.A.
Current Profession	:	Immigration Consultant PTE, IELTS and OET Trainer, Las of Attraction Coach & NLP Trainer
Age	:	37 years
E-mail ID	:	**86radhika@gmail.com**
City/ Country	:	**Punjab, India**

Radhika Devgan is a well-established business woman. She started her career as a global language trainer in 2016 and continues in this role. Apart from her academic qualification in MCA, she pursued her interest in spiritualism and completed a Reiki Master Course in 2020-21. She is also a member of FICCIFLO Amritsar. Recently, she completed a basic level hypnotherapy course. As a science student, she had a great interest in science, particularly biological and chemical reactions in the body. Because of this, she is studying NLP and providing training to international students. Her aim is to educate everyone on how they can heal their own bodies and manifest all their dreams.

Keywords : Patience, Nurture, Relation, Partnership, Soul

Successful marriage is just like a tree, to enjoy the fruit of married life, there is need to nurture this relation with plenty of patience and faith for its actual growth. It's possible, only when both partners will spend time with each other and scrutinize the each other's perspectives. As the time move ahead, they can experience a true Love or affection and they feel there is a incompletion of something when one of them is absence. To reach this pinnacle, there is no need to hold this beautiful relation very tightly, no one is here perfect, just release it and accept from heart, and in this moment they can experience a majestic life.

Marriage is not a meeting of two person together, its meeting of two soul together, that may be separate from each other's may be hundreds of years before, the meeting of two souls come is not happened by a chance that is preplanned by the supreme power. We can say it's a greatest blessing that is just created by the God for creating the path of our life very simple to fulfill our dreams.

Unfortunately, today's generation don't know the value of this knot, because they highly impacted by the foreign culture, where there is no definition of soul mate, they don't give it a value more than a cloth, that they can change any time, when get fad up, as per mine perspective they are right somewhere, because nowadays to fall in love is very easy because of this digital era, previously it was very hard to talk with a person with whom they had a crush. It's a universal truth, thing that is available in the huge quantity, its value drops automatically.

As per my personal experience, all fingers are not same in size always, everyone must have to loyal because husband wife is the only relation that survives till the last breath, to nurture this relation there is need to put extra efforts from both sides.

I personally implement one simple rule that really works for me even that is FRFL=Love. There is a need of four ingredients to build a strong foundation of any relation. F stands for Friend, R stands for Respect, F for Faith and last L is Loyalty. All these work like a strong pillar of building/ relationship, without that enjoying successful married life is hard to imagine for everyone. If husband and wife will share their responsibility or respect each other's likes and dislikes, then rest two faiths as well as loyalty will give strength to others two. Now it should be our moral responsibility to take care of these pillars of life, wherever their eyes will turn they will experience the heaven.

The Joy of Wedded Life

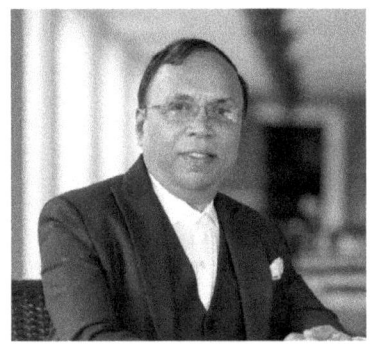

Author's Name	:	Raghunandan Chowdarapu (Raghu NC)
Qualification	:	B.A. – Triple Maths
Current Profession	:	Chairman of Magnifiq Group Companies
Age	:	63 Years
E-mail ID	:	**ncraghu@gmail.com**
City/ Country	:	**Hyderabad, India**

Raghunandan Chowdarapu, with over four decades of experience in building businesses and fostering financial independence among entrepreneurs, has established himself as a seasoned expert in the industry.

He holds multiple Master degrees in Mathematics and has undertaken numerous personal development courses, continually evolving his skills and knowledge.

As the founder of **Magnifiq Group Companies**, Raghunandan leads a conglomerate of successful enterprises. His unique expertise as a Master Practitioner in Graphology, combined with his profound knowledge in Astrology and Numerology, has empowered countless businesses to achieve remarkable growth. Raghunandan's holistic approach, blending scientific analysis and metaphysical insights, offers innovative strategies for personal and professional success. His dedication to financial awareness and entrepreneurial empowerment underscores his commitment to driving positive change in the business world.

Keywords : Emotional Well-being, Communication Skills, Conflict Management, Personal Growth, Loving Always

Now I am 63 years old. I still remember, the year was 1979, a time of youthful exuberance and boundless dreams. On a fateful day in June, I got married to Padmaja – a union that shaped our future in ways unimaginable. I was staying in Hyderabad studying engineering and my wife was studying 8th Class.

I was 18 years old, my wife Padmaja 16 years old. We were dependent on our parents. I was fearful to my father, whatever he says I used to follow and oblige. Though I was not keen on my marriage at that age, but had to follow, because of fear and no escape.

I was so shameful in inviting my friends but invited two of my high school friends they were close to me and they attended also. Got married and I returned to Hyderabad for to pursue my engineering and she has gone to her parents place Metpally to pursue her studies.

My wife cleared 10th Class. I got the job in 1982 and started living from September 1982 onwards in Hyderabad. Our village is 200 kms from Hyderabad. Balancing the demands of academics and married life was no small feat, yet together, me and Padmaja forged ahead with determination and resilience.

My wife Padmaja just 19 years and I am 21 years. She speaks only Telugu language. I have two friends they are Kameshwar Rao and Parthasarathi. I used to go to work in the afternoon and used to drop my wife Padmaja at Parthasarathi residence and his mother Sridevi garu like my mother also used to take care my wife and taught her everything about life and shaped up my wife. Today my wife speaks good English and Hindi also. We both delved into the realms of knowledge, eager to carve out a future that was bright and promising.

We are blessed with two sons in 1986 and 1991. My wife is my life and she learnt lots of things from Sridevi garu and she manages whole family now. I started my business in 1985 and grown successfully. I had some challenges in my business from 1999 to 2002 but bounced back and doing very well now. My sons are fond of each other and very closely connected. By looking at their closeness I thought of getting them married to two sisters and used to say in the family, when they were just 10 years old. We performed our sons' marriages and the daughters-in-law are two sisters. It happened the way I thought. We all are staying together now I have two lovely grand-daughters. My sons and I do business together having 100plus employees running few companies successfully.

I realize that my marriage has been a journey of self-discovery, growth and forever love.

Ultimately, marriage is a testament to the enduring power of love. It teaches us about patience, forgiveness and the beauty of staying together. It is a beacon of hope, guiding us through the years with the commitment of a life enriched by the presence of our beloved partner. In its truest form, marriage is a lifelong adventure, filled with excellent opportunities for connection, happiness and profound fulfilment.

I am grateful to my friends Kameshwar Rao, Parthasarathi and particularly Sridevi garu used to call her Amma. She crafted my wife. Expressing loads of gratitude to Sridevi garu and her family.

Gratitude to my friends Kameshwar Rao and Parthasarathi.

Gratitude to my Gurus

Gratitude to Divyaa, she is the instrumental in writing this information.

Finally, I am grateful to my parents, my In-laws and My wife Padmaja,

My sons Rahul & Ratul and my daughters Sathyavathi & Sravani

My grand-children Esha and Devalekha

|| ॐ ||

Marriage is a Toss

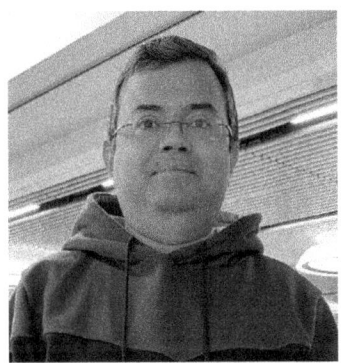

Author's Name	:	Rahul Churi
Qualification	:	B.Sc.
Current Profession	:	Assistant Professor in English
Age	:	50 years
E-mail ID	:	**aashwa@yahoo.com**
City/ Country	:	**London, UK**

Rahul Churi is an IT Consultant for 25+ years, belongs to Indian family. He loves to write and healthy discussion on the topic of relationship and society.

Keywords : Friendship, Involvement, Prarabhdha, Karma, Couple

To say in a book anything about relationships in a few pages will be an audacity where centuries of poets from Kalidasa to modern lyricists have all but only managed to open the topic of relation can be. There is a nice line in a movie "Umrao Jaan", "Doston ko nahi Dosti kaa naaZ", it roughly translates that friends don't value the friendship but when you have no friends you realise the longing.

'Marriage is a friendship and what works and what does not, is something even a toss cannot predict.'

I see marriage from a different perspective. It becomes holy when you have children at stake and it becomes an institution when you are grandparents. Then the "prarabdhas" come to dance and the "Karma" fights back and then rest is history as it says.

One fact I remember is and it has even mention in our culture about "Shringar Ras" but beautifully put my Hollywood. "Couples that sleep together, stay together". And funnily enough the reason for marriage failures is lack of physical intimacy.

Guys and Gals might be all excited about relationship but in the end its eventual giving up from both sides that lead to what we now know as "Modern Marriage"

Stress of all sorts and too much involvement of the so-called Friends plays its own role in this. Man is a social animal and yet he moves to place of nuclear family and then tries to find long lasting friendships in unknown people, if ridiculous only had a scale.

"Taali ek haath se nahi bajti" and it means you cannot clap with a single hand. A successful marriage is a work of two souls who work in tandem. And souls come with baggage of prarabdhas and they cannot escape and there is nothing one can do when the path is set with these two souls, but in my opinion it's a mother which runs the house, where a woman is not able to become a mother emotionally the marriage is out for a break.

This is a story of my friend, who was 180 degrees opposite of me and was proud of his wife, they had a nice family with their son, but as fate would be his wife passed away suddenly due to Pancreatic Cancer. This is his story. My marriage was fantastic and as our patrika/ chart joined for 21 points it remained and then my wife left us forever. But she hasn't left my heart, even when I moved to different place and I still remember where to keep things, she had great art in arranging the kitchen as my job meant we kept on changing houses. My job was only to find the house and get the TV working rest of the things happened automatically, it never occurred to me the kind of work she put in.

My memory of my wife is her presence in the house. When she was there my son was quietly doing his work. She taught our son to talk and took his studies. She was just the most perfect woman one could get. But I had my anger issues and the stress of money meant that we started parting away from each other. Our relationship just meant that I was always demanding things from her. I became the child in the marriage whose only objective was to work and get food on table. I still miss all my wife cooking of Chinese food and her curries were simply fantastic.

But in all these days I never said I love you but I truly loved her very much. As our marriage went into monotonous form, I realised that neighbours stared entering in our life more and more and to an extent realised that my wife was more comfortable in talking with my neighbours than me.

It was during this period I learnt that my wife had fallen in love with my neighbour's husband. My neighbours was very odd, for her money was everything and she was not interested in her husband and she was ok for her husband to have affairs and in that she had beautifully trapped my wife initially, later on decisions taken by my wife were her own and I could imagine that she was enjoying the attention she got from our neighbours husband.

I was totally not aware of these happening behind me but only noticed that distance my wife maintained with me. She stopped talking completely with me and there was a marked change in her mood when she met the neighbours. Them 3 were a couple and I was third man out.

My other friends kept on warning me about this, and I kept on ignoring saying that all is fine and that my wife is of very high character.

I realised something was missing when she started ignoring my son and taking care of neighbours' children more, her whole dynamics changed dramatically over the period of time and I kept on reacting as my anger knew no bounds, our communication dropped to only extreme frustrations with no talks.

And then the news came of her cancer and the neighbours stopped coming and my wife kept on crying, and I was thinking she was crying because of her cancer but then she told me the story of her life. It left me totally shocked, and I refused to believe that what she was telling was truth as I thought she had lost her mind or her Chemo was doing wrong things. There are drugs which make the patients very happy and that could be the reaction of that but I was wrong.

I never confronted our neighbours as my wife's health deteriorated and we had to move her to an hospice where her last days she spent in sub-conscious state and when she passed away at night in sleep I was not there.

Her death brought too many emotions all contradicting, I don't know how to remember, miss her or forget her.

I did not perform her last rites and I managed to send her last remains to India to her family whilst I and my son remained here in UK.

|| ॐ ||

Marriage is a Boon

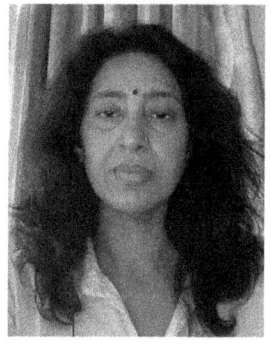

Author's Name	:	Reva Sarangal
Qualification	:	M.Sc. (Chemistry), M.Sc. (Ecology and Environment), B.Ed.
Current Profession	:	International Educator
Age	:	50 years
E-mail ID	:	**sarangalkakshi125@gmail.com**
City/ Country	:	**Mohali, India**

Reva Sarangal is an online International Educator with passion of teaching. Teaching gives her immense satisfaction. Even teaching for hours won't make her tired. She tries her best to motivate young minds to make their lives beautiful, happy and inspirational.

She believes –

IF YOUR PASSION BECOMES YOUR JOB THEN YOU ARE NEVER TIRED OF WORKING.

Reva believes that-make use of time as you cannot touch again the same water in the stream, so work hard to achieve your goals.

Keywords : Compromise, Memory, Soul, Relationship, Family

Life is too short; make it memorable, so that when looked back one should be contended and proud of it. Every individual has some role to play on this Earth and he does the same as destined by God. Once an individual leaves for ever, he/ she leaves a void, which never get filled. The lines of this song never appealed so much, but now every word means a lot and appears so true ;

Phool khilte hain, log miilte hain.

Phool khilte hain, log miilte hain,

Magar pattajhad men jo phool murajha jaate hain,

Vo bahaaron ke aane se khilte nahin…

Kuchh log ik roz jo bichhad jaate hain,

Vo hazaaron ke aane se milte nahin,

Umr bhar chaahe koi pukaara kare unakaa naam,

Vo phir nahin aate, vo phir nahin aate…

Marriage is a boon, if it is between two right individual at the right time otherwise it is just an adjustment.

RIGHT means two individual, who value the presence of each other and automatically it develops the feeling of LOVE and CARE.

Presence of any one of these qualities won't make marriage work. RUNNING marriage on any one feeling is a COMPROMISE. Marriage is a beautiful thing in a couple's life. It makes you live life more lively creating memories and cherishing them in future. The bond between the two becomes stronger with the passage of time. A SUCCESFUL marriage is always the one where the husband loves his partner more than her.

Mine was a beautiful marriage. Among siblings I was the middle one. My parents thought of marrying me first. I was still studying and completing my post- graduation, when I got engaged. He was the eldest among the three siblings. We had a courtship period of 5 months, the best time. It was the first marriage in both the families. The level of excitement was beyond explanation as my family I mean my brother and sister my parents we all were very excited as we had hardly witnessed any marriage in the family. It was more like a great festival. I n my husband family also as he was the eldest so it was the same. I got married in the beginning of my second year of studies. Managing two things side by side was quite difficult lt b b brings smile on my face when i remember those days .When you had someone who supported you. I learnt many things in life from him. We too had quarrels. Sometimes he used to shout at me but within a gap of few seconds he would talk to me as nothing happened. Many a times i thought of extending our fight for more than one day but it never happened. This is marriage where you fight over small things and then life again become normal because there are some bigger important things that overpower small issues.

He had a very busy and stressful life as he was at a very responsible position in his job, where there is more of social and political stress. I never understood this as for me office work is just that's get done in office and when you are at home it should be all a family life.

It took me many years to understand the complexity of his job. I stopped complaining then knowing this is how life works. I was busy raising my kids giving them my all attention, while he was busy in his office and field responsibilities. One more thing I learnt that if you are at a higher designation then you have more responsibilities. I was a housewife. Life was going good. We both were busy doing our duties. One best quality he had was he knew how to maintain relations. He was there in every function of relatives or his social gatherings and was keeping a humble and affectionate personality. We shifted to different locations due to his job and the higher studies of children. He used to come on weekends and sometimes in between also. I realised one thing that both the parents should stay together and raise their children but our case was different I always wanted my daughter to be more attached to her father and my son to be attached to me. But staying at different regions never built that bond. He used to complain some times that kids are more attached to me. I was staying with my daughter as she wasn't keeping well. My son had to join an institute and me, my husband along with a family relative went to drop make my son join an institute. This was the last time when we stayed together for 3 days. I left to see my daughter the next day. He came to drop me to airport. He picked up my suitcase down the stairs for the first and last time as I never made him pick my luggage. I dove to the airport as he came late the previous night and hardly slept for 2 hours. That was the last time I saw him. I was with my daughter, my son was in institute. After a gap of 14 days he met with a tragic accident along with his 2 friends.

We got the news on phone. Our lives that were running so smoothly and tension free because of him got completely shakened till date we can't believe that he is no more. As we were staying at different places for 15 years till date we feel that he is busy doing his job and will visit us soon.

The only thing a learnt is make your married life beautiful by staying with each other, raise your kids with good values. We miss him always. I feel bad, when I see my kids as they are not called by their name by their father. I feel bad as he is no more to see his kids growing and fulfilling his dream.

Life is beautiful if two beautiful souls stay together for a long.

|| ॐ ||

Journey to Bliss

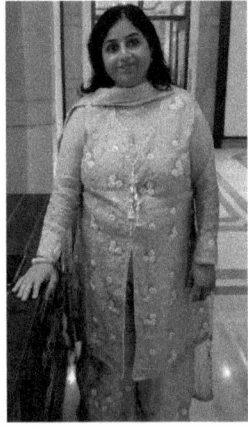

Author's Name	:	Rita Sehgal
Qualification	:	Graduate
Current Profession	:	Professional Vastu Consultant, Certified Numerologist Astrologer, Tarot Card Reader, Dowsing Expert, Certified Published Author, The Owner of Lions Den lounge
Age	:	54 years
E-mail ID	:	**ritasehgal18.rs@gmail.com**
City/ Country	:	**Kolkata, India**

Rita Sehgal is here to serve her soul mission of helping and transforming lives through her expertise in occult science and intuition. She has over seven years of experience in this field and has consulted clients globally, offering them profound knowledge and insights.

Keywords : Sacrifice, Trust, Love, Support, Mutual Respect

Marriage is about finding true happiness and joy in a lifelong partnership, where two souls come together, to share their dreams and joys. It is a journey of growing together built on trust, respect and unwavering love while navigating the challenges that come with it. For some couples marriage is filled with moments of joy, laughter and deep emotional connection while for some it is a prison of shattered dreams where love turns to bitterness and every day is a struggle.

This is the story of a cheerful 21-year-old college girl Ananya. She lived with her parents and three elder sisters. She was close to her third elder sister Madhvi and her brother-in-law Dhruv. Madhvi had a 3-year-old son, Saurav and was expecting her second child. Ananya was a carefree and lively girl who was very playful and spirited. She often used to visit and stay at Madhvi's place. She loved playing with Saurav and he also adored his aunt very much.

A few months later Ananya's life took a tragic turn. Madhvi passed away after giving birth to her baby. The entire family was plunged into grief and darkness. Ananya's parents were heartbroken. Losing a young daughter was a tremendous loss for them. Dhruv was devastated by his wife's death and there was no one to care for him and his children, as his parents had died, when he was a young boy. Every day he was lost in thought about what to do next.

Ananya's father, finding no other solution asked her to marry Dhruv. He explained that this way, the children would have a mother and Dhruv's family would be complete. On hearing this Ananya went into a state of shock. Even the thought of getting married to her brother-in-law was beyond comprehension. In college, she had fallen in love with a boy whom she had dreamt of getting married to. No one had thought about her desires. Her dreams of a loving marriage seemed to be slipping away. Overwhelmed by despair she retreated to another room where she sobbed uncontrollably. After much reflection, Ananya felt a sense of guilt. She wondered if she had become so selfish that she might ruin the children's lives for her happiness. She realized that no one else could love the children with the same affection she could as an aunt. She put her feelings aside and agreed to the marriage.

The marriage took place in a very simple manner. On the wedding day, she was adorned with a red bridal bangle set [Churra] a symbol of a newlywed bride. However the next day she took it off thinking about what people would say about a mother of two children, still wearing bridal bangles. At every turn, Ananya felt she was sacrificing her happiness for the marriage. Accepting her brother-in-law as her husband was very difficult for Ananya and she struggled with the adjustments. Dhruv meanwhile, lived apart and was still unable to move on from Madhvi's loss. Dhruv had a friend named Kavita, whom he regarded as a younger sister. Kavita supported Dhruv during difficult and emotional times. Kavita visited Dhruv almost every other day, which Ananya did not like. Doubt started creeping in her mind about Dhruv and Kavita's friendship to be something more, making her even sadder. This doubt became a source of conflict between Ananya and Dhruv. One day things got so bad, that Dhruv in anger took the children and dropped Ananya at her parent's house telling them to return only, when she grew up in her behaviour.

Ananya felt as though her life had reached its end, all her adjustments and sacrifices seemed in vain. Overwhelmed by despair she wept uncontrollably, consumed by her thoughts. Time passed Dhruv kept calling her, but she stayed distant. When her family advised her, she realized that Dhruv was also very hurt. Perhaps he could not openly talk to her and needed a shoulder to lean on, a friend with whom he could share his sorrows and feel lighter. Keeping this in mind she decided to give him a chance to take her home.

A few days later it was Dhruv's Birthday. Kavita sent him a birthday cake that said "Happy Birthday Brother". After reading it Ananya realized that she could have been misunderstanding them. Giving Dhruv the benefit of the doubt, she decided to trust him.

Day by day the children's responsibilities were increasing. Ananya no longer had any peace, feeling like a bird trapped in a cage instead of flying freely. Ananya's dream was to become a teacher and open her own school. She thought of fulfilling her dreams by giving wings to her ambitions. She managed to both study hard and take care of her house. Soon she became a teacher at a reputed school. One day Ananya slipped at home and the doctor prescribed 15 days of rest for her. Dhruv's difficulties increased as managing the children the house and the office seemed nearly impossible. That day he felt the weight of Ananya's sacrifice. Gradually Dhruv felt in love with her and started respecting all that she had done for this marriage and the family. He helped her to transform her dream into reality by opening a school for her. He not only fulfilled her aspirations but also became a pivotal part of her success. Their story is a beautiful example of love and mutual respect.

"TWO SOULS UNITED, LIVES JOURNEY SHARED, IN EVERY MOMENT, FOREVER PAIRED"

॥ ॐ ॥

The Epitome of Love and Togetherness

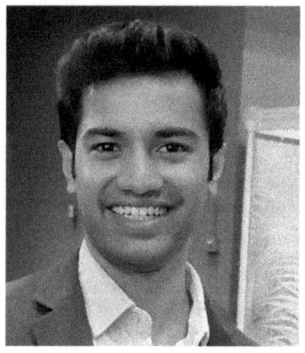

Author's Name	:	Rohan Jain
Qualification	:	BBA, MBA
Current Profession	:	Business
Age	:	26 Years
E-mail ID	:	rohan@texcarp.com
City/ Country	:	**Pune, India**

Rohan Jain is based in Pune and lives in a close-knit family with his wife, parents and grandparents. A management graduate with a specialization in marketing, he joined his family business in 2019 after completing his studies. He aspires to build on the foundation that his father has set up and diversify the business into new verticals. To reinforce this goal, he has also completed his masters in family managed business. A strong believer in work life balance, he loves to spend his free time with his family, reading books and playing table tennis.

Keywords : Union, Love, Companionship, Balance, Responsibility

Between the divine miracle of birth and the inevitable embrace of death lies a pulsating and vivid flow of time, actions and memories- life. This is the journey that every human being embarks upon, and it is the choices and decisions which they make that determine their fate. One such pivotal decision, perhaps the most important one, is the one to get married. Until this point in life an individual predominantly navigates life according to their own beliefs, thoughts, actions and interests. However, marriage is a confluence of two such individuals and if you're based in India, usually their families too. Life as they know it undergoes a complete transformation. Whether it changes for the better or for the worse depends entirely on how people walk the tight rope of balancing their individuality, their past, and emotions in one hand and the expectations, feelings and desires of their partner in the other. For each one, marriage could mean different things but one question that intrigues every person yet to embark on this journey is this- Whether marriage is a curse or bliss.

Imagine you're doing something that interests you, something that fills your heart with joy. Maybe that could be taking a relaxing walk, watching a new movie or maybe sipping your coffee on a lazy Sunday morning. Now for a moment just think if you had someone by your side to share these little moments of bliss with, to cherish the joy that you feel and to add to the warmth of emotions that you feel. This is just a small glimpse of how marriage can enrich your life. Whether one is an extrovert or an introvert, the need for companionship and the desire to be loved constitutes one of the basic human needs. And marriage is instrumental in the fulfilment of that need. Your partner doesn't just add to your happiness but also stands by you like a rock to weather every storm and overcome every challenge in your life. For instance, recently my grandfather suffered a major thigh fracture and was bedridden for a month. It was heartbreaking for all of us to see him in that state for he was immensely active until then. My wife not only motivated him with positivity and humour every single day but also helped me remain afloat amidst all the stress and pressure. She did this tirelessly and without any complaint.

Marriage is a blessing, but it is also one of the biggest responsibilities of your life. The unwavering support and love that you get must be respected and valued. You must consciously take into consideration their needs, emotions and expectations along with yours and sometimes even before yours. You must give them this assurance through your words and actions, the latter being more impactful. Be it saying a simple I love you, partaking in shared activities that you both enjoy, complimenting them, just listening to them without always giving your opinion and perhaps the most important one- holding them close when they say they need you and closer when they don't say anything at all. These small yet thoughtful gestures will go a long way in cultivating a relationship characterized by love, trust and openness.

So yes, I believe with all my heart that marriage is bliss. It does have its share of ups and downs, trials and tribulations. However, these are mere waves in the vast ocean of growth, togetherness and lifelong love and happiness. Yes, every marriage is different and not all marriages work. But believe me, you have to make a marriage work. A wedding is for a day, but marriage is for life. Be prepared to give it your all and you will be rewarded with someone who will never let go of your hand no matter how difficult the path, who will be the brightest light in your darkest nights, who will wipe away every tear and make your eyes water with laughter, someone who will fill your heart with so much love that it cannot comprehend but can only rejoice in. You will be with someone not just for your entire life but with someone who will become your entire life.

I feel that having open discussions about marriage is the need of the hour. It is imperative that we educate and enlighten the next generation about how to navigate the nuances of their new relationship and prepare them to overcome any obstacles that may come their way. Moreover, having 108 authors from varying age groups and such diverse backgrounds providing their perspective about marriage will help a wider audience relate to the content that they read. This anthology is sure to leave a lasting impression on the readers' minds and provide a guiding light in times of need.

|| ॐ ||

Marriage Can Become an Obstacle to the Spiritual Path

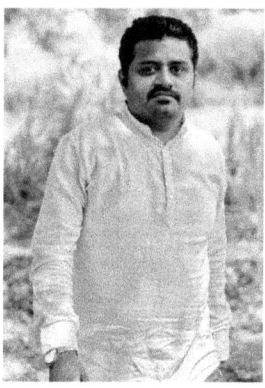

Author's Name	:	Rohet B Kummbar
Qualification	:	B.Tech. (Chemical)
Current Profession	:	Consultant and Organiser
Age	:	34 years
E-mail ID	:	**rohitkumbhar31@gmail.com**
City/ Country	:	**Kolhapur, Maharashtra, India**

Rohet B Kummbar studied B. Tech in Chemical and worked as a Production Engineer for 2 years. Since he did not like a bonded job, he associated himself with network marketing to start his own business. Due to his interest in studying spirituality, he participated in meditation camps and satsangs. For the past 4 years, he has established an educational and consultation academy by the name of Sadhna Healing Hub, where through his experience many people are getting trained in occult sciences and spirituality. He is a Professional Numerologist and Vastu Consultant; due to his interest in occult sciences, he remains engaged in new research.

Keywords : Acceptance, Balance, Spirituality, Goal, Surrender

Whatever is happening in our life is the result of our wish or what we choose.

So in the same way marriage is also a bond chosen by our choice. Marriage is a bond of union of two minds, emotions and souls of two persons. So whether it is blissful or a curse depends on many things. In which the way of living life of both, understanding of mind and emotions, social system and economic status are important. Apart from this, various other reasons are important, which include our karma, respect for each other, freedom, acceptance of life, love for each other, trust and loyalty.

My experience of marriage has been somewhat different. I have learnt that marriage is based on each other's wishes and understanding. This is useful for living a worldly life but in my life, I want to move ahead in worldly life i.e. to move ahead with spirituality, so marriage can support you well in this also, when your and your partner's wishes and understanding of mind are in sync, then it can work. But my experience is that if we cannot handle our own feelings, aspirations and needs i.e. our own mind, then it can be a little difficult to handle someone else's mind.

So if two people have the same dreams and resolutions, then marriage can be a boon for them, but if there is no compatibility between those two people towards life, then it can become an obstacle.

I think marriage is an important process to fulfill our worldly needs. It also helps us in fulfilling our social, mental and emotional desires. So we consider marriage as a means to connect with the outside world and it is also necessary to live life.

My Marriage Experience:

I met my wife during my college days. We first became good friends and then we felt in love with each other. We knew each other for about 5 years before marriage and we wanted to live a spiritual life together. So we decided to get married, but there was a hindrance in the marriage due to family differences, but we chose to marry against the family.

If we are tied in the holy bond of marriage, then it is also important that we have love for each other. If we love each other, then married life can be pleasant and full of love.

We chose to get married to move forward with spiritual life, but our life after marriage was going through a lot of problems. Our families did not want to see both of us together because we were moving forward with spiritual life. So due to opposition from wife's parents, gradually negative feelings were developing towards each other in our married life. We started feeling that marriage is hindering our spiritual growth, so we started living separately as per our wish and after few months we decided not to continue our married life. We both chose to live our life as per our wish and after 2 years we got separated from marriage legally. Our separation was done after considering our wishes and goals.

So, I am separated from marriage for almost 4 years and I feel that marriage is a hindrance to spiritual growth and even today I don't want to get married.

Title of the book is very beautiful; and I really appreciate the initiative about the book, where we are free to share our opinions as per own experience.

Marriage can be both a bliss and a curse depending on many factors. It helps us to fulfill our physical, mental, social and economic needs, but it can also be a hindrance to moving forward on the spiritual path.

Ultimately, whether marriage is a bliss or a curse depends on individual circumstances, communication and the quality of the relationship. A healthy, loving and supportive partnership can bring happiness and satisfaction, while a troubled or toxic relationship can cause suffering and stress.

So the best way to live is to live with understanding and acceptance of what we find on the path of life.

|| ॐ ||

A Blessing Disguised as a Curse

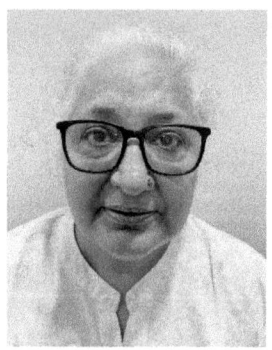

Author's Name	:	Romi Maakan
Qualification	:	Graduate
Current Profession	:	Law of Attraction Coach and Healer
Age	:	62+ years
E-mail ID	:	**contact.thesoulradiance@gmail.com**
City/ Country	:	**New Delhi, India**

Romi Maakan is a renowned Gratitude and Law of Attraction coach with over 25 years of experience in helping people transform their lives through healing practices and manifestation techniques. She holds multiple certifications including Ho'Oponopono Healing, Chakra healing, NLP and life coaching.

She's the founder and CEO of The Soul Radiance, an organization dedicated to holistic healing and self-empowerment. Her 30-day gratitude challenges and workshops have gone global and set the agenda for framing positive mental well-being and personal growth. Passionate to develop self-love, resilience, and compassion, Romi further inspires people to have gratitude and lead richly fulfilling lives.

Keywords : Blessing, Challenge, Feeling, Struggle, Pain

"*A successful marriage requires falling in love many times, always with the same person."* – Mignon McLaughlin.

This quote speaks directly to what my heart believed, when I got married. At 18, I felt hope and excitement, giving shine to my eyes and warmth to my heart, marrying the man I deeply loved. It felt like a dream finally coming true—having a wonderful, supportive family and the man I loved treating me like a queen. At that point, my marriage was a blessing and I thought I had everything anyone could ever wish for.

But life has its own ways of testing our limits, my dear. Over time, I discovered that my husband had past relationships, including two women whose impact had persisted. What once felt like a dream soon turned into a complicated and tough situation. My husband, the love of my life, was torn between these relationships and me, making me feel as though I was getting in between them. The blissful marriage I once had now felt like a curse.

For some people, marriage can sometimes feel overwhelming, especially when faced with challenges. It's easy to look at tough times and feel like you've made a mistake or that your life has taken a wrong turn. But throughout my journey, I've come to accept that marriage is full of ups and downs. The journey of two people being together evolves, and with every challenge, it feels different—sometimes a curse, and sometimes a blessing.

It's important to understand that challenges in relationships should not be seen as curses but as lessons. In my case, the challenges came unexpectedly. The complications in our bond, my partner's sadness and his dependency on alcohol almost made me give up on the life. Walking away or resigning myself to a life of bitterness would have been easy, but I couldn't stand the idea of seeing my marriage as a failure.

I will always be thankful for the teachings in *"The Power of Positive Thinking"* by Norman Vincent Peale. I had learned at a young age to always look for the shining light. Each obstacle in my marriage became an opportunity to grow. Within the hardships, I fell in love with my husband more and more each day—not because he was perfect or because the problems went away, but because I believed that with every struggle, I was learning something new and good.

It wasn't easy. My husband, pressured by his own demons, turned to alcohol and his unhappiness deeply affected our relationship. But, as always, I kept holding onto hope. I believed the next day would bring better situations and that the love we had would eventually help us overcome everything. Maybe he loved me less than I loved him, but I never let that change my thoughts about him or my efforts in our marriage.

As time went by, I realized that every struggle made me stronger and more resilient. The teachings of Rhonda Byrne's *"The Secret"* and *"The Magic"* introduced me to the Law of Attraction and the Power of Gratitude. These readings transformed my perspective on life, allowing me to see my marriage not as a curse, but as a blessing.

What once seemed like a painful chapter, ended up being a stepping stone towards my own self-improvement. I began to understand that my husband and I had a karmic connection and the challenges we faced were somehow helping us grow. This understanding didn't come easily—it took years of reflection. It wasn't until my husband passed away in 2009 that I fully grasped the meaning of our journey together.

What I want others to understand from my story is this: Marriage, like life, is full of phases—some blissful, some painful. But none of these phases should be seen as curses. Every difficult scenario is an opportunity for growth, for learning, and for deep self-reflection. It's easy to label bonds like marriage as curses when things don't go as planned, but in reality, those tough times are like the pressure that forms a diamond—they make the bond special, shiny, and everlasting.

If you're struggling in your marriage, know that it's only a phase. Don't give up on the belief that your marriage is a blessing. The obstacle you face today is shaping you into a stronger, more understanding, and more positive person. As you navigate the tough times, remember never to think of anything as a curse. With the right perspective, every problem can lead to something greater.

In the end, my marriage—with all it's ups and downs—made me who I am today. The love, the heartbreak and the challenges all helped shape me into the person I am now—a coach, a healer and someone who understands the beauty of forgiveness and the power of gratitude.

So, I leave you with this thought:

No matter how hard it gets, nothing is a curse. In every struggle, there's a chance to win; in every problem, there's hope; and in every phase, there's a blessing disguised as a curse.

|| ॐ ||

Tying the Knot: The Ebb and Flow of My Marriage

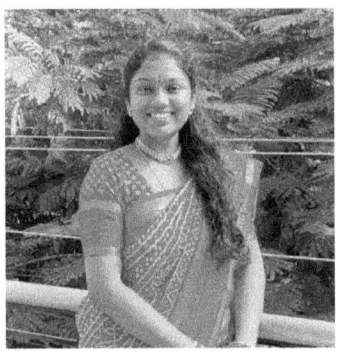

Author's Name	:	Sadhana Athinamilagi
Qualification	:	B.E Instrumentation Engineering
Current Profession	:	Lead Software Engineering
Age	:	28 years
E-mail ID	:	sadhanaathi77@gmail.com
City/ Country	:	Trichy, India

Sadhana Athinamilagi, an Engineering Graduate turned Data Engineer, is a passionate advocate for lifelong learning and personal development. Inspired by the transformative power of literature, she embarked on a journey to establish herself as a writer with the goal of making a meaningful impact on people's lives. What sets her apart is her unique approach to exploring these topics, continuously evolving as she delves deeper into her craft.

Beyond her writing endeavors, Sadhana is also an avid explorer of diverse interests like Art and Craft. She finds joy in delving into Yoga and practising meditation. As a mother, Sadhana aspires to be a source of inspiration for her daughter, imparting not only wisdom gained from professional and personal experiences but also a sense of wonder and curiosity about the world.

Keywords : Marriage, Ultimate, Relationship, Happy, Journey

Marriage is often envisioned as a significant milestone, the ultimate dream of many people's lives. The idea of finding a better half, starting a life together, building a family, and leading a happy, peaceful life is appealing. However, does marriage always go as expected? Not always. Just as the best views come after the hardest climbs, marriages also face ups and downs that need to be navigated. The reality of marriage goes beyond the romantic portrayals in media and literature. While opposites often attract, understanding the complexities behind this dynamic is crucial. Here is the story of my marriage, illustrating this journey.

My marriage was a typical arranged marriage that took place amidst the COVID-19, Pandemic. We had only met once before the wedding and talked sporadically for a month beforehand. I was quite clueless about my spouse, but the initial stages after the marriage were good. We had great moments together, laughed a lot, and joy filled the air.

However, beneath the surface, significant issues were brewing. We lacked understanding, shared goals, proper communication, boundaries and quality time. We had substantial differences in our ways of living, career ambitions, and life goals. I started wondering, how I had entered this marriage without truly knowing the person I had married. It was a rough phase of my life and I was clueless about how to come out of it. But I knew this didn't mean it wouldn't work. Maybe we needed some additional support and we both agreed to work on ourselves and the relationship to keep it alive.

We took relationship counseling, which helped in many ways. It not only helped us explore our relationship and understand the phases of love and conflict resolution, but it also showed me the importance of self-love and inner work. Communication plays a crucial role in marriage and how partners interpret each other's needs matters immensely. One needs to show empathy and always put themselves in their partner's shoes before making big decisions.

We learned to appreciate each other for the little things, started planning finances together and spent time understanding each other's needs. This changed the bond and strengthened it. We began planning vacations and dedicating time to quality interactions. These efforts led to a renewed sense of connection and mutual respect, reinforcing the foundation of our marriage.

In my opinion, the marriage has a dual nature i.e. Bliss & Curse and the key to a successful marriage lies in the ability to adapt and grow together. It is essential to recognize that both partners will change over time and that the relationship must evolve accordingly. Communication, empathy and mutual respect are vital in navigating the inevitable challenges that arise. While the journey is not always easy, the rewards of a strong, supportive partnership are immense. Embracing both the joys and struggles of marriage can lead to a deeper, more resilient connection that stands the test of time.

My marriage, like many others, has been a journey marked by both bliss and challenges. The ebb and flow of our relationship have taught us valuable lessons about love, commitment, and resilience. By understanding and accepting that marriage involves both highs and lows, we have learned to appreciate the beauty in our shared journey. Ultimately, the quality of a marriage depends on the ability of both partners to nurture their relationship, address conflicts constructively and support each other's growth. Through the ebb and flow of our marriage, we strive to build a partnership that can weather the storms and celebrate the triumphs, tied together by the enduring knot of our love.

|| ॐ ||

Embracing My True Self
Uncovering My True Path

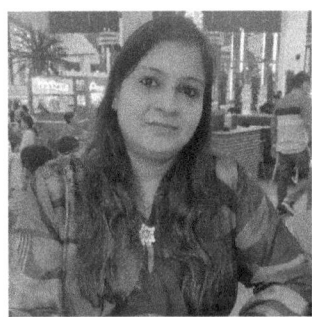

Author's Name	:	Sapna Gaurav Gupta
Qualification	:	B.Com.
Current Profession	:	Teacher, Counselor and Coach
Age	:	47 years
E-mail ID	:	**sgdream22@gmail.com**
City/ Country	:	**Mumbai, India**

Mrs. Sapna Gupta is a Cheerful and Passionate Educator with an impressive 25 years of experience in teaching and guiding students. Beyond conventional teaching, she has excelled as a mentor, helping students improve their handwriting skills as an expert graphologist, thus playing a pivotal role in grooming their personalities and boosting their confidence.

In addition to her expertise in graphology, Mrs. Gupta is a professional numerologist, logo analyst and designer, wristwatch analyst, and drawing analyst. These diverse skills have allowed her to provide comprehensive guidance and support, enriching the lives of thousands of individuals. Her profound knowledge in these areas has enabled her to add tremendous value to people's lives, helping them achieve personal growth and success.

Mrs. Gupta's influence extends beyond her professional life. She is also an avid traveller who finds joy in exploring new places and immersing herself in the diverse cultures and traditions of each destination. Through her extensive experience, diverse skills, and personal interests, Mrs. Sapna Gupta continues to inspire and positively impact the lives of many, leaving a lasting impression in the field of education and personal development.

Keywords : Imperfect Souls, Compassion, Trust, Jeevan Saarthi, Shiv-Shakti

Marriage is a sacred bond of two **IMPERFECT** souls who find solace, **companionship**, and **endless love** in each other's embrace. It is a bond of **friendship**, **trust** and **understanding**, respecting each other's desires and decisions. Marriage is care, compassion, and compatibility between the two partners.

The year ending month of 1999, was my first encounter with my soulmate – a charming dashing young man who arrived on a sleek bike, donning a stylish cap. In an instant, he captivated my heart and soul with his irresistible personality.

My heart resonated with certainty, affirming that he was indeed my life companion, my "**JEEVAN SAARTHI**" in this so-called journey LIFE. My sceptical eyes waited for his validation, yet he graciously reciprocated, agreeing to embark on this journey together.

The year 2000 marked a profound turning point in my life. Like a budding flower ready to unfurl its petals, I was on the brink of transformative journey just at the age of 22, leaving my countless aspirations and dreams behind. We both tied a knot while taking the seven feras (circle around the fire) considered as a beautiful gesture to put the two Indian lives into a pure companionship, wherein, we promised to respect, trust and support each other. It was our commitment to nurture the long-term relationship.

Being brought up in a nuclear family it was a struggle to adjust in a joint setting which extended beyond us. But after countless efforts and a lot of compromises, my husband and I decided to move out together before our relations became bitter. Since then, we continue to maintain healthy relations between us and the extended family.

We settled into our new apartment with limited though satisfying resources. The year 2002, blessed me with a beautiful soul-my daughter. I forgot all my pains, my emptiness was filled with a feeling of motherhood, my loneliness was overcome by a new purpose, I channelised my unfinished dreams towards her bright future.

Days and years passed by. My daughter grew up into a beautiful maiden, who now embarked on her own journey of dreams and aspirations. Husband remained busy with his passion of upscaling his business. I started feeling myself stuck with responsibilities and clueless life ahead. I shifted my energies towards my husband's business with a purpose of supporting his endeavours. Still felt a void with in me. Arguments, discussions and conflicts became a daily chore. The internal turbulences kept me upset and disheartened all the time. I now looked for the lost identity which I believed was overshadowed by marriage and motherhood.

I spoke to my husband and daughter about my unfulfilled dreams. They became my backbone and guided me towards my personal and professional growth. I started teaching, which was always my passion since childhood. Meanwhile, I also upgraded my skills in Graphology, colour therapy, drawing and doodle therapy, wristwatch therapy, logo designing, kept adding countless feathers to my cap. Thus, adding value to more than 200 students for their academic achievements in a span of 13 years and guiding over 500 people with my skills of graphology and parallel modalities under the name of two brands **SAPNA TUTORIALS & GRAPHO STUDIO**.

This journey has been challenging, but I am proud of where I stand today. I have discovered my soul's purpose, and I have no intention of stopping. The satisfaction I feel in myself and my story is immense, and my husband will always be the main character in it.

In the pursuit of my goals and visions my husband backs me up as a strong support, a loving companion, and my biggest source of motivation. Embarking into the 25th year of marriage today I look myself as a pillar to my family standing bold both emotionally and financially looking forward to guide and create differences in the lives of 10000 people in the next five years.

Marriage is thus a bond of **'Shiv-Shakti'**, a balance of actions and emotions, Shiv being an action and Shakti, the emotion. If this balance is maintained and valued, marriage can be **a BLISS**. Certainly, coming out of marriage or not accepting a marriage is easy but staying in a marriage with adjustments and compromises is indeed difficult but in a way it's a feeling of wholesome as well as building a strong support system for each other.

On the contrary, if the partners don't respect each other's likes and dislikes leading to often heated arguments due to lack of understanding will make a life hell for both. Such marriages then become a **CURSE**.

In conclusion, marriage is like a Shadi ka Ladoo (an Indian sweet): whether you eat it or not, there's always some regret. So, it's better to eat the Ladoo and experience the regret.

|| ॐ ||

A Journey of Acceptance

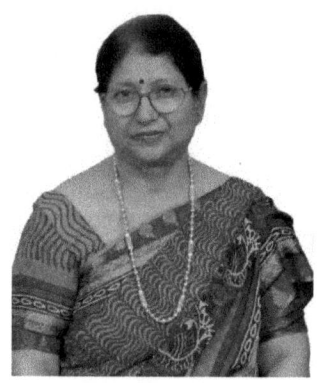

Author's Name	:	Sharlet Seraphim
Qualification	:	M.A, B.Ed.
Current Profession	:	Retired Teacher
Age	:	68 years
E-mail ID	:	**sharlet.seraphim@gmail.com**
City/ Country	:	**Gurgaon, India**

Sharlet Seraphim is a retired educationist. She has taught humanities to senior secondary students in Bihar Government for 33 years impacting lives of around 5000 students during her professional journey. She specializes in national and international history of modern era. She has keen interest in current affairs and is an avid reader. She has two daughters and currently lives in Gurgaon. As a retired professional she is currently pursuing her passion of cooking, baking, travelling and spending time with grandchildren.

Keywords : Acquired, Companion, Friend, Honest, Unity

Marriage is a bond of two souls with body and mind united together.

I got married to late Sudhir Seraphim in December, 1978. Marriage for me was just a responsibility of parents transferred to a very unknown person. Being an arranged ceremony, everything was new for me. It was a big change and I felt my world got transformed. Though we were of same community and same culture, it took a lot of time to adjust in the new environment. Gradually, I embraced the expectations of my spouse as I understood him well. I realized that I got married to a very kind and genuine person who was extremely devoted to his mother and his family. Soon, I became a mother of two lovely daughters. My husband welcomed his two angels as blessings from the almighty. This was the most beautiful part of my married life.

It is said that marriages are made in heaven. Within the norms of a social contract the families and couple accept each other. Marriage is considered to be a unification of two people with blessings of the families, however there are some exceptions where it become a curse. I have seen people suffer mental and physical abuses. Reference to this, I recall an instance about one of the known families, where the woman had a very torturous life resulting in the end of her tragic marriage. A teenage girl in close acquaintance, married to an elderly man. For a long time, she had succumbed to inhuman and torturous behaviour. Coming from a very sophisticated family, she did her best to save her family but all went in vain .Finally, she had to take a tough decision to end her marriage. It was another night, when she was again assaulted and beaten brutally but this time she had to flee her house with her two little kids to save herself and her children. In the midnight, she arrived at her widow mother's house. Her mother welcomed them with a broken heart. The woman suffering from torture and humiliation for years was finally free. Her mother stood by her side like a pillar. She started building upon her carrier all over again, which was left behind due to her forceful marriage. Time passed on and she got a government job. Things started changing. The nightmare was finally over.

Now, if someone would ask her, whether marriage is bliss or a curse, she will definitely choose it to be a curse. This could be diverse perspective of another married woman with an unpleasant experience.

There is another example of a man I knew, who wanted to live a simple and contented life but he was always mentally harassed by his spouse, because of her continuous aspirations and demands. The relationship became so tensed that the marriage ended up with deep grief and sorrow.

These series of experiences have led me to believe that marriage is a gamble. Future has been so unpredictable. Some time we see that the consequences might be very different even for similar situations. It also depends a lot on the resiliency of the couple and support from family and friends.

However, we should generally consider marriage as a strong bonding of mind and body where two people share their joys and sorrows for the whole life. Despite their different background, many ups and down in their journey, the couple remain united and nurture a beautiful family. When the God is kind enough, they get to celebrate their silver and golden jubilee as a testament of their togetherness and commitment.

Unfortunately, these days marriage is not considered to be a very serious affair. The commitment, faithfulness and loyalty is often very questionable. Are we going in the right direction? Are we diluting the marriage as an institution which has so far created generations and provided safe nest and love to most of us? Are we ready to pause, reflect and fix or just let go to a free world, where the price of freedom could be very high for the generations to come.

Marriage is a blessing. It is a gift of God and the society. We must respect it.

|| ॐ ||

A Beautifully Created Real Bliss

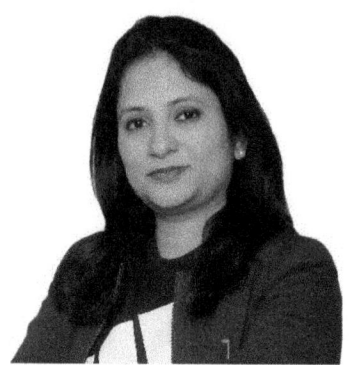

Author's Name	:	Sheetal Pratik
Qualification	:	BE (Electronics and Communication) BIT MESRA MBA (Systems) – IMT Ghaziabad
Current Profession	:	Director Engineering – Data and Analytics
Age	:	44 years
E-mail ID	:	**Shietal.paratik@gmail.com**
City/ Country	:	**Gurgaon, India**

Sheetal Pratik is a Data Leader, who has enabled organizations to deliver business values from data. With around 20+ years of experience in data related technologies at large organizations and start-ups, she has held various roles architecting and delivering data platforms across companies such as Oracle, Colt, NaviSite, Syntel, Mphasis, Reliance Jio Payments Bank, Saxo Bank and Adidas.

Currently she is working as Director Data Engineering, Data and Analytics at NatWest.

She holds a B.E. degree with distinction, from BIT Mesra in Electronics and Communication and is also a postgraduate in Business Administration from IMT Ghaziabad.

She has authored two research papers on data mesh and her paper on "Data Mesh Adoption: a Multi-case and Multi-method Readiness Approach" has won the Best Overall Paper award in December 2023, at EMCIS (European, Mediterranean and Middle Eastern Conference on Information Systems) The British University in Dubai.

She was interviewed for her work in 2022 by Harvard Business review on 'Creating Business Value with Data Mesh' for rolling out one of the early federated data governance platform.

In 2022, she received Indian Achievers Award 2022 by Indian Achievers Forum.

Keywords : Bond, Communication, Happiness, Respect, Values

"Marriage is not a bed of roses but it's a Garden that goes through all the seasons. It has flowers, thorns, stems and leaves and looks beautiful together, with all of it."

The concept of marriage has been made so delusional by the phrase "Happily Ever After", that when people enter a marital bond, they expect a perfect life, a perfect partner and a perfect family. This need of perfection becomes suffocating. In real life this does not happen and this is where dreams crash and so does life. The life is real yet beautiful. When we are born into a new family, there is no pre-conditioning unlike marriage. We accept everyone in our birth family, as they are and most of the time we love our families. If this was extended to marital construct, the world would be a different place.

My Marriage has been a **beautiful journey** of learnings and acceptance. I got married two years after my engineering at the age of 25 years, to my classmate and friend, Nishant Pratik. It was a love marriage, formally arranged by our parents and very well accepted. However, I soon realized that it was not a bed of roses. But it was neither a bed of thorns. All were nice with good intentions, but the prick of pre-conditioning did not spare us as well. This is when I met a friend, who had lost her spouse. She told me something which I could never forget – "I have decided to be happy no matter what". Being a single mother, she had much to deal with. I met her at the right point of my life, and I started counting my blessings. I have someone who I could fight, demand and share my achievements. Nishant gave me a secured family to which I could get back to everyday, a family who would take care of me no matter what, and where I could be always myself.

My next stage of marriage was, revelation, when I decided, to keep myself and all around me happy. It was in these years, that I attended a retreat where the priest said in a sermon "it's all inside us". Our relationship and the happiness and the success of it is inside us. My whole attitude towards people changed. I moved from first me to first us. However, being an ambitious woman, I could articulate clearly about what was important to me and why, and what help I needed. So, communication was important. Marriage does not mean burying your wishes. It is about gives, take, and ask.

Few years later, I met another Italian priest in a couple retreat in the U.S. who explained the spirituality around marriage. He Said – *"The very reason of divorce is the reason for Marriage. Separations and Divorce happen because the couple think they are incompatible and different. However, marriages happen to complete our learnings in this life and make us more complete souls. We are surrounded by people and often married to partners who might be very different than ours."*

It is rightly said *"A great marriage is not when the 'perfect couple' comes together. It is when an imperfect couple learns to enjoy their differences."* – Dave Meurer

We grew and evolved here-on, we started seeing every difference and every disagreement to being our teachings that is meant to help us grow and become a better human and an evolved soul. From here on, life has been beautiful. I kept sharing my learnings and perspective to my husband, my tonality changed, and my messages were better comprehended. We started enjoying things which we had never explored earlier, because of getting confined to our own personalities. We need to also use our intuition, intelligence, wisdom, and experience to analyze the situation and people, and act accordingly.

For me value alignment has been important. My journey was possible, because there was a core value alignment between us, and our families. Recognizing the importance of communication, respect, shared values, and personal well-being can help in navigating the complexities of marital life. Ultimately, the perception of marriage as bliss or curse is shaped by individual experiences and the dynamics within the relationship.

"The real act of marriage takes place in the heart, not in the ballroom or church or synagogue. It's a choice you make – not just on your wedding day, but over and over again - and that choice is reflected in the way you treat your husband or wife." – Barbara De Angelis

Sheetal Pratik wants to express her heartiest Love and Gratitude to her husband, Mr. Nishant Pratik, for standing always as a strong pillar of life positively. Both are blessed to live together and their marriage is a successful journey with full of Bliss.

॥ ॐ ॥

Freedom in Relationship

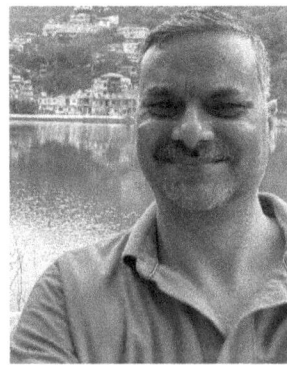

Author's Name	:	Shelaj Kant
Qualification	:	M.Sc. (Chemistry), B.Ed. Diploma in Naturopathy and yoga
Current Profession	:	PGT Chemistry
Age	:	47 years
E-mail ID	:	**Shelajssis@gmail.com**
City/ Country	:	**Dharamsala, India**

Shelaj Kant is Post Graduate Teacher in Chemistry. He has done his Master Degrees in Chemistry with speciation in Organic Chemistry. Worked more than 20 years as PGT Chemistry in reputed schools in India and UAE

He has completed three years Diploma in Naturopathy and Yoga.

Shelaj Kant`s current area of focus is Trigonum Numerology and is exploring extensive reading of books and research papers.

He loves to spend his leisure reading, cooking and exploring mountains.

Keywords : Independence, Cooperation, Relation, Expectation, Situation

"All you need is love." I personally disagree this I may be wrong but many marriages today are ending in divorce because love alone is not enough. Love is very important but love is not the only criterion for successful marriage. After marriage main complaint is my husband do not love me, where is that love goes suddenly. Wives needs love and what about husband he also needs love and one more important thing he needs that is respect. Respect is missing nowadays from relationship and this is the major cause that most beautiful relationship nowadays becomes curse. Everyone wanted independence in each aspect of life like social independence, financial independence. Azadi slogans are very famous these days in JNU and same slogans are coming to our relationship through social media. Azadi from each other, Azadi from Parents and Azadi from all relationships. Is this the real meaning of independence? Our interpretation of the term Azadi is wrong somewhere

Independence in marriage means you keep your own hobbies interest and sense of self and passion. That means do not lose your identity. Both husband and wife should have the space to grow and develop personally. When both partners are growing the relationship will evolve in positive manner. Open and honest discussions about your needs, boundaries and expectations. Clear communication helps to prevents misunderstanding. Mutual respect and support strengthen the relationships. But we are more influenced by the slogans in social media AZADI AZADI AZADI from expectations of each other.

I got married at the age of 29 and things are going smooth my wife was house wife in the beginning. We are living in extended family. My parents retired from government job. My younger brother and his wife also working. After some time, we were blessed with a baby boy and my wife got government job. We are living in extended family so she was able to join government job without hesitation that who will look after baby. When my son was in 4th standard, I got opportunity to work in Dubai so I left India and shifted to Dubai alone. Things were going great but suddenly my life makes U turn. My mother was hospitalized due to some nerve issues and she was totally bedridden within three months. My wife got promotion and transferred to Chandigarh she along with my son shifted to Chandigarh. My son was in Grade 10 at that time. My brother is also posted away from my native place so he cannot come every day he is coming to home on weekends only. My father is taking care of my mother, my father around 82 years old at this age he is not able to manage everything alone. So, I decided to quit my Job and come back to India. I cannot leave my mother and father in that stage alone. People may think I am a hero but I don't see myself that way. You know from where I got this courage to leave my job and come back to India without hesitation. I got this courage from my wife. For me Marriage is Bliss not curse. I am able to look after my mother because my wife is taking care of my son. If she doesn't support my decision, I could not manage things. I am not, she is my hero. I have never said it loudly and openly but I don't want to let this moment pass without saying thank you. You mean the world to me. We all family members helping each other in one or other way in this challenging time.

If we respect each other's decision marriage is bliss.

I want to conclude my thoughts with a small story, though I am not sure if it's relevant, but I still want to share it

It was the coldest winter ever, and many animals died because of the cold. The porcupines, realizing the situation, decided to group together. This way they covered and protected themselves; but the quills of each one wounded their closest companions even though they shared their heat with each other.

After a while, they decided to distance themselves one from the other to stop being wounded.

As they did this, they began to die… alone and frozen. So, they had to make a choice: either accept the quills of their companions or disappear from the Earth. Wisely, they decided to go back to being together. This way they learned to live with the little wounds that were caused by the close relationship with their companion, but the most important part of it, was the heat that came from the others that enabled them to survive the coldest winter ever.

What is the moral of story???

Please share the moral of story after reading this chapter.

Marriage is bliss, when you got emotional support; you share your laughter and memories with each other. Build your life through ups and down. Only ups and down makes your life beautiful. In good phase of our life, we generally do not bother about relationships. We value our relationship when we are going through hard time.

Marriage becomes curse when you have conflicts due to communication breakdown. Unrealistic expectation "Mujhko Chand la ke do ….. Mujhko Tare la ke do" gives disappointments in relationships. Life is not a move of three hours.

Ultimately whether marriage is bliss or curse depends on individual perspectives and experiences. Marriage has been a blissful experience for me. One should learn from others experiences too so enjoy this amazing relationship as bliss doesn't make your marriage curse.

|| ॐ ||

A Beautifully Created Real Bliss

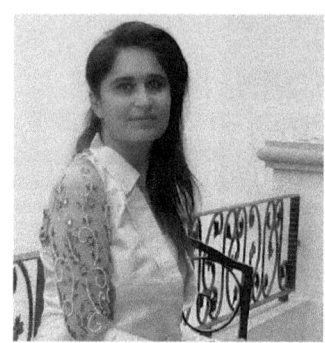

Author's Name	:	Shelly Arora
Qualification	:	Graduate
Current Profession	:	Consultant and Counselor in Occult Science
Age	:	42 years
E-mail ID	:	**anantadrishtishelly@gmail.com**
City/ Country	:	**Amritsar, India**

Shelly Arora is a co-founder of Anantadrishti Infinity Eye of Shiv. For over five years, she has dedicated herself to the world of occult practices. Her expertise spans a variety of disciplines, including healing, numerology, tarot card reading, rune reading, angel therapy, Akashic reading and glass ball gazing. As an award-winning rune reader, she has been recognized for her deep understanding and application of ancient wisdom. Shelly's work as an NLP coach and life consultant allows to guide individuals toward their true potential, helping them overcome obstacles and achieve their personal and professional goals. At Anantadrishti Infinity Eye of Shiv, aim to provide holistic guidance and support, empowering the clients with the knowledge and tools they need to lead fulfilling lives.

A thought-provoking question! Marriage can be both a blessing and a challenge, depending on various aspects of life. Here is a balanced perspective:

Bliss :

- Emotional support and companionship

- Shared experiences and memories

- Personal growth and self-discovery

- Building a life together

- Unconditional love and acceptance

Curse :

- Conflicts and disagreements

- Compromise and sacrifice

- Loss of independence

- Financial stress

- Potential for emotional hurt

Ultimately, whether marriage is bliss or curse depends on:

- The individuals involved

- Their communication and relationship skills

- Shared values and compatibility

- Efforts to maintain a healthy and loving relationship

Marriage is a journey, not a destination. It requires work, commitment and understanding to navigate life's ups and downs together. What are your thoughts on this?

I am sharing a real incidence of one of my friends situation as per promise her real name is not going to be revealed. So the characters' names are Jaya and Raj. Here's a story based on the characters and dynamics you described:

Raj and Jaya were married, but their relationship was far from perfect. Raj's ego and dismissive nature had created a rift between them, and Jaya felt like she was walking on eggshells around him.

One day, Raj's arrogance led him to make a reckless business decision, which put their entire livelihood at risk. Jaya tried to caution him, but he refused to listen. As the consequences of his actions unfolded, Raj was forced to confront the damage his ego had caused. Jaya, with her calm and wise demeanour, helped him see the error of his ways

Despite Jaya's efforts to make their relationship work, Raj's insecurities and ego continued to drive a wedge between them. He became increasingly possessive and accusatory, often making Jaya feel guilty for no reason.

"Who were you talking to on the phone?" Raj would ask, his tone laced with suspicion.

"No one, just my sister," Jaya would reply, trying to reassure him.

"Don't lie to me! I know you're having an affair!" Raj would shout, his accusations escalating.

Jaya tried to reason with him, but Raj's mind was consumed by his own paranoia. He began to monitor her movements, questioning her every action.

Jaya felt suffocated by Raj's behaviour, but she didn't want to give up on their relationship. She tried to be patient, hoping that Raj would eventually see the error of his ways.

But as the accusations continued, Jaya started to feel like she was walking on eggshells, never knowing when Raj's temper would flare up again. She began to doubt her own sanity, wondering if she was indeed doing something wrong.

One day, Jaya realized that she had had enough. She couldn't take the constant guilt trips and accusations anymore. She decided to confront Raj, to make him see the damage his behaviour was causing.

"Raj, I've had enough of your accusations," Jaya said, her voice firm but calm. "I'm not having an affair. I'm tired of being made to feel guilty for no reason. You need to trust me, or we're done."

Raj was taken aback by Jaya's assertiveness. For a moment, he saw the hurt in her eyes, the toll his behaviour had taken on their relationship. But his ego quickly took over and he lashed out again.

So,

- A loving partnership can bring immense joy, support and companionship.

- Shared experiences, laughter and adventures can strengthen the bond.

- Marriage can foster personal growth, understanding, and empathy.

- A healthy relationship can provide a sense of belonging and security.

- Unrealistic expectations, lack of communication and unresolved conflicts can lead to unhappiness.

- Incompatibility, infidelity or abuse can cause immense pain and suffering.

- Marriage can also bring financial stress, compromises, and sacrifices.

- Individual freedom and autonomy may be compromised.

Ultimately, whether marriage is bliss or curse depends on:

- The dual-quality of the relationship

- The individuals' willingness to work together and grow

- Effective communication and conflict resolution

- Mutual respect, trust and understanding

Marriage is a journey, not a destination. It requires effort, commitment and dedication from both partners to navigate life's ups and downs together.

॥ ॐ ॥

Husband is a Powerful Pillar
It's a Two Way Path of Life

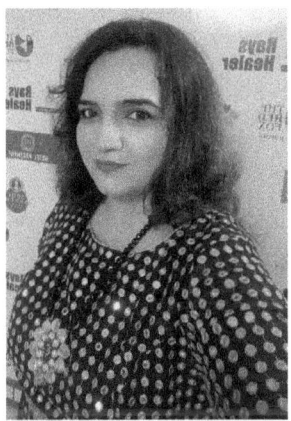

Author's Name	:	Shetall G Desai
Qualification	:	M.Com.
Current Profession	:	Practice in Occult Science
Age	:	42 years
E-mail ID	:	**sheetalgauravdesai81@gmail.com**
City/ Country	:	**Mumbai, India**

Shetall G Desai is a renowned Tarot Counselor, Numerologist, Candle Healer, Fengshui Consultant. She has clients all over the globe. She has won many awards for different modalities. She has learnt more than 20 modalities in occult science. She has not only changed her life but has changed lives of people around the globe. Serving society and helping them is the main goal of her life.

Keywords : Adjustment, Compatibility, Harmony, Love, Respect

Marriages are made in heaven as we all know. To marry a right person is every girl's or boy's dream. Marriage is a ritual where a boy and girl are binded together by vows to be with each other always. Apart from being a ritual it's a Union of two souls. It is a relationship which has been already planned before we are born and also that we come together because most of the times we have some karmic ties, pacts, connections and agreements to be with each other. It also helps the other souls to fulfill their destiny. Sometimes it is believed that we are brought together because we have a pact to birth souls together who then are born as our children, because these souls have to be born out by the union of two souls. Our marital partner is from our soup group and our biggest teacher in life. We have been together even before in many lifetimes. Just that we keep changing our relationships.

To make a Marriage a Bliss or a Curse is completely in the hands of the couples. My marriage has been an adventure filled with love, learning and growth. Marriage works on Adjustment not on Compromise, because compromise comes from one side, but adjustment comes from both the ends. It has been building a life together where both happiness and challenges co-exist. But what makes my marriage a blissful journey for us is the deep companionship it brings. This companionship isn't just about having a partner to share your life with but it's all about having a best friend, a confidante and a pillar of support, rolled into one. A successful marriage is falling in love many times, always with the same person. My marriage is not about the wedding, but it's about the years we are growing together as individuals and not giving up on each other. One of the most important thing in our marriage is we respect each-others differences. Instead of changing each other, we focused on understanding and adapting. This acceptance formed the foundation of our relationship, teaching us vital lesson. We see these quirks not as barriers, but as opportunities for personal and mutual growth. We always look out for prefect soulmate while getting married. But we don't understand that even moon is not perfect, it is full of craters. The sea is incredibly beautiful, but it is salty and dark in its depths. Similarly sky is also infinite, but often cloudy. So everything that is beautiful isn't perfect, but it's special.

So it is very important to understand in a relationship that both individuals can be perfectly imperfect. It's all about embracing each-others flaws and imperfections and understanding that they are the part of what that makes their relationship special and unique. As its always said that behind a successful man there is a woman but in my case I am very fortunate enough to say that behind my success lies a very "Powerful Pillar My Husband". I can describe our relationship as a real relationship which has helped to achieve ones goals in life, support each other when one has broken down, push each other to be successful, shower on each other the positive vibes, compliments each other on regular basis, never leave each other at bad times.

So remember the perfect marriage doesn't exist. However a fulfilling, harmonious and loving relationship is not just a lofty dream, it's a possibility crafted through effort , understanding and endless love. As we continue to walk on path of marriage , lets choose to focus on building bridges, celebrating love in its many forms, and supporting each other through trials and triumphs. Here's to marriage, a beautifully complex journey that is worth every step. Two heads (and wallets) are often better than one! Marriage can offer financial stability as me and my husband pool resources, share responsibilities and work towards mutual goals. This teamwork extends beyond finances, touching every aspect of life, from household chores to decision making, enhancing life's quality and reducing the burdens on each individual. The bliss found in our marriage isn't mystery or a lucky chance. Its real mutual respect, understanding and effort. Embracing each-others imperfections, cultivating shared interests, maintaining open communication, supporting each-others dreams and facing challenges together are the pillars of successful marriage.

It's truly said that **"A GOOD WIFE IS CROWN OF HER HUSBAND"**.

|| ॐ ||

Will Meet Again…
Phir Milenge…

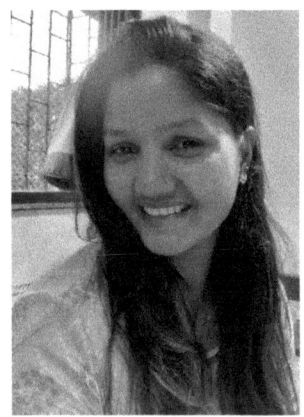

Author's Name	:	Shikha Meher
Qualification	:	H.S.C
Current Profession	:	**Tarot Card Reader, Numerologist**
Age	:	43 years
E-mail ID	:	**sheekhameher3@gmail.com**
City/ Country	:	**Mumbai, India**

Shikha Meher is a professional renowned for her expertise in tarot card reading, numerology, candle magic healing, crystal healing and remedies. With 6 years of dedicated experience in the occult field, she has positively transformed many people's lives through her accurate and insightful tarot readings. Her work in this field has guided individuals towards clarity, healing and personal growth.

In addition to her occult practice, Shikha has been a pet groomer for 15 years. Her extensive experience in pet grooming has allowed her to care for and enhance the well-being of countless pets. This dual expertise in both human and pet care highlights her commitment to improving lives, whether through spiritual guidance or practical grooming skills.

Keywords : Caring, Growth, Togetherness, Trust, Sharing

Hi, I would like to share a beautiful real story of my one of the clients, who trusted me to share it with all of you :

She got married in December 2007. Blessed by her parents, relatives and friends, it was an incredibly happy moment after 5 years of being in a relationship. They both were very happy. In 2008, she was blessed with a baby boy, which felt like a miracle for both of them. They were extremely happy, sharing everything with each other. Writing this story brings back a flood of memories and tears to my eyes, just thinking about how a marriage that was once so blessed could one day feel like a curse.

As their son grew, after he turned 3 years old, she started noticing many changes in her husband's behaviour. The first fight stemmed from her wanting to be financially independent. They began to argue over small things, and her husband started hiding everything from her. Eventually, she discovered that these changes were due to the influence of a third person, who had made their life hell. They were continuously fighting with each other for no reason.

She wants to continue her relationship with her husband; she doesn't want to break it. However, the influence of the third person has been so damaging that they have separated many times, and come back together again. Currently, they are separated, but she is doing her best to reconcile and be together again.

'This all happen because no communication with each other and no communication means no solution.'

Whatever happens, no matter we should talk to each other and most importantly give respect to each other so the other people also respect and learn something from you.

Marriage is not one celebration, marriage is what you give & take from each other. Most important is love, respect, trust in each other, without this your marriage will not work in long term.

The message in this story is clear; Marriage is between two people and no one else should interfere in their lives. Once someone else enters in your personal life and if have bad intension. It can destroy your world, which had created by both of you and it's not easy to fix again. To third parties, friends, relatives, in-laws, or siblings: do not destroy someone's life and do not create bad karma for yourself. Remember, karma comes back tenfold.

Third party interference is good, but only for betterment, not betterment. I hope you remember this story as someone have gone through this situation and had experience all this, when you read this story you'll know what step should take before taking any actions.

Thanks to everyone !!!

|| ॐ ||

Our Marital Journey
Love, Trust and Mutual Respect

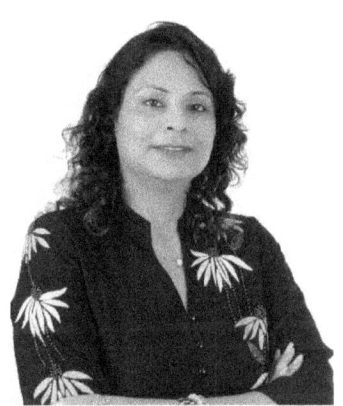

Author's Name	:	Shipra Goswami
Qualification	:	B.Com., M.B.A
Current Profession	:	Team Lead Business Development
Age	:	47 years
E-mail ID	:	**shipragoswami123@gmail.com**
City/ Country	:	**Gurgaon, India**

Shipra Goswami is a senior revenue development professional at Forrester, based in Gurgaon. She is responsible for managing India operations from last 11 years at Forrester. She has been awarded with many awards for her contribution in the field of excellence. She has done her graduation from Panjab University, Chandigarh and M.B.A from Delhi. Along with having a successful career she is a caring mother of twins and a dotted wife. Strong believer of God and Good Deeds.

Keywords : Life together, Marriage, Partner, Mutual respect, Wedding day

My marriage is a true haven of happiness and fulfillment. It all began with a deep connection and understanding between my husband Raj and me, which blossomed into a beautiful friendship. We shared a strong bond, built on mutual respect, trust, and a sense of humor. As we grew closer, I was constantly impressed by Raj's kindness, intelligence, and zest for life.

The Magical Wedding Day :

Our wedding day was a magical celebration, filled with joy and love. As I exchanged vows with Raj, I felt an overwhelming sense of bliss and contentment. The ceremony was a reflection of our unique bond and the promises we made to each other. It was a day where we were surrounded by family and friends, all there to witness the beginning of our journey together. The atmosphere was electrifying, with every smile, every tear, and every cheer echoing the love and support we felt from our loved ones. I will always cherish the memory of walking down the aisle, seeing Raj's eyes filled with emotion, and knowing that this was the start of our forever.

Building a Life Together :

Over the years, our love has only grown stronger. We are true partners, supporting each other through life's ups and downs. We make decisions together, rely on each other for strength, and celebrate each other's successes. We approach challenges together, finding solutions as a team. Raj's unwavering commitment to our relationship is something I deeply appreciate, and I strive to do the same for him.

Our everyday life is a blend of shared responsibilities and mutual respect. We both understand the importance of balancing our individual careers and personal aspirations with our commitment to each other. Whether it's discussing our financial plans, planning our next big adventure, or simply deciding what to have for dinner, we ensure that both our voices are heard and respected. This has helped us build a foundation of trust and understanding that supports our relationship.

Adventures and Memories :

Our life together is filled with laughter, adventure, and new experiences. We love to travel and explore the world, creating lifelong memories. From hiking in the mountains to relaxing on sandy beaches, each trip is a new chapter in our story. We also prioritize quality time for just the two of us, whether it's a romantic dinner, a cozy night in, or a weekend getaway. These moments help us reconnect and strengthen our bond.

Navigating Challenges :

Of course, no marriage is perfect, and we've had our share of challenges and disagreements. However, we've learned to communicate openly, compromise, and approach conflicts with empathy and understanding. We've grown together, becoming more patient and forgiving. Each challenge we face only reinforces our commitment to each other and our relationship.

Gratitude and Growth :

Raj's kindness and positivity are infectious. He has this incredible ability to

see the good in every situation and in every person, which has taught me to approach life with a similar mindset. His unwavering support during my career transitions and personal struggles has been my rock. Whenever I doubted myself, Raj was there to remind me of my strengths and capabilities. This mutual support has been the cornerstone of our relationship, enabling us to grow individually and as a couple.

Looking Forward :

As I reflect on our marriage, I am filled with hope and excitement for the future. I hope to continue growing as individuals and as a couple, facing life's challenges hand in hand. I look forward to many more adventures, shared dreams, and moments of joy. Our story is far from over, and I am excited to see where it takes us.

In summary, my marriage with Raj has been a beautiful journey of love and growth. Our marriage is not just a union of two people; it is a celebration of love, trust, and mutual respect. It is a partnership where both individuals are committed to bringing out the best in each other, supporting each other's dreams, and facing life's challenges together. I look forward to the future with Raj by my side, knowing that no matter what life throws our way, we will face it together, hand in hand, with love and laughter.

|| ॐ ||

When Handled Right, A Dynamic, Else A Dynamite

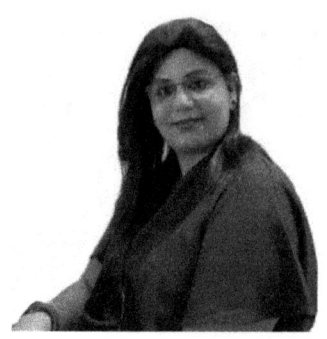

Author's Name	:	Shweta Singh
Qualification	:	B.B.A., B.Ed., M.B.A.
Current Profession	:	Consultant and Advisor
Age	:	45 Years
E-mail ID	:	**shwetasingh.vastugyan@gmail.com**
Phone/ Whatsapp No.	:	…
City/ Country	:	**Mumbai, India**

Shweta Singh is a renowned Shree Vastu Consultant and Certified Vedic Astrologer. She has done her Master Degree in Business Management and worked as Event Coordinator and a Teacher for many years in different schools in Gurgaon. She expanded her horizon of work and came into occult sciences to solve problems behind the scenes through Sanatan Principles of working such as Vastu Shastra, Vedic Astrology and Dousing.

She also is a creative spirit, who loves to paint, sketch and write. She coaches budding artists to fine tune their desire of expression through portraying on paper.

Keywords : Experience, Backbone, Connection, Dynamic, Loyal

His work schedule is mostly chock-a-blocked with a lot of travelling while mine is flexible & mood-driven in the comfort of my home. We truly justify Linda Goodman's work on zodiac signs where he is a Taurus; stubborn, routine and loyal and I'm an Aquarian; curious, unpredictable and humanitarian.

I understand my marriage like a treasure trove of countless heart touching gestures, shared experiences in small fleeting moments.

All this, reflects a deep seated longing for each other and this serves as the backbone for my connection. .

As a couple we share similar ideologies for most of the life's aspects yet we have our individual approach. This contrast makes us edgy sometimes but we have learnt to deal with it with simple necessary fights over a declared war.

"Marriage : When Handled Right, A Dynamic, Else A Dynamite"

In the poetry of our shared moments when I'm singing Asha ji's melodies, he is beating his drums of logics, I'm talking about the vastness of sky, dreamy stars and how they may be interacting with us, he is watching Narcos for the 5th time.

He is in love with Pablo Escobar's Plata or Plomo, can't blame him, who wouldn't want to sleep on a bed of money and feel like God.

If he could he would have lectured Pablo on poor leadership, he thinks Escobar lost the track and derailed his business empire running after power when I think Pablo needed to upgrade his moral standards.

He enjoys thriving in the quietude of the wee hours, made me my first tea of the day with elaichi (Cardamom) and poured in my cherished cup. (gosh! I miss this when he is travelling)

My enthusiasm to start a day leaving the warmth of the cosy comforter kicks only after my morning indulgence. With each sip my mind and body prepare to fold the comforter and open the doors and windows of the room and of my heart to offer gratitude to everyone and everything.

At breakfast when he is deep into affair of states, I slyly sneak in one more chilla in his plate (oatts of course! He will kill me otherwise he's following a diet) and also his favourite green chutney to the side.

He's an avid listener of political podcasts, while he is embroiled and fascinated by relevant facts aired in the ongoing exchange of views , my help and I have packed his lunch with a lot of food, oh ! he is very proud of his food choices and loves to flaunt it and share.

We had spent the entire Covid period watching other people eating food from across the globe and realised that at forty plus glaring others eating interesting food is equally satisfying to our senses without adding any extra pound to the body.

Over decades of cat-dog fights and cold-nuclear wars we now sit as equals at 180°. Neither of us is bothered about more respect, blind trust or unconditional love, it's all there and if it's not, we don't care.

We have understood that by hook or by crook, we have to make it to the end of this tunnel to see the light. As aging together we now often support each other's choices. A win-win.

In the game of Ludo in the evening, when I miss on purpose to kill his token he becomes upset with my strategy and mentors me how I shouldn't have overlooked the opportunity of beating him in the game, while I am enjoying the pleasure of shared time, his attention and exchange of dialogues after a long day at work.

We are aware of our difference and have become humble, ingenious & kind to each other with passing time and add more value to our lives collectively.

"We love to fight and we fight to love". As Keanu Reeves puts it 'if you are a lover you got to be a fighter, if you don't fight for your love what kind of love do you have? No it's not easy in marriage, it takes a lot to settle for an unsaid promise that keeps two as a couple for the rest of their lives.

In one's life marriage is an important aspect and it reflects on virtues of strength of character & sharing. This dynamics is the building block of our society which preserves and nurtures our rich cultural linage. In Geeta, Krishna says our Soul purpose is to evolve as a human in this life. Marriage provides a stage where we enact & emulate emotions and play different roles which empowers us to gain prowess over our weaknesses as a being.

॥ ॐ ॥

Sapthapadi
Bliss or Curse

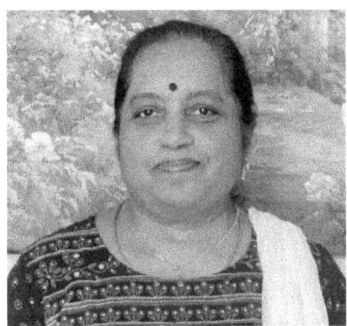

Author's Name	:	Sri Rajeshwari Devi
Qualification	:	M.A.(English), M.A. (Counseling Psychology)
Current Profession	:	Counseling Psychologist
Age	:	63 Years
E-mail ID	:	**authorsri60@gmail.com**
City/ Country	:	**Bangalore, India**

Sri Rajeshwari Devi is a Counseling Psychologist, Life skill Coach, Graphoanalytical Therapist and an Author. She has done her Master Degrees in English and Counseling Psychology, Diploma in Community Mental Health, Diploma in N.L.P and Certificate in Career Counseling. She has more than 16 years of experience as a Counseling Psychologist.

She is a Certified Career Counselor and Tarot Card Reader. She spends more of her leisure time reading, writing, traveling and giving emotional support to Cancer Patients and their relatives. She has published some of the articles in international science journals.

> **Keywords :** Acceptance & forgiveness, Love & Care, Commitment & Communication, Mutual Respect & Responsibility, Patience & Personal Boundaries

santuṣṭo bhāryayā bhartā bhartrā bhāryā tathaiva ca yasminneva nityaṃ kalyāṇaṃ tatra vai dhruvam ||- Manusmriti

It means that in the family where the husband is pleased with his wife & the wife with her husband, happiness will assuredly be lasting.

Marriage is like an institution, which has got its own positive and negative things. When procreative organs become active, animals crave for a companion to fulfill one's own biological needs which is free for them. Human beings cannot be like that. Marriage is important bond made for companionship and family to grow. It requires care, love, trust effective communication, respect to one another and committed relationship, to improve physical & mental health. If marriage provides good companionship, emotional support and sense of well-being, then that marriage can be a bliss otherwise it might become a curse.

"May this marriage be full of laughter, and everyday a paradise. May this marriage be a seal of compassion, for here and hereafter. May this marriage have a fair face and a good name May this marriage be as welcome as the full moon in the night sky."- Rumi

In this 21st century, most of the woman experience Independence and equality. Even then there are still so many women who are facing numerous complex challenges such as violence, gender inequality, the gender pay gap, limited reproductive health care and work-family balance. Since now a day so many married couple are working, they are unable to give their valuable time to each other, Some of the women who are career oriented are not interested in getting married or not interested to become mother. Some of the present generation people prefer to live in together rather than getting married, due to fond of over Independence or fear of taking responsibility. It might lead to some complications later in life, if one of them betrays another.

Marriage is like roller and coaster with so many challenges. Even I faced so many hurdles. Sometimes we feel we are on the cloud nine and sometimes we may feel that we are struck under the ground. Married people like us understand about our spouse and their families gradually day by day. By accepting each other's flaws, setting boundaries, forgiving, sharing responsibilities, giving respect to each other & validating feelings our marriage became a bliss.

The ritual 'Sapthapadi' in Hindu marriage symbolizes seven rules for happy family in the journey of life. This is a list of the seven promises of marriage:

1. Accept of responsibilities towards each other's families
2. Work towards a richer mental and spiritual self-existence together.
3. Earn wealth with honest means.
4. Understand, respect and trust towards each other and take care of each other and their respective families.
5. Seeking blessings from God for a healthy, and virtuous children ahead.
6. Healthy and long life filled with joy and peace.
7. Promise for a committed and honest long-lasting relationship.

Each and every one will have their own upbringing, their own personalities, their own passion, their own habits and their own responsibilities. If there is domination vs caring, infidelity vs commitment, responsibilities vs addiction to anything like gambling, alcohol then entire family has to suffer. Some people who are perfectionists or people with high expectation or not having flexibility or adaptability will not be satisfied even though they go on divorcing and marrying multiple times. They feel that the marriages are curse. The reason for this is nobody is perfect and not every situation will be perfect. If someone is addicted to drugs, alcohol, gambling or any other such things, has violent behavior, unable to take care or take responsibility, then marriage will be a curse, not only for their spouse but for entire family.

Marriage is the foundation of family, and family is the fundamental unit of society. Marriage is not only union of two individuals but of two families. Anyone who gets married without proper understanding of marriage, then that marriage can become curse for them. Most of the time the criteria for selection of bride or groom are made within the boundaries of caste, religion, money, social status, looks. Like mindedness, likes and dislikes, compatibility are rarely considered. Whether the marriage is a boon or curse, depends on whom they marry. Recent research has indicated that married people are not only happier than unmarried people, but also healthier. If marriage provides emotional support, companionship, sense of belonging, loving and committed relationship, it improves one's mental and emotional health.

Here are few tips for marriage to be a bliss-

1. Accept the things that you cannot change about, build trust, learn to forgive & spend some valuable time together.

2. Khalil Gibran gives marriage advice in his 'PROPHET', mentions love is not bondage. According to him there should be space in togetherness of the couple like a moving sea between the shores. Means that individuality is of great importance in a relationship.

3. Try to repair conflicts skillfully with effective communication & stop blame game. Commitment offers couples a sense of being part of a team.

4. A respectful partner will be responsible, built trust, understand and empathize with other's feelings, support spouse's emotional well-being.

5. Patience helps to listen & understand each other. Healthy boundaries lead to healthy marriages.

The Seven Sacred Vows of Unity and Love

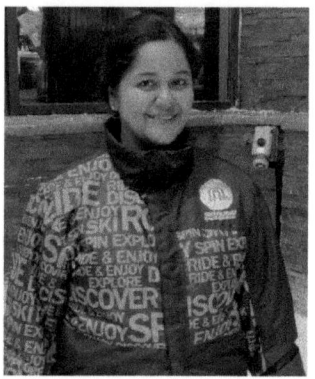

Author's Name	:	Sudha Krishnan
Qualification	:	B.Com.
Current Profession	:	Healer and Handwriting Analyst
Age	:	56 years
E-mail ID	:	**krishnansudha9@gmail.com**
City/ Country	:	**Hyderabad, India**

Sudha Krishnan, originally from Mumbai and now residing in Hyderabad, has 24 years of experience in a Nationalized Bank. She is a Healer and a trained Handwriting Analyst, utilizing her unique skills in handwriting therapy and various healing modalities to help others achieve personal growth and well-being. Sudha is also deeply committed to animal welfare, a passion that began in Tamil Nadu, where she started caring for stray dogs. Now, she dedicates time to feeding and providing medical care for strays in her community.

Sudha balances her professional life with being a mother to two grown-up children and a devoted caregiver to her beloved dog, Cookie.

Keywords : Blissful Marriage, Clear Communication, Gratitude, Partner, Saptapadi

My marriage has made me smarter, stronger and a better human being. My life partner is the most admired and respected person in his industry and I have witnessed his journey from a Senior Manager to an Executive Director through sheer hard work, passion, and dedication.

The comforts and luxuries that come with my partner's success have allowed me to take voluntary retirement from my job when I truly wanted to be at home for myself and my children. This freedom has enabled me to be there for my parents whenever they needed me and to take care of them in every way.

During times when my husband was busy or traveling, I learned to manage the household and handle things independently. We have two lovely children who are now well-educated and have taught me to be cool, calm and independent. Through our journey, I have made wonderful friends who are an important part of my life. They supported me during difficult phases, and now we always cheer ourselves up by recollecting our past and celebrating how strong we have emerged.

My experiences in marriage have taught me to be grateful for what I have rather than complain about what I do not. I have learned the value of gratitude, writing affirmations, manifestation and the law of attraction. This growth has made me happy, content and able to love myself for who I am.

Strengthening my bond with my creator has been another significant outcome of my marriage. During tough days, a dear friend and colleague introduced me to a Saint who taught me to be a giver of love rather than a beggar of love. I came to understand the 'Power' above all of us and the importance and beauty of surrendering and doing my duty without attachment to the results.

Starting my journey as a wife, I was a weak, immature, innocent girl. Over the years, the experiences and learnings have made me responsible, smart, forgiving, more loving, and more connected to the supreme power and all living beings. Welcoming a stray dog into our family, who has become a best friend and an important member of our household, has deepened my love for animals and brought joy to our lives.

Independence, strength and taking charge of everything are qualities I have developed through my marriage. I learned to ask for help from others outside our family, be there for them when they needed me, and feel safe and secure in my own way. Paying attention to important things and aiming and thinking big, rather than being held up by small hurts and misunderstandings, has been a valuable lesson. Realizing that my negative emotions were blocking my growth has been a blessing for my personal development.

Clear communication, gratitude, trust, forgiveness, couple time, compromise, commitment, and romance are all keys to a blissful marriage, but these cannot always be present in every marriage, every moment. That doesn't mean marriage has become a curse.

Whenever I felt a lack of something, I cried, fought, felt bad, shared with my close friends and parents, heard their perspectives, done some introspection, and then healed myself, sometimes talking it out with my family and other times silently. When the pattern kept repeating, I took mind power sessions, worked on myself, and emerged brighter and stronger.

After all these years, sharing, learnings, and healing sessions, I understood that whatever condition I am in is my own creation, attraction, and responsibility. I realized that the change has to come within me. It's up to me to feel happy or keep sulking, take responsibility and become powerful, or blame others and keep playing the victim. I can call my marriage bliss and work to make it blissful, or call it a curse and give up on myself and my family.

Therefore, I proudly declare that my marriage is a bliss and to keep it so, I will always be blissful. I will maintain positive body language, always vibrate at a high frequency and work on my feelings, thoughts, beliefs and actions, because words have power and I want mine to be always positive and powerful.

|| ॐ ||

Union of Two Souls Embracing Each Other's Imperfections

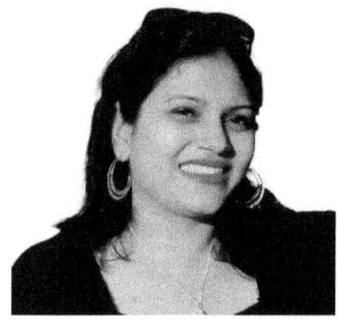

Author's Name	:	Suvigya Seraphim Raj
Qualification	:	MBA (Human Resources and Marketing)
Current Profession	:	Sr. HR Consultant/ Talent Advisor
Age	:	42 years
E-mail ID	:	**contactsr21@gmail.com**
City/ Country	:	**Toronto, Cañada**

Suvigya Seraphim Raj is a Sr. HR Consultant working with a top US global recruitment process outsourcing company. She holds a Master's Degrees in Business Administration from Mount Carmel Institute of Management, Bangalore, India. She is deeply committed to helping clients discover top IT/ Engineering professionals for consulting engagements. Her unwavering dedication revolves around the genuine well-being and success of both consultants and clients alike.

Keywords : Love, Realisation, Values, Understanding, Embracing

"Marriage, a timeless institution, is the beautiful journey of two lives woven together, each thread representing shared dreams, laughter, and the promise of tomorrow. It is not just a contract; it's a shared adventure where love is the compass, understanding is the map, and trust is the guiding star."

I have been married to my husband Manish Raj for 17 years and it was arranged by our respective parents. When I met him for the first time, I felt that we both had a basic thing in common (family love). He was simple decent and pure hearted soul (still holds true till now with a lot more additions).

I've learned that when we come into marriage, we all have our own expectations and ideas about how the ideal marriage should work. We all want the same thing—a good marriage, a happy marriage, a lasting and fulfilling marriage—but we have different ideas on what gets us there.

One person even said there is no ideal marriage, but "adventurous experiments."

My husband and I didn't really talk about this before we got married, and it was years into our marriage before we began to do so. We got married and just went on expecting things to end up "happily ever after" because that's what we both wanted, even though we didn't discuss it. Nope, didn't happen.

We soon began to realize the things I thought were most important and essential for our marriage to work weren't always the things he saw. After plenty of mistakes, many frustrations, and much counsel we began to grow in this area and eventually learned what made it possible for us to have that good, happy, lasting and fulfilling marriage.

In the spirit of reflection, I thought it'd be special to sum up the lessons I've learned in our marriage that I think can apply to any partnership. I really enjoyed reflecting on this, and it made me realize just how much my husband and I have grown together in these years.

In the face of inevitable challenges, your values are your compass. When I think about the challenges that popped up in our marriage, our values are what guided us and helped us find our footing.

It's important to both of us that we can do what we want, and we know our trust is what makes that possible. And because we both value independence, we encourage it in each other.

Both of us work to become better today than we were yesterday. We are passionate about growing as people and about growing our impact and our careers.

I think about how many times the transition felt so daunting to me and how Manish encouraged me to step outside of my comfort zone and chase the thing my heart was calling me to do. I was always anxious about settling in the new country (Canada) and adapting to the new environment and culture. I honestly don't think I would have had the courage to go for it—and to *keep* going for it—if it weren't for his support. It's become very clear where his strengths are and where mine are not and at some point, when my strengths come in, *I* can carry us.

My point is that there are things that are important to discuss and work through, and there are things that you choose to accept and embrace. The more that I understand the areas where I need to grow and the more, I work on those areas, the more beneficial it is for our marriage.

Acceptance is a powerful pillar of marriage and lays the foundation of a happy marriage. Unless you practice acceptance, your relationship will seem unfulfilling to you.

Usually, apologies are taken as a sign of failure or acceptance of failure. In the marriage, it is a crucial pillar of a happy and successful marriage. It establishes that you care for the relationship more than your ego.

"Throughout the course of the marriage, the couple grows, learns, and evolves. When you live with the person, they uncover us to various perspectives we otherwise remain unaware of. We grow with our relationships and these lessons of marriage help us evolve better and handle relationships well."

|| ॐ ||

Children vs Marriage Wed-Lock

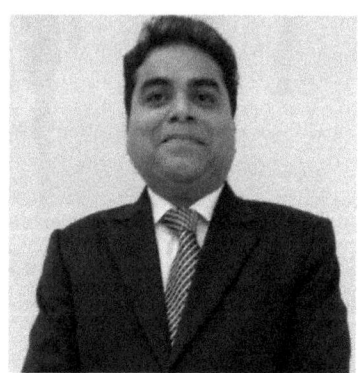

Author's Name	:	Suyog Patil
Qualification	:	Bachelor Degree in Science, M.B.A.
Current Profession	:	Entrepreneur and Consultant
Age	:	48 years
E-mail ID	:	**suyog_p2@rediffmail.com**
City/ Country	:	**Mumbai, India**

Suyog Patil is an Entrepreneur, Consultant, Graphologist, Face Reader, Angel Therapist, Akashic Reader and a Writer. He has done his Graduation in Science and Masters in Business Management. He has worked for 22 years in Seven Companies including Corporates like Pidilite and MNC's. He is a Partner with Ariel Engineering and Technologies and Proprietor of Standard Vacuum Industries.

Suyog's Father and Grandfather had their own Photo Studios, but His Passion since Childhood was to join The Indian Airforce, but couldn't make it and opted for his second carrier choice of completing Masters in Business Management. Had decided to get into full time Business only after gaining sufficient Rich Work Experience and designated his carrier in that Path.

He is a Happy, Joyful Person who believes in Spirituality and Practices the same.

Keywords : Bonding, Marriage, Trust, Differences, Communication

Marriage is not just a Bonding of Male and Female couples but it is a Bonding between Two Families. It is a new relationship development between Groom's Family members and Bride's Family members. Marriage is an institution which is governed by certain Rules and Regulations which every Couple needs to follow for a Successful Married Life. Marriage involves adjustment not only for Bride and Groom but also for Bride's and Groom's families, Groom but also for Bride's and Groom's Family. Deep understanding is required by all during the arise of a Situations. Husband and Wife should be given full freedom to resolve the issues and challenges they face without interference by both Parents. In many cases interference by either Parents in Situations leads to turmoil in Married Life and Strained Relations between Couple. Only if the issue or Situation goes out of control than the interference of Parents is required to some extent and should avoid the blame game.

This is the real story of one of my close friends. He was not getting a proper bride as his Horoscope was getting rejected. He got married almost 5 years of searching through a newspaper advertisement. He and his Parents agreed to go ahead as he was fair and handsome and the girl was fair and beautiful and parents looked cultured as per their behaviour. Immediately after marriage my friend and his family members were suspicious with Bride's behaviour relating with her mental health. Moreover, she used to go to her parent's house almost every weekend and used to join her office directly on Monday Morning though her office was hardly 5 mins walking from her In-Laws house. Due to her conditions, there was a continuous interference of her parents in the married life and with their influence she started ill, treating her husband and mother-in-law as she was guided by her parents to take control of entire finances and property of the boy's family. She used to casually inquire about investments and Gold ornaments.

After few months, in the due course of married life, the bride became pregnant and her parents insisted to take her to their known Gynaecologist. Shortly my Friend and his Father accompanied her to the Gynaecologist and as per her demand dropped her at her parent's house as she insisted on resting on weekend. Next day some complications were developed in her health and she continued to stay with her parents for better care during the pregnancy period.

After 8-1/2 months a baby was born and after the birth, she refused to return back to stay with her husband. My Friend had a heated argument with his Wife and In-laws at their home as they too were not ready to send her back and my friend tried to resolve the issue through her relatives and his family- friends, which went in wain so he convinced his wife that they should visit a professional marriage consultant, who was a qualified Psychiatrist. They completed all the sittings with the Psychiatrist, who advised and concluded that both should stay together in Groom's parents' house and should visit him again after six months. But she did not follow the counselor's advice. The counselor told he will not discuss the case, either Parents, Relatives or Family-Friends involved, but surprisingly after receipt of Psychological reports, he had a closed door discussion with bride's parents. During this discussion my friend entered the discussion room as he required a diaper for their baby. To his surprise, he saw 2 prescriptions written by the Psychiatrist on the table. The Psychiatrist hide the 2 prescription papers from my friend and asked him to take the diaper bag and immediately leave his discussion room. As recommendations by elders and family friends, my friend insisted the Psychiatrist to hand over him his wife's Psychological reports to which the Psychiatrist refused to hand over.

My friend was hoping the situation will improve, but after some years, surprisingly, he got a message from one of his In-laws friend to agree for a Divorce with mutual consent followed by huge alimony in crore or else all of them would be framed in false criminal case. My friend and his parents could not meet the undue demand, so they were framed in false criminal case followed by a divorce notice. My friend and his parents were acquitted by The Hon. Court against all the criminal charges as they had strong evidence and for divorce, they had to take a loan to settle the Divorce Petition.

As per my understanding and opinion, this marriage took place between a Matured Groom and Immature Bride. The bride's parent lacked maturing, as they did not implement the advice of their relatives and counselor to send their daughter back to her In-laws house. It seems that due to some mental health issues the parents of the bride did not have much control on her behaviour. My friend and his parents' mistake was that they neither involved any relatives or family-friend, while arranging the marriage, nor did they take any effort to find the details about the bride and her family. Also my friend and his parents were not able to handle the aroused situation on their own and involved their relatives and family-friends in that critical matter only after things went out of control.

As per my understanding the approach to resolve the issue by my friend and his parents was not as per requirement to handle immature parents of a bride with some mental issues. On the contrary my friend had a dirty fight with his in-laws, which made the matter worst. The communication between parents of **Groom and Bride** came to a halt after the bride started staying with her parents. During this period there aroused a misunderstanding, between both the families and more-over the bride's parents in their egoistic approach wanted the groom's parents to ask them how long will the bride be staying with them.

Never take Marriage lightly. Any triggers after Marriage should not be kept hanging and should be sorted out amicably by keeping ego aside in Desired Time Frame. The communication is very important for a married life to survive and grow. If the communication between the couple comes to a halt than there are chances of the married life going into turmoil. Before fixing a **Marriage**, apart from **Horoscope**, it is also important to find out the **History** of Groom and/ or Bride and their family. During final meeting of fixing a marriage it is important to involve qualified and/ or experienced relatives and/ or family-friends. All terms and conditions of marriage should be finalised during Final Meeting/ Talk. The children born out from Marriage Wed-lock should not be the sufferer for others deed.

If differences arise in a Married Life Path,

Children should not be the Sufferer.

|| ॐ ||

A Bliss or Burden?

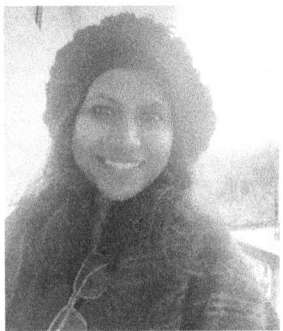

Author's Name	:	Tanvee Kakati
Qualification	:	M.A. (Sociology) Visharad in Vocals, NLP, Ho'oponopono healing, LOA and Energy Coaching, CBT, Happiness coach, Reiki, Mental Health counseling, Meditation Teacher
Current Profession	:	Consultant, Energy coach and Singer
Age	:	35 years
E-mail ID	:	**harmonywithtanvee@gmail.com**
City/ Country	:	**Guwahati, India**

Tanvee Kakati, originally from Guwahati, Assam, is rooted in a culturally rich family of artists. She graduated in sociology from the prestigious Hindu College and the Delhi School of Economics, University of Delhi. She has also cleared the UGC- NET and has been invited as guest speaker in colleges. With nearly a decade of experience, Tanvee has worked as a researcher, consultant and program manager on social impact projects for esteemed non-profit organisations and research institutions like MIT (USA) and the University of Surrey. She has led initiatives funded by organizations such as UNDP, the US Embassy, DFID. etc in some renowned organisations. Additionally, Tanvee is a passionate trained singer, with her regional songs featured on AIR Guwahati.

Besides this, her love for human development has guided her to specialize in positive psychology and energy healing, utilizing techniques like CBT, reiki and NLP. She has studied under notable teachers, including Eckhart Tolle and Deepak Chopra. Currently, she is pursuing mind and energy coaching, believing that life is an art. An avid traveller, Tanvee views the world as her home and seeks spiritual growth through her journeys.

Keywords : Choice, Independence, Spiritual, Perception, Inner work

Is marriage a blessing or a burden? This question has lingered in my mind, much like the saying, "Shaadi ka laddoo: jo khaye pachtaaye, joh na khaaye woh bhi pachtaaye."

As a grown woman, I reflect on my teenage dreams of love and family, inspired by Hindi romantic movies. I once believed I would marry "THE ONE AND ONLY" for a happily ever after, but reality proved more complex. While romance can be fleeting, marriage extends beyond romanticism.

In this article, I'll share my perspective on marriage based on my studies and experiences.

As stated in Sociology, marriage emerged as a social institution to create order in the society. French ethnographer Arnold Van Gennep described it as a significant "rite of passage". Yet, this sacred practice is now often questioned: Why marry at all?

Through my work with women in India and globally, I found many feel trapped in roles that diminish their value. Many women married out of limited choices or not knowing any better, asking, "Agar itna aata toh shadi karti kya?" Today, as women seek financial independence, they ask, "Why should I depend on anyone?" This shift invites us to reconsider the purpose of marriage in contemporary life.

As we navigate these complexities, I reached out to my esteemed spiritual teachers Eckhart Tolle and Kim Eng, to get more clarity. Eckhart, in many of his books, emphasizes that we marry not just for joy, but for growth. When I asked this to Kim Eng, she share her view on marriage as a spiral of ascents and descents, that allows us to reach new heights in our spiritual evolution.

In spiritual terms, the world is a mirror and our partners reflect the hidden, unaccepted parts and limiting beliefs within us. By embracing the idea that our partners are mirrors of ourselves, we can transform marriage into a profound journey. While it may be daunting, this exploration can lead to lasting bliss, revealing marriage as both a blessing and a challenge.

How to experience the bliss?

To experience bliss in marriage, we must shift our focus inward rather than fixating on perceived flaws or actions. Ask ourselves what aspects of our own being is our partner may be reflecting? This introspective approach can transform struggle into harmony. Awaken to the divine within us; clean the metaphorical mirror to gain clarity and discover the richness inside. This journey mirrors the spiritual union of Shiva and Shakti, balancing masculine and feminine energies within us all. Embracing both aspects of ourself , shifting perception, can foster deeper connections and genuine love.

Hence, I can say that marriage can prove to be both bliss and curse, mainly with the following poetic comparison:

Marriage is bliss when it feels like a choice,
A curse when seen as a rule with no voice.

It's bliss when "we" stand hand in hand,
A curse when "me" and "you" struggle to understand.

Bliss arises from shared challenges faced,
A curse when hearts feel out of place.

It's bliss in warmth, respect, and grace,
A curse when it is competition and a race.

Marriage teaches worth and the need to appreciate,
It shows us how to cooperate, navigate, and create.

Marriage teaches awareness, a journey to share,
Together we grow, learning to truly care.

Today, the traditional view of marriage as essential is losing its validity. Instead, marriage should be a conscious choice rooted in self-awareness and inner work. As we evolve, shifting our focus inward allows us to appreciate our duality, finding bliss in understanding both our light and shadow. Embracing these aspects fosters deeper connections and authentic love. This journey reflects the spiritual union of Shiva and Shakti, balancing the masculine and feminine energies within us, aligning with universal laws. Ultimately, meaningful relationships arise not from obligation but from a genuine desire to connect and grow together.

By accepting our shared humanity, we enhance our relationships—not through asceticism, but by recognizing life's duality of joy and sorrow. The choice to awaken and embrace this truth leads to lasting bliss. Ultimately, we must ask ourselves: what aspects are we willing to embrace, and what will we choose?

When two people are willing to play their parts and take 100% responsibility, that's the deciding factor. That's when marriage can be a bliss.

So, do you choose bliss or curse?

|| ॐ ||

From Despair to Healing : Embracing Obstacles as Blessing

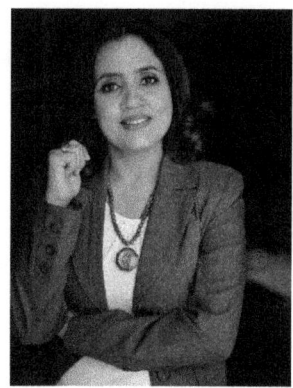

Author's Name	:	Tejjal Bhanshalii
Qualification	:	Nutritionist 20 Yrs Practice
Current Profession	:	Psychic and Holistic Healer
Age	:	42 Years
E-mail ID	:	**tejuritu5454@gmail.com**
City/ Country	:	**New Delhi, India**

Tejjal Bhanshalii is a passionate advocate of holistic healing through a variety of modalities. Her practice encompasses Access Bars, intuitive healing and distance healing, each designed to dissolve energy blockages and foster mental clarity. She specializes in chakra balancing and aura cleansing, essential for maintaining energetic harmony and vitality. Through talk therapy and word energy techniques, She facilitates emotional release and mental well-being, guiding individuals towards inner peace and resilience.

Tejjal's mission is to empower individuals on their healing journeys, helping them discover the interconnectedness of mind, body, and spirit. With compassion and expertise, She strives to create a supportive environment, where healing and self-discovery flourish.

Keywords : Blessing, Healing, Holistic, Journey, Obstacles

From Despair to Healing: Embracing Obstacles as Blessings

"How My Journey from the Brink of Suicide Led Me to Heal Others"

Life often throws unexpected challenges our way and how we perceive and respond to these challenges can shape our destiny. This is a story of a journey from the brink of despair to a place of healing and hope. It is about overcoming obstacles, not by avoiding them, but by embracing them as blessings in disguise. My story is one of transformation—from contemplating suicide to becoming a holistic healer, who now helps others find the light within their darkness. There was a time when life felt unbearably heavy. The weight of my struggles, compounded by the overwhelming sense of failure, pushed me to the edge. I stood at the precipice, ready to give up. Suicide seemed like the only escape from the relentless pain. But in that darkest moment, a small, inexplicable spark of hope flickered within me. It whispered, "This is not the end." I began to see my obstacles not as curses, but as opportunities for growth. Each challenge, each painful experience, became a lesson—a stepping stone on my path to self-discovery. The more I embraced my struggles, the more I realized that they were shaping me into the person I was meant to become. Instead of being consumed by despair, I allowed myself to feel the pain, to understand it and ultimately, to transform it. My healing journey was not easy. It required me to confront my deepest fears, to forgive myself and to rebuild my life from the ground up. But through this process, I discovered the power of holistic healing—an approach that nurtures the mind, body and spirit. As I healed, I felt a profound calling to help others who were suffering as I once had. Today, I am a holistic healer, guiding others through their own journeys of transformation. I have turned my pain into purpose and my despair into a source of strength. I believe that every obstacle we face is a blessing in disguise, a chance to grow, evolve and ultimately, to help others heal

The idea that obstacles can be blessings resonates deeply with me. It is a concept that has not only saved my life, but has also given me the strength to save others. My journey from the brink of suicide to becoming a holistic healer is a testament to the power of perspective. When we choose to see our challenges as opportunities, we unlock a path to healing and growth that we never thought possible.

Life's challenges are inevitable, but how we respond to them is within our control. By embracing our obstacles as blessings, we can transform our lives and the lives of those around us. My journey is a living proof that even in our darkest moments, there is hope. And with that hope, we can heal, grow and help others do the same.

Arranged Marriage: An Unexpected Recipe for My Life
My Journey in a Nutshell with my Ever Smiling Spouse

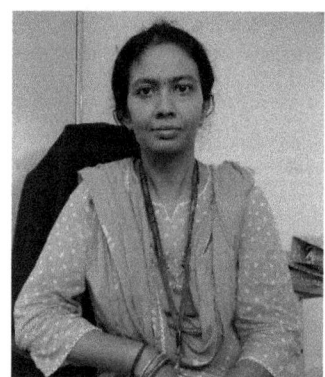

Author's Name	:	Trina Kanungo
Qualification	:	M.Sc. (Maths & Computing-IIT Dhanbad)
Current Profession	:	Scale 2 Officer, ECGC Ltd, under Ministry of Commerce
Age	:	31 years
E-mail ID	:	…
City/ Country	:	**Mumbai, India**

Trina Kanungo, hailing from Hind Motor, West Bengal, a Postgraduate in Mathematics and Computing from IIT Dhanbad, currently serves as an Assistant Manager (Scale 2 Officer) at ECGC Ltd. in Mumbai, under the Ministry of Commerce and Industry, Government of India. Beyond her professional role, Trina's passions lie in Indian Fine Arts, Yoga and Literature.

Trina's literary contributions shine brightly, being a co-author of numerous anthologies in English and Bengali literature. Her literary prowess has been recognized through multiple awards and accolades. She has been awareded Honorary Doctorate on "Peace and Meditation" by the Grace Ladies Global Academy , USA, in the year 2022 for her tireless contribution to the society towards fitness goals through yoga and meditation.

Keywords : Arranged Marriage, Adjustment, Dependence, Trust, Unconditional Love

Arranged marriage, a cultural practice in many societies, involves families selecting spouses for their children based on various factors like compatibility, social status, and family ties. While it may lack the romantic allure of love marriages, proponents argue that it fosters stability, respect for tradition, and familial harmony.

Today, our generation is actually afraid of arranged marriages. But I was determined to go for arranged marriage, as I had complete faith on myself.

On 17th of January 2020, I legally and socially executed my marriage process with my better half and ultimately stepped into the "Married Club". So this narration is basically my own journey.

Right after our marriage, I realised that during courtship period, the interaction which I had with my parent-in-laws was so useful. You get to know about their lifestyles and get used to it automatically, and vice versa too, they also get to know about your lifestyle.

My husband is a Research Officer (Grade B, Economics Cadre) in Reserve Bank of India. He was then struggling with his PhD. thesis submission on one side and his office assignments on the other side and it was a tough time for him. Right after marriage, we went to Andaman for a vacation. There I got to know that he is a pure travel soul, has a great hunger for historic research, whatever he explores. After we returned to Mumbai and joined our respective offices, something worse was waiting for us. On March 22, 2020, national lockdown was declared by Government of India, due to the deadly COVID-19 attack and our life was shattered. Our family got stuck in Kolkata. both of us were in Mumbai. Covid-19 had brought frightening disaster to every family, our family members too got infected. Some got admitted to hospitals in Kolkata. During the second, third and fourth wave, my husband got tested positive thrice consecutively. Basically, COVID-19 trauma brought stress and adversity to everyone's life, but I strongly believe, it was this phase that both of us developed that strong bonding and trust between us. During this Covid adversity he completed his PhD. He carried out his office assignments, he received the prefix title "Dr." before his name and honestly, the journey was marvellous. Due to the struggles that were faced, we became inseparable soul mates today. We cannot imagine life today without each other.

During that phase, we have fought together, we have seen food crisis in Mumbai, we had cash in hand but no food to have. We had embraced each other and confronted every crisis. We had shared a single meal box together, took strolls together, he learnt to chop vegetable for me, as I used to cook our meals during lockdown. At times, I used to feel low, but he became my strength and stood by me that actually helped me march ahead and overcome all hardships in our married life.

Today mostly relationships break due to ego clash. For me, I always try to disallow ego from entering our relationship. Both of us are different individuals. We both have different views for life and that complements our lives. We both try to nullify the negative force that comes in our ways. We are transparent to each other. I have always been an introvert person, but when it comes to my spouse, I am always open to him. Marriage is a journey and not a competition. So completion of this journey is vital.

For me, my marriage is undoubtedly a boon. I am blessed with such a talented and honest person, who understands me every time without any expectation. His smile always provides a positive vibe to my struggles and I move ahead with courage to face my hardships with ease. Trust, Love, Reliability, Dependence, Honesty and Friendship is what makes my marriage the biggest blessing in my life, with my husband, my best half, my smiling Economist, Dr. Ranajoy Guha Neogi, PhD, M.Sc. Economics, ISI Kolkata. I am blessed to be his spouse, and by God's grace, we wish to live every minute of this journey called *"MARRIAGE"* together till infinity and eternity.

|| ॐ ||

Essential Base of Life and Happiness

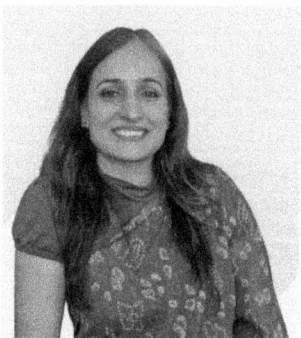

Author's Name	:	Uman Hooda
Qualification	:	M.C.A.
Current Profession	:	Microsoft Corporate Trainer and Consultant, Motivational speaker
Age	:	43 years
E-mail ID	:	**uman.kumari@gmail.com**
City/ Country	:	**Gurugram, India**

Uman Hooda is a Microsoft Certified Trainer (MCT) & Microsoft Certified Data Analyst. She has experience of working with Power BI, Power Platform, MS Dynamics and Azure. She has trained professionals and done consultancy projects around the globe.

She has previously worked as a Software Quality Analyst in multinational companies. She is a very impressive motivational speaker as well. She has motivated lots of people by listing their problems, doubts and giving some guidance to change and become better at living a happy life with peace.

Keywords: Appreciation, Forgiveness, Honesty, Love, Respect

Marriage—what is it really? Is it essential? What are its fundamental principles? How will my life change once I'm married? How will my partner and their family treat me? What role does marriage play in our lives? These questions frequently arise when we contemplate marriage. Today, many young people are uncertain about the meaning and values of marriage. With both partners often working, there is less time for understanding and communication. We observe a variety of examples around us: some couples are happily married, some are struggling, and some choose not to marry at all. Marriage is a profoundly pure bond in life. It is the core value of both life and family. We should uphold its principles and strive to enrich each other's lives by nurturing a healthy relationship. Happy couples will raise happy children and happy children create a happy world to live in.

The real story is about a couple, Neel and Dolly, both from middle-class families. They grew up in similar environments and closely observed their parents' marriages. Neel firmly believed that a happy marriage is crucial for children's well-being. Dolly, on the other hand, decided at a young age that when she married, she would act maturely, strive to understand her partner, and be happy in all circumstances. She was inspired by observing various married couples in her family and friend circle.

Neel was diligent and worked hard to secure a good job, eventually joining a multinational company. He hoped to marry a confident woman from the same profession. Meanwhile, during her graduation, Dolly's family started looking for a suitable match for her. She convinced them to let her focus on her studies, and they agreed, allowing her to complete her graduation and pursue a master's degree. Dolly was not ready for marriage as she wanted to start her career first, but she couldn't force her parents to wait any longer as they had already given her enough time.

Eventually, Neel and Dolly met for the first time through an arranged marriage setup. Neel wasn't excited about Dolly, though his family approved and left the decision to him. Dolly also hoped that Neel would decline the match, which would buy her more time. They ultimately got married. In the beginning, their relationship was quite formal, as is common in many arranged marriages. Due to Neel's job transfer, they moved to a city far from their hometown. Dolly felt that Neel was very sophisticated, while she saw herself as lacking confidence and not suitable for him. Their conversations were limited, and their relationship remained distant. Dolly didn't want to have kids until they had a strong understanding and bond, and she wanted to secure a job before having children. Their differing expectations led to misunderstandings. At one point, both were unhappy in their marriage, and then Dolly suggested divorce. However, Neel disagreed, emphasizing their commitment to their families and their marriage. This conversation shifted Dolly's perspective, and she began thinking about how they could make their marriage successful. With patience, forgiveness, understanding, and trust, they worked towards improving their relationship. Now, after 18 years of their marriage, they have reached a point where people often ask if they had a love marriage. Their journey wasn't easy, but they believed in themselves and understood the importance of finding happiness in whatever life brings.

In my opinion, marriage is bliss. Marriage provides a lifelong companion with whom you can share everything and face all ups and downs together. The first step is to have understanding and respect for each other. You need to accept each other's good and bad traits, giving space and freedom to each other. Initially, avoid setting big expectations; understand each other's nature and convey your points of view through healthy discussions. Gradually, you will understand each other's expectations. The path isn't easy; you will face hurdles and challenges, but you need to work together to make your marriage successful. If you have both tried everything to make your marriage work and still can't stay together, then, in my opinion, you should separate. If you can't live a happy life together and can't provide a happy environment for your kids and family, it's better to part ways.

For a successful and happy marriage, it is essential to avoid ego and negativity at home. A fulfilling marriage is built on appreciation, forgiveness, honesty, love, respect, understanding, and loyalty. We may not always get everything we want, but it is important to learn to be happy with what we have. While happy marriages are not easy, they are certainly achievable, focus on maintaining a good relationship and finding happiness together.

|| ॐ ||

A Beautiful Journey of Learning

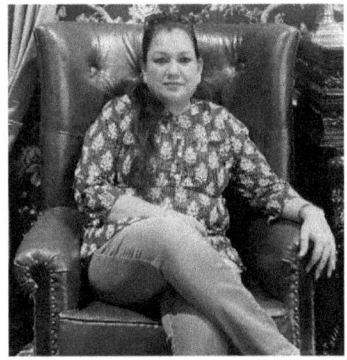

Author's Name	:	Vaishali S Iyer
Qualification	:	M.A. (English Literature)
Current Profession	:	Freelance Interlocutor for Cambridge Exams
Age	:	43 years
E-mail ID	:	**vaishali.s.iyer@gmail.com**
City/ Country	:	**Ahmedabad, India**

Vaishali S Iyer is a homemaker, a Freelancer and a Vastu practitioner. She has rich experience in Human Resources and content writing with more than 10+ years of experience in different domains. She works as a Freelancer for multiple organisations. Along with her Master's degree, she also holds various certifications from Cambridge Language Tests and has certificates from Vastu Shastra, Numerology and many more. Her love towards occult science has inclined her towards learning more about the subject and is still diving deep into other occult modalities.

Keywords : Journey, Belief, Soulmate, Companion, Give & Take

'Life is a journey and becomes more beautiful if you have a companion.'

- **Vaishali S Iyer**

Marriage is a beautiful journey of two souls. Two souls living freely in their lives unaware of where their destiny will take them. But destiny has already decided their future and their union. It is said that marriages are made in heaven and this is true. I feel that we do not cross paths just like that, there's a purpose for meeting people and coming into our lives. My belief became more strong when I met my soulmate – my partner. We were different in many ways, nothing was common between us. He comes from a South Indian family and I come from a Gujarati family. The traditions, rituals, food, language everything is very different. But what reassured us to get married was the understanding for each other and probably the qualities we were looking for in an ideal partner.

We usually forget that it is not just two people who are responsible for making a marriage successful, there are other members involved too. It's not just two of you, but two families are involved when you tie a knot. We tend to forget that, and that's where all problems arise. Situations change and so do people. Things are not always the same as you expect. Once you get married, there are more and more expectations from you; unfortunately, you have to stand by that and if you fail to do so, you're constantly being judged and criticised. As time passes, with that comes more and more responsibilities. At this stage of life, more understanding is required from both individuals. A couple must understand each other in difficult times and stand by each other's side whenever needed. After all, both are humans and need love and support in tough times.

Here, I would like to emphasise knowing/understanding your partner's concerns and addressing them unbiasedly. We as humans get carried away with the emotions of our parents/relatives and sometimes take harsh decisions or have arguments with our partner, just because our parents/relatives don't like it. That's wrong! Things become worse when we try to please everyone. We cannot please everyone at every stage. Our commitment towards the relationship should be more than just pleasing. Marriage is not just about expanding your family by having a spouse and kids. It's much more than that. A lot of emotional and mental support is required by both partners. A lot of cooperation and understanding is required from other family members also, but usually, it does not happen (especially in Indian families). Families in which elders and other family members are understanding and supportive, these couples will generally counter fewer issues than others.

My Journey:

When I look back, I find that there were a lot of struggles which we as a couple went through. Emotionally, mentally and financially had turbulence in life. The challenges we faced in relationships due to different cultures were tearing us apart. But we sailed through it with courage and patience. There were times when we felt that it was enough and we couldn't move further, but then we thought it was always easy to quit. But it takes more courage to stay together and face the challenges that life throws at you. Eventually, we discovered that "letting go", keeping our egos aside and just being calm when the other person is furious worked well.

Staying calm most of the time helps to figure out the real cause of the problem, it also helps to solve the problem healthily. Basically, what life taught us in these many years is to "let go", have "patience", last but not least "love and respect" for each other.

Who will stay with you?

When we come into this world we have a family – mother, father, brother, sister and then we have spouse and kids. At one point in time, everyone goes away. Parents as they age are no longer with us. Siblings have their own family and their own life. After a certain number of years, even the children have their own family and live their lives.

The person who stays with you till your old age is your spouse, taking care of you in your good and bad times, looking after you when you are unwell. Remember, your partner will always remain by your side in good and bad times, your highs and lows. We should always be grateful for having them and value our partners as they are the only ones who will be there for us always.

Take Away:

My advice to the young generation is, do not fall for flashy lifestyle, money, power or beauty. Look for a true companion, a true company with whom you would love to spend your precious life. Discuss your expectations and your beliefs, your future plans/goals before you get married, this will allow you to understand each other in a better way. Marriage is a give-and-take relationship where you have to give more and take less. Life is much better when you have someone to walk with you in this beautiful journey called "marriage". My marriage is bliss. It is a blessing in disguise, as it changed my whole perspective towards life.

"The greatest marriages are built on teamwork, mutual respect, a healthy dose of admiration and a never-ending portion of love and grace."

— Fawn Weaver

|| ॐ ||

Marriage : The Gamble of Love

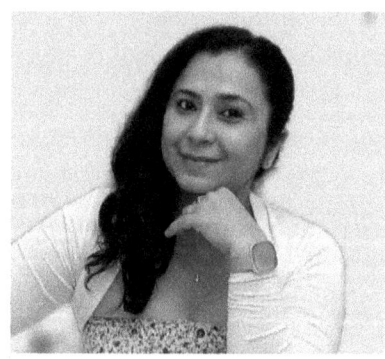

Author's Name	:	Veena Chugh
Qualification	:	B.Com, MBA
Current Profession	:	Author, Coach, Public Speaker & Entrepreneur
Age	:	46 years
E-mail ID	:	**chugh.veena@gmail.com**
City/ Country	:	**United States of America**

Veena Chugh is a multifaceted professional with a deep passion for personal growth and storytelling. She is the author of A Pink Rose and Other Short Stories, a collection inspired by her spiritual journey and reflections on life. With two decades of corporate leadership experience, including roles as Head of HR, Veena has guided teams with her expertise in organizational strategy and people development.

In addition to her corporate career, she is a certified yoga instructor and coach, promoting holistic practices for mental health and personal well-being. Veena is the founder of Arthaa Advisors, a consulting firm specializing in wealth planning and legacy management.

Residing in Conshohocken, Pennsylvania, with her husband and son, Veena draws from her life experiences to write compelling narratives and share insights through public speaking engagements. Her work reflects her belief in resilience, growth, and the power of second chances.

Keywords : Awareness, Growth, Honesty, Marriage, Relationships

Marriage is often romanticized as a sacred bond, a seamless merging of souls. But for me, it was a dice roll—an uncertain gamble. My first marriage was fleeting, lasting only a few months. The promises of eternity dissolved, leaving me adrift in heartbreak and self-doubt. Yet, from this pain, I emerged stronger and wiser.

The support of my family became my anchor, urging me to risk love again. When I met my current husband on a matrimonial site, something in me hesitated, but his kindness and honesty broke through my reservations. With him, I chose to take a leap of faith, a gamble that has brought me the joy I once thought I'd lost forever.

My first marriage was a storm that I never saw coming. Our promises unravelled in months, leaving me grappling with questions I couldn't answer: *Was it my fault? Did I not know myself enough to choose wisely?* Divorce is a heavy word, a heavier reality, and in those days, it felt like an unbearable weight.

The end of that marriage wasn't just the end of a relationship; it was the beginning of my reckoning. I looked in the mirror and saw not failure but opportunity. Slowly, I began to sift through my wounds, finding lessons amidst the pain.

My family—my brother and mother—played a pivotal role. They saw the spark in me that I had forgotten and urged me to trust again. With their support, I took the unlikely step of signing up on a matrimonial site. There, I met the man who would change the course of my life.

His kindness wasn't grand or showy; it was in the small things—the way he listened, his quiet honesty, the consistency in his actions. In a world that felt chaotic, he was calm and steady. Our courtship wasn't without its moments of uncertainty; after all, love is never a sure bet. But something about him told me that this gamble was worth it.

This second chance at love wasn't just about finding the right partner; it was about becoming the right partner. Marriage is a reflection—of your fears, your strengths, your willingness to grow. It is not the easy romance of songs and fairy tales. It is work, often hard and unrelenting, but deeply rewarding when both partners are willing to grow together.

With my husband, I've found a relationship built on respect, honesty and shared dreams. We don't gamble with each other; instead, we take calculated risks for our family, our community, and the legacy we want to leave behind.

In my understanding, marriage is neither a guaranteed jackpot nor a game rigged against us. It is what we make of it—an intricate dance between love and effort. My second marriage taught me that the success of this gamble depends on honesty, communication, and a willingness to confront our own imperfections.

For arranged marriages, especially prevalent in the Indian context, I believe that investing six months to a year in building understanding is essential. No facade can last that long. This period allows couples to discover the depths of each other, avoiding the heartache and stigma of a hasty union or a rushed divorce.

Time and patience are the keys to nurturing any relationship. Marriage becomes blissful when both partners are willing to invest not just in each other but in the growth and evolution of the relationship itself.

Marriage is at its core, an act of faith. It is a gamble, yes, but one that can lead to immense joy when approached with integrity and self-awareness. My journey from heartbreak to happiness showed me that marriage isn't about perfection; it's about persistence.

In the end, love's gamble is not about winning or losing—it's about the courage to roll the dice, to take the chance, and to grow through the experience. Today, I am grateful for the second chance that brought me to a fulfilling partnership. It's not the end of the game but a beautiful continuation of life's unfolding story.

॥ ॐ ॥

A Journey of Efforts and Blessings
A Blissful Lifelong Partnership

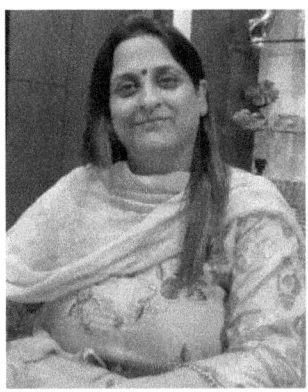

Author's Name	:	Veenu Mehendiratta
Qualification	:	Graduate
Current Profession	:	Occultist (veenumero)
Age	:	45 years
E-mail ID	:	**veenumero@gmail.com**
City/ Country	:	**Gwalior, India**

Mrs. Veenu Mehendiratta is an Occultist by passion and profession. She is a Numerologist, Tarot Card Reader, Dowsing Expert, Fortune Teller by Dice, Switch Words and Healing Codes Master. Have an expertise over Mind Money Mastery, a certified Life Coach and a Reiki Grand Master. From being a teacher turned into an industrialist, then from there, she moved towards being a home maker and devoted her time in growing kids and now at this phase, she has started her journey of being an Occultist. She always believes that whenever a person approaches any Occult practitioner, he or she is looking for the guidance and consider us the mediator that whatever we are going to tell him is the message from universe for him/ her, So, She always believes in showing the right and positive path to the native.

Mrs. Veenu feels blessed as universe has chosen her for the same.

Keywords : Compassion, Love, Support, Togetherness, Trust

Once I read marriage is a bliss for man and curse for a woman.. ohh! Is it? I would like to reframe the statement as *"Marriage is a mix of joy and challenges for everyone, regardless of gender."* It's a beautiful journey, where both the partner's efforts can make it fulfilling. No couple is perfect and accepting each other's flaws works like a magical ingredient of a successful marriage. Instead of focusing on imperfections, try to nurture your relationship. There's no rulebook for a blissful marriage, but putting in efforts can make it wonderful. Marriage is an album of both good and bad times. To ensure that good times outnumber the bad, avoid involving others in your conflicts. Resolving issues together is essential, and it's important to listen to your partner's emotional needs rather than imposing your own decisions. I strongly believe we have the power to decide how our marriage turns out—whether it becomes a happy, fulfilling life or a difficult experience."

"My marriage has been a mix of joy and challenges and making it truly blissful has been tough for both of us. The reality is, no marriage is perfect, including ours. We've had our share of fights and regrets, but it's been a blend of both highs and lows."

"At its heart, marriage is what we make of it and always needs ongoing effort and adjustment. We both had our own challenges and strengths, and there was no set formula for a successful marriage. Each day often started with new arguments and ended with a stack of complaints. I always heard the advice to never go to bed angry, so I tried to resolve our issues each night. There were times when we stayed up late talking, especially since he never admitted being wrong and always thought he was right. It was hard to balance my self-respect with fighting for my emotional needs. Looking back, I think that letting go of my pride actually brought us closer together."

"I was 19 and he was 25 when we got married and getting married at such a young age helped me build a strong bond with him. I was open to adapting and accepted him as the one with more experience and wisdom. Being younger to him made it easier for me to adjust and meet his needs. It was like growing with him to make a solid foundation for our future. However, getting married early also brought challenges, like gaining maturity and life experience.

"Adjusting to a new family was tough. I went from a family of three siblings in a busy city to a big family of a small town with four of his siblings and his parents. Looking back, I see that trying to mediate between my husband and his family was a mistake. He didn't admit his faults and was often blunt, which caused differences with his family. I always appreciated him for who he is, even though he was not sugar coated or great at pretending to be sweet.

Marriage involves connecting with both your spouse and their family. My husband also had to get used to my family, which sometimes made things more complicated. Many of our arguments were about family issues rather than problems between us. It took time to resolve these conflicts and getting him to see his mistakes was hard.

I wanted to keep our arguments private, but it was difficult and at times became embarrassing. Though he was not good at showing affection but was very expressive when he was angry, which made our problems more visible. Looking back, I see that these challenges made me stronger and eventually helped him understand things better. Today, many people focus only on their relationship with their spouse and overlook the importance of getting along with each other's families. Adapting to each other's families is key to a happy marriage."

"Through all the ups and downs, we were blessed with a wonderful daughter and son. By this time, we had become inseparable after facing many challenges together. Having children brought new struggles, from early arguments to learning how to care for them. Dreaming about their future and wanting the best for them helped us grow more mature and responsible.

As time went on, we grew closer, sharing both good and bad times. We laughed and cried together, and enjoyed a period when he was successful and working hard for our family. We had learned to understand and meet each other's emotional needs. However, good times don't last forever, and we faced many difficult moments. We fought most of the time, and our constant fighting started to affect our children.

One thing that stayed the same was that we always slept in the same bedroom, no matter how tough things got. This kept a spark alive between us. Many people think that physical intimacy is the only measure of a successful marriage, but that's not true. A strong marriage is built on emotional connection and how partners support each other every day. It's about sharing responsibilities, offering emotional support, and building a life together with mutual respect and love."

"Reflecting on my 25 years of marriage, I can say it has taken a lot of effort and patience from both of us. We've had many joyful moments as well as challenging times. Despite everything, our commitment to each other has stayed strong. Difficult times, even the very tough ones, actually helped us build a stronger relationship. There were times when it was just the two of us facing challenges together, and we had no one else to rely on.

We also had conflicts with our families, the bond had weakened over time which was very hard. When happy times end, it ends with collateral damage and so as ours which took all our siblings and families emotionally away. During a particularly tough period, my husband fell into severe depression and needed treatment. Through it all, we were each other's main support.

Our marriage has been a mix of good times, bad times, hurdles, love, romance, and arguments. It was like a platter with many different elements, and we had to decide what to focus on. With each passing day, we grew closer and developed a deep love for each other—not just the romantic kind, but a love of being truly incomplete without one another. I'm proud to say that with all our efforts, we've made our marriage a joyful and lasting journey."

In conclusion, marriage is a complex relationship that can be both wonderful and challenging. It requires effort, patience, and mutual respect. Whether it feels great or tough at times, how we handle and care for the relationship makes a big difference. Trust is essential for a successful marriage. Without trust, it's hard to have a healthy and fulfilling relationship. It's not just about believing in your partner but also about being confident in each other's support and understanding.

Maintaining a strong bond takes care and attention. It's not just about big gestures but also the small, everyday actions that show love and commitment. Both partners need to be dedicated to making the relationship work, and this dedication should be shown through their actions and attitudes.

This year we celebrated our **Silver Jubilee** and I'm sharing some lines, which I had written for him :

तुम्हारे साथ शादी को बीत गये यु पच्चीस साल

लो आज तुम्हें बताती हूँ अपने दिल का हाल

मेरे नाम की माला जपते हो

अपना हर काम मुझसे करवाते हो

वीनू वीनू वीनू, तुम्हारी आवाज़ पे चिड़ जाती हूँ

पर मन ही मन इठलाती हूँ

कि मेरे बग़ैर तुम्हारा एक पत्ता नहीं हिल सकता

और इन्ही तानो बानो से चलता है हमारा रिश्ता

पतझड़ सावन बसंत बहार

यु तो होते है मौसम चार

हम दोनों ने देखे हैं

बदलते वक़्त के मौसम कई बार

मुझे गर्व है की हर बार हुई तुम्हारी जीत है

और यही तो हम दोनों के प्यार की असली प्रीत है

क्यूँ सोचते हो क्यूँ घबराते हो

कभी कभी मुझे भी डरा देते हो

पर ये मत भूलो जानेमन

वी हैव बेस्ट डॉटर एंड सन

और यही दोनों है हमारा असली धन

माना के दौर बुरा है

देखना ये भी बीत जाएगा

जाते जाते हम दोनों को

और मज़बूत बना जाएगा

मुझे नहीं परवाह कोई क्या कहता है

में तो इतना जानू मेरा संजू चोखा हीरा है

जैसे असली हीरे को अफ़्फोर्ड करना हर किसी के बस की बात नहीं

वैसे ही तुम्हारे दिल को समझना हर किसी के लिए आसान नहीं

तुम्हारे साथ शादी को बीत गये यू पच्चीस साल

और बस यही था मेरे दिल का हाल ||

|| ॐ ||

The Blissful Beginnings

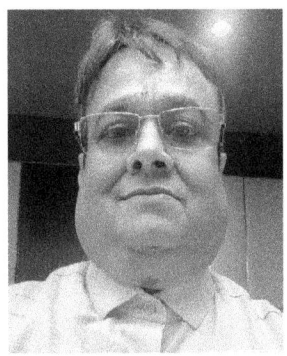

Author's Name	:	Vijay Jain
Qualification	:	B.Sc.
Current Profession	:	Astrologer and Vastu Consultant
Age	:	58 Years
E-mail ID	:	**vijayjain731@gmail.com**
City/ Country	:	**Kolkata, India**

Vijay Jain is a distinguished Astrologer, Vastu Expert, Graphologist and Pyramid Vastu Expert. Renowned for his profound knowledge and expertise, he has been honored with the prestigious Best Vastu Expert Award by the Economic Times and Dr. Jiten Bhatt, the esteemed founder of Pyramid Vastu. With a passion for enhancing lives through ancient wisdom and modern insights, Vijay Jain has dedicated himself to serving communities across the nation. His holistic approach and commitment to excellence have made him a trusted name in the field, empowering individuals and organizations to harness positive energies and achieve their fullest potential.

Keywords : Journey, Challenges, Perfect, Arguments, Understanding

Marriage is often seen as a journey filled with both joyous highs and challenging lows. My own experience with marriage has been a testament to this reality, showcasing both the bliss and the curse that can come with this lifelong commitment.

The Blissful Beginnings :

When we first got married, everything felt perfect. We were deeply in love, excited about our future together, and ready to face any challenge as a team. Our days were filled with laughter, late-night talks, and shared dreams. Cooking dinner, watching our favorite shows, and even doing mundane chores together brought us closer. We were each other's best friends, partners, and confidants.

These early days were the epitome of happiness. We celebrated our differences and embraced our similarities. Life was simpler, and our relationship felt unbreakable. The joy we found in each other's company was genuine, and we believed nothing could ever change that.

The Emergence of Challenges :

As time went on, the honeymoon phase began to fade, and real-life challenges started to creep in. Financial pressures, career demands, and family responsibilities tested our patience and resilience. The differences that once seemed charming began to cause friction. Misunderstandings became more frequent, and communication required more effort than before.

Arguments over small things turned into bigger disputes, and our once effortless connection started to feel strained. We struggled to find the balance between our individual needs and our commitment to each other. The pressures of life began to weigh heavily on our relationship, and the cracks started to show.

The Descent into Darkness :

At our lowest points, marriage felt more like a curse than a blessing. The person who once made me feel whole now seemed to be the source of my frustration and pain. Our arguments grew more intense, and the emotional distance between us widened. I felt isolated and began to question whether we had made a mistake in getting married.

The sense of companionship and support that once defined our relationship was replaced by resentment and disappointment. We were both struggling, and the love that had once brought us so much joy seemed like a distant memory. These dark times were incredibly hard to navigate, and the thought of giving up crossed my mind more than once.

The Path to Reconciliation :

Despite the difficulties, we both knew that our marriage was worth fighting for. We sought help through counselling and made a conscious effort to improve our communication and understanding. This process was not easy and took a lot of time and patience. But slowly, we began to heal.

We learned to listen to each other without judgment, to compromise without resentment, and to appreciate each other's efforts. Rebuilding trust and reconnecting emotionally was a long journey, but it was worth it. We rediscovered the love and respect that had brought us together in the first place.

The Duality of Marriage :

My marriage has shown me that it is both a source of immense joy and significant challenge. It has taught me that marriage is not about constant happiness but about weathering the storms together. The blissful moments are precious and should be cherished, while the tough times are opportunities for growth and strengthening our bond.

Marriage requires effort, patience and a willingness to face challenges head-on. Despite the struggles, the love and connection that can be rebuilt make the journey worthwhile. My experience has taught me that marriage is a complex and dynamic relationship that, with dedication and love, can bring deep fulfilment and joy.

This anthropology book **"My Marriage : Bliss vs. Curse"** by Mr. Abhishaik Chitraans and his wife Mrs. Rainu Mangtani, offers a profound exploration of the dual nature of marriage, highlighting its potential to be both a source of immense joy and deep challenges. This topic is highly meaningful as it resonates with everyone, who has experienced or witnessed the complexities of marital life. The book delves into the blissful moments that bring partners closer and the darker times that test their patience and commitment. It emphasizes that marriage is not merely about happiness, but about enduring hardships together, growing stronger through understanding and compromise.

Their insightful analysis provides a realistic view of marriage, breaking the myth of everlasting perfection and encouraging couples to see challenges as opportunities for growth. The narrative serves as a guide for navigating the ups and downs of marital relationships, making it an essential read for anyone interested in understanding the human experience of marriage.

॥ ॐ ॥

An Unique Experience of Joy & Sorrow

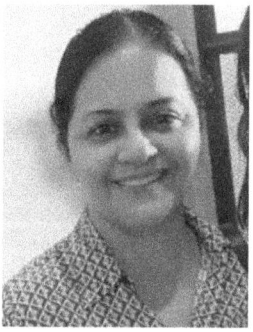

Author's Name	:	Vijayshri Panchikal
Qualification	:	Graduate
Current Profession	:	Counselor/ Therapist
Age	:	52 years
E-mail ID	:	**viji.panchikal@gmail.com**
City/ Country	:	**Bangalore, India**

Vijayshri Panchikal is a certified counsellor and founder of The Wisteria Centre, an emotional and mental wellbeing space, and the beacon, a career and college counselling venture in association with Proventus India. She brings years of rich experience and training in various other therapeutic modalities to this space. She is certified in Art therapist, a Therapeutic Dance in Education practitioner, an EFT Practitioner and is trained in NLP and Gestalt.

Vijayshri is an amateur artist and has held exhibitions successfully. She is also a published author.

Keywords : Companionship, Joy, Laughter, Respect, Trust

My own experience with the institution of marriage has not been very great. But I've been fortunate enough to witness some truly blessed ones; unions that were made in heaven, solemnized on earth and couples who were uniquely made for each other. Of course, nothing flourishes or grows without nurture and care and marriage is no exception. In marriage, like in all other relationships, I feel authentic compassionate communication is the key to unlocking impasses in interactions thus creating an atmosphere of freedom and honesty within the marriage. Everything starts with love but only love is by no means enough to make a marriage work. Respect, friendship, humour, attraction, trust, etc. all play an equally important role in the longevity of a marriage.

Looking at marriages and how they are today I feel now that our forefather's kind of knew what they were talking about when it came to choosing someone who's compatible for oneself and one's family. As a counsellor what I've observed is that most marriages break down due to a lack compatibility and shared values and goals. There is of course so much that goes into making a marriage, or any relationship for that matter, work. Everything is important; time, effort, trust, financial responsibilities, children, parenting styles, families and their roles in the marriage, affection, attraction, faith, values, etc. However, one thing no one really talks about is past personal trauma that an individual can carry into a marriage and how that presents itself in the landscape of the relationship. Is it held safely by the partner? Is it discussed? Communicated? How is it resolved? Is it ridiculed? Is it further abused and neglected by the spouse? What roles do the families play here? For me personally I see this from the lens of a counsellor as I've seen how, if unaddressed, these issues can definitely break down a marriage. Honesty and communication here is of course key as only then can a spouse understand what the affected partner is going through and then be able to offer help, solace and understanding. Now, of course, slowly, couples are becoming more aware of how mental health issues can affect the nature of the marriage and are actively seeking out help to heal, evolve and grow both individually and in their marriage.

When I was much younger, being free spirited, I never really felt faith played that big a role in marriage. Now, many years later, my views on this have changed. But more than having a shared belief system or faith, I feel what's more important is how a couple expresses that faith to each other and in their homes with their children. The consistency and compatibility in this expression of faith can bring a lot of stability, peace and harmony in the home and can bind the couple together strongly.

Last but not the least, definitely, I feel it's so important for a couple to know what gives each other joy. We live in a very fast paced, harsh world today (at the risk of sounding fatalistic, but for the most part it is true) and for a couple to know what brings their spouse joy and how can they put a smile on the others face can be extremely heartening at the end of a tiring day. Doing little things, and maybe sometimes big things too, to bring laughter love n happiness into the relationship can make all the difference.

Marriage is by no means an easy institution, but it is a unique one and hence not to be taken lightly. I have seen marriages fail badly and succeed amazingly too, and I don't think anyone is really to blame here if it does fail, unless of course there is some drastic misconduct or abuse. However, having said that it would definitely be wise to think things through thoroughly before getting married to someone and in my opinion, among all the various other factors, compatibility is definitely way up there as a criterion when it comes to choosing a partner for marriage.

The topic of this anthology book has been extremely challenging, because it's so vast and so culturally and socially dependent. I had a lot to say and had to in a sense condense it into that which I felt was most important, when it came to marriage. A marriage can be bliss and yes it can also be a curse unfortunately and how we handle ourselves through both possibilities is what will truly define, who we are as human beings.

The union of a marriage is a beautiful one. There are hopes and expectations, fears and misgivings, love and a future together and it's up to us who we choose and what we choose to make of it. So, choose wisely and live a life free of regrets!

|| ॐ ||

Clues to be a Cheery Couple

Author's Name	:	Viji S
Qualification	:	M.A., M.Phil., B.L.I.S.
Current Profession	:	Guest Lecturer
Age	:	36 years
E-mail ID	:	…
City/ Country	:	**Tamil Nadu, India**

Viji is a budding author and an educator. She is always curious to learn new things. She is a good listener, detail-oriented person, self motivated, hardworking person with positive attitude towards her life and career. During her leisure time she enjoys listening to music, reading and drawing.

Keywords: Communication, Ego, Forgiveness, Intimacy, Prayer

Marriage can be characterized as a secured commitment between a man and a woman, which strongly unites couples together along with their two families.

There are certain elements like love, trust, quality time, communication, intimacy, respect, support and friendship influencing a blissful marriage life. Use all these oars to create a smooth sailing marriage life. Marriage is the celebration of the divineness of the union. To celebrate it divinely, first make it divine and never intervene any third-party in between.

Marital matters are emerging prominent due to the hiking rate of divorce, which makes a great impact on the society. So, this article is all about the hacks to gel with your beloved.

Ever wondered what makes a marriage strong? When I sit and ponder over my marriage life, I realised that communication, forgiveness, intimacy take the most pivotal role.

Communication is one of the essential ingredients in marriage. Couples should talk and listen to each other empathetically very often. The worst part of communication is assuming your partner knows, what you are thinking or feeling, moreover never expect your spouse to assume too. Most of the women do this blunder in their marital life, which would end up negatively most of the times. Instead tell your spouse openly what do you want and how you feel even if you are frustrated with each other and struggling to express your emotions verbally. It is indispensable to communicate your needs without hurting the other besides giving each other a strong feel that you could tell your spouse anything you want to share without having the feeling of being judged.

When your spouse communicates with you give an undivided attention by putting down your phone, laptop or anything which grabs your attention. Communication is the golden key opener to a blissful marriage and also paves the way to intimacy.

Marriage does not work without intimacy. Emotional and physical intimacy separates marriage from every other relationship and binds us together with our spouse. Marital intimacy, the most vital part of marriage, certainly turns the relationship to the next phase. However, intimacy does not always mean sexuality. An often forgotten aspect of intimacy is the emotional one.

If you are not emotionally available, it is likely to worsen the partnership. Ignoring your partner's pain is a form of emotional neglect and incredibly turns toxic and indicates the other that their pain does not matter to you at all that agonize your partner even more alongside gives the most dangerous feeling of being alone.

If you are deprived of emotional intimacy instead of stepping out of the relationship, try to screw your ways to chain with your partner on a deeper level. Additionally couples can find emotional intimacy through forgiveness.

As the saying goes human is err, almost everyone commits mistakes or hurts anyone at one point of time. So, one must learn to forgive others. As a couple hurting each other's feelings is quite normal. However, strong couples use powerful forgiving tool. When you make a mistake never hesitate to apologize to your partner.

The worst and silliest part of fighting is giving a silent treatment and argue over the past issues recurrently in every subsequent fight. If you do, it may lessen the love between you. Though forgiving your spouse in all scenarios is really tough, yet it is the most prime virtue in marriage, since no one is perfect.

Marriage is a heavenly bond. To make it a heaven, ego should not play a vital role, but unfortunately now a days ego plays a crucial role, which results in divorce. Substitute the most egoistical question "Why should I" to "Why don't we?" We must understand explicitly that relationships are not winning or proving who is stronger, but it's about losing in each other to relish it's real essence.

If I had known all these things then what I know now, my marriage would not have ended. But honestly no worries at all, though my marriage ended up fruitlessly, I would never suggest that marriage is futile and no longer meaningful, because I still believe in marriage.

We must live in each other to keep our relationship healthy. How exercise is to keep a healthy body, similarly there are some determining regular exercises like communication, forgiveness, intimacy, trust, and an unconditional love to keep a healthy marriage and it takes both the partners collaborating to attain this blissfulness.

Above all believe in Almighty and pray for an unconditional love, which grows deeper and stronger to transcend our life entirely blissful.

|| ॐ ||

Marriages are Made in Heaven

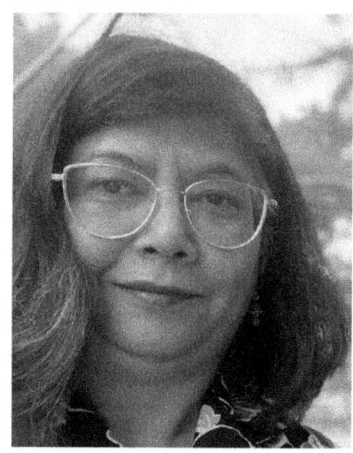

Author's Name	:	Vinieta
Qualification	:	B.E. (Electrical), M.B.A
Current Profession	:	Information Technology Services
Age	:	56 years
E-mail ID	:	**vinieta00@gmail.com**
City/ Country	:	**Gurugram, India**

Vinieta is a Meditation Teacher associated with Ananda Sangha and is a disciple of Paramhansa Yogananda, author of Autobiography of a Yogi. She has been sharing her guru's teachings through offline/online classes in Hindi and English. She is a Certified Ananda Yoga Teacher.

She is an engineer, currently working in the field of Information Technology in a reputed Petroleum sector Consultancy. She did her M.B.A. from University of Ljubljana, Slovenia. An avid reader and enthusiast traveler who has visited number of European, African and Asian countries and various cities in India.

She loves playing Badminton, Carrom and Chess and has been representing her company in Carrom and Badminton in various tournaments.

She has been working towards upliftment of and spreading awareness amongst the downtrodden.

Writing poetry is her passion along with chanting spiritual chants - mainly of Paramhansa Yogananda and Swami Kriyananda, direct disciple of Yogananda and founder of Ananda.

Keywords: Devotion, Educated, Fulfilling, Knot, Forgiving

Marriages are definitely made in Heaven. This got proven to me again and again when my husband, Dev appeared at our residence unannounced time and again whenever there were talks for my marriage. With no mobiles and rare landlines, how Dev got to know is incomprehensible. Daughter of a Municipal Commissioner in Delhi in British Raj, I wore latest fashion apparel so I and my sisters nicknamed Dev, a clown who came wearing bell bottoms and a hat. He still managed to look handsome though.

My father liked him but my mother was apprehensive due to Dev's humble background. She agreed to my marriage only because he became a cop and she realized he was sincere.

I got married at the age of 21 without completing my education, but thanks to Dev, I completed my graduation after marriage and children. Dev was well educated, aristocratic, firm and always supported women education.

In spite of the ups and downs in our nomadic lives, I say that because almost every other year we moved to a new place, there was *not a single moment of marital insecurity*. These uprootings and interactions with new people only made us mentally strong and free of fears of unknown.

Dev was ever eager to help the needy. I was in awe of him as he had an aura of magnificence around him. Very disciplined, he would be up at 4am and went for a walk irrespective of the weather. A sportsperson to the core, he would get a badminton court built near our house wherever we went.

Had loving, affectionate and intelligent children who completed me as a woman and mother. I doted on them and for them we were a combination of a very strict father and a very loving mother. I couldn't scold them for anything except when it came to being anything but respectful to their father.

With a house full of relatives, days were buzzing with life. I did not mind their presence as I love to be in the company of people. Though there were quarrels, bickering, jealousies around but never felt throttled. *Surprising! how a simple knot can give one so much strength to face the whole world of negativities and still remain unscathed.* There were times when we had around 20 people for days together and we had meals in three batches. I enjoyed them as I also liked cooking and had a lot of help.

I accompanied him almost everywhere he went, supporting every decision he took. He never took any decision related to the family without consulting me. He was not praying types nor temple-going types and I never ventured alone but amazingly, I have seen all famous temples and places of worship all around the globe. He visited them as a tourist and I, went with devotion in my heart.

Once we went to Banaras for a wedding. Dev was sitting in the train with the whole group going for the event but I and my daughter got late. He thought we will not be able to make it, so he got down with the luggage. When we reached the platform right in time, there were shouts of joy from the whole group and we were hurriedly pulled inside the coach along with our luggage.

This trip was life changing as Dev met someone who brought him on to the spiritual path. Earlier he was disciplined and helpful but now he had compassion and a drive to work hard to help the downtrodden. Also, he became forgiving. I am yet to meet a person who is more forgiving than him. Although he could have easily punished a cyclist for badly injuring our daughter, he forgave the culprit when he appeared on his own and asked for forgiveness. The culprit was advised to approach

Dev and seek forgiveness by some police man also shows Dev had gained the reputation of being a good human being.

He was also blessed with an ability to read palms. People thought he was practicing palmistry but I gradually realized he told people things in a meditative state. I am yet to meet two people who were told same things by him. His favourite quote was "*Banat Banat Ban Jaye.*" He said it was spoken by a Mahapurush.

He connected well with children too. I loved the way he took care of our youngest daughter when she was unwell. With a partner at my side, who had all qualities of a perfect soulmate, *I feel blessed and even more grateful for my fulfilling married life.*

I promise you my love without any boundaries,

And accept what you believe in, as if it is my own;

Happiness, sorrows, ups and downs not known a moment ago,

I face all bitter challenges our life together, brings forth.

I go with you however, wherever you go,

I smile when sun is shining and even when, tide's low;

Your presence is God's blessings, as a straw to take me ashore,

Through drowning stress and hurdles, our love keeps us afloat.

A fulfilling married life I've lived with you and children,

An integral part of our lives, The Almighty we adore;

His blessings of abundance made us humble, forgiving and whole,

Everyone is worth loving and is our very own.

Anthology on *My Marriage: Bliss vs Curse* is collection of poems and stories which reflect various perspectives under one umbrella. Pearls of diverse views, opinions and experiences are creatively interweaved in one garland, a book. It has the essence of one's married life outlined with different interpretations and learnings.

When the writer treads down the memory lane, penning down in words what the person went through, in words, the writer too experiences a therapeutic effect along with enlightening the reader. A sense of freedom and release of a tension engulfs the author surrounding the writer with inner peace.

Married people are bound to relate to one or more stories because everyone in this world faces similar situations with a twist here and there. It is not the happenings or negative interactions that cause pain but one's reactions to the situation. A source of inspiration for all – married, unmarried, about to be married or not wanting to get married… It is a bridge for all ages, encompassing different type of thinking patterns and genres.

The Bliss Called Marriage

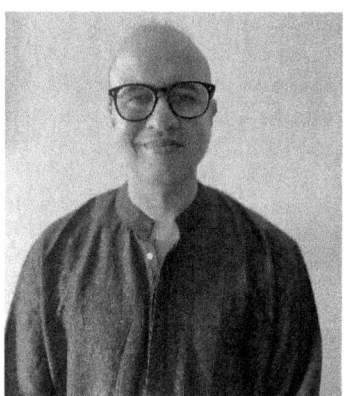

Author's Name	:	Vishal Sachdev
Qualification	:	Post Graduate in Personnel Management
Current Profession	:	HR Consultant, Yoga Trainer, Numerologist & Tarot Card reader
Age	:	49 years
E-mail ID	:	**vishals65@hotmail.com**
City/ Country	:	**Bangalore, India**

Vishal Sachdev is HR Professional turned Numerologist & Tarot Card Reader.

He has over two decades of experience in the IT industry handling Talent Acquisition. He is a post graduate in personnel management & business administration. He has worked with several MNC s like HPE, SAP, IBM etc.

Vishal is a certified Numerologist & Tarot Card reader. Qualified in Vaastu Shastra & is a qualified practicing Yoga Trainer.

Keywords : Marriage Bliss, Successful Marriage, Soul, Give & Take, Partnership

These are my thoughts in poem form on my experience of marriage. I have also shared the few points on what makes a marriage work and what bliss does marriage provides in life.

"The Bliss Called Marriage"

Two Hearts one Soul,

Together we rule the world,

Give & Take ; Take & Give,

Partnership of love behold.

The Teamwork of marriage is

T for Togetherness

E with Empathy

A for Affection

M with Mindfulness

Space, love and tenderness are the recipes for successful venture called marriage.

Happy marriage is ongoing conversation, which seems too short.

Great marriage is each for the other and two against the world.

It's always "us" against the world & not against "each other"

It's the union of two souls

In the rhythm of life

Music of two bodies entwined in time as one

That keeps you from growing old

As we are always told

I become yours & you become mine

Till the end of time

Marriage is a promise

Marriage is an agreement

That two hearts engage

Promise to be authentic

Courage to reveal your real self

Patience & Tolerance are key

To ensure you are not just you but we

Learning and unlearning happens

If you give love a chance

In the union called marriage you see

Marriage is the mirror

That exposes your flaws

Marriage is the space where you share it all

Marriage is gift of togetherness

License bestowed by the Gods

Treasure It

Don't Measure It

It's a fortune that you hold

No wealth or treasure can buy a True marriage of Souls…

॥ ॐ ॥

Blurb

In the pages of *'My Marriage: Bliss vs Curse,'* embark on a journey that delves deep into the intricacies of one of life's most profound institutions – Marriage, where love's sweet melodies harmonize with the dissonance of life's challenges. This anthology uncovers the nuanced essence of wedlock, painting a vivid portrait where the sweetness and bitterness of married life intertwine, revealing profound insights into the human experience.

In this anthology, you'll encounter tales of undying love and unyielding devotion, where the bonds of matrimony serve as a source of unending bliss. From tender moments shared under starlit skies to the profound joy found in building a life together, each story celebrates the unparalleled beauty of marital harmony. The pages embark on a journey through the highs and lows of marital bliss, where each story is a testament to the resilience of the human heart. From the euphoria of newfound love to the sobering reality of conflict, these narratives capture the essence of the marital bond in all its complexity. Experience the intoxicating aroma of passion as couples navigate the exhilarating highs of romance, where every glance is a promise and every touch ignites a flame. Yet, amidst the ecstasy, lies the shadow of adversity, where misunderstandings brew and trust is tested. Explore the depths of despair as marriages confront trials, grappling with loss, infidelity and the weight of unfulfilled expectations.

'My Marriage: Bliss vs Curse' is more than just an anthology or a collection of stories—it's a culmination of 108 perspectives in the form of a mirror reflecting the multifaceted nature of human relationships. It celebrates the joy of companionship while acknowledging the struggles that accompany it. Through laughter and tears, triumphs and tribulations, these tales offer a poignant reminder of the importance of love, forgiveness and perseverance in the journey of marriage. Whether you're embarking on your own marital adventure or simply seeking insight into the human condition, this anthology is a compelling exploration of the ties that bind us together—and the profound impact they have on our lives. So, immerse yourself in these stories and discover the enduring beauty of *My Marriage.*

|| ॐ ||

Gratitude to Readers

Thank you for taking the time to delve into *'My Marriage : Bliss vs Curse'*. This anthology is a collection of reflections, stories, articles and moments that speak to the universal experiences of partnership, resilience and sruggledd growth of the married couples. Your willingness to journey through these pages means the world to us, as each story was crafted with honesty and care by each co-author of the book.

To our readers, thank you for choosing to embark on this journey with us. It is your curiosity, empathy and desire to explore the depths of marital relationships that make this anthology meaningful. We hope that these stories/ articles touch your hearts, challenge your perceptions and perhaps even provide a sense of comfort or camaraderie approach to your marital life.

We are truly grateful for your support, and hope these stories bring you comfort, inspiration or simply a sense of deep connection between authors and readers. Thank you for being a part of this journey.

With heartfelt appreciation and gratitude,

Rainu Mangtani

Abhishaik Chitraans

(ईष्ट कृपा एवं गुरु आशीष)

॥ ॐ ॥

Kindly Connect with us and Share Your Feedbacks/ Reviews

---

 ankakshrmiracless@gmail.com

Full Name :

Nick/ Popular Name :

Name of Spouse :

Date of Birth :   Date of Marriage :

Profession :

WhatsApp Number :   Social Media handle :

Email ID :

City/ Country :   Pincode:

Reviews/ Feedback :

Thanks for your Time & Efforts

|| ॐ ||

List of Books

Books written by Abhishaik Chitraans:

1. **Sex**: A Complex Intersection of Physical Need and Mental Well-being
2. **Life**: A Dance of Light and Shadow
3. **The God's Tender**: Love & Care
4. **Mobile Addiction**: 21 Simple Techniques to Remove or Reduce Mobile Addiction in Children/ Students and Adults
5. **P³**: The Triple Power of Alphabet–P (Proud, Pain, Prayer)

Books written by Rainu Mangtani:

1. **The Height of Life in 24 Rains**: An Inspirational Auto Biography
2. **Today's Corporate World**: A Robotic Mechanism of Youth
3. **Ladder of Success**: Best 15 Ways to Achieve Your Goals

i) **Deep Secrets of Name :** A comprehensive book on advanced Name Numerology based on Chaldean System & an extensive research based on real life case studies. The best book on Name Numerology by 3 eminent Indian authors in Google search, launched at Pragati Maidan, New Delhi in World Book Fair 2024.

Mr. Abhishaik Chitraans is as main Author/ Guide of the book with the two renowned authors and research scholars of Numerology namely Mrs. Rainu Mangtani (Numerologist & Graphologist) and Mrs. Jyotsnaa G Bansal (Astro-Numerologist).

ii) **Women Empowerment and Economic Developments :** An anthology/ articles collection of 51 Co-Authors, lunched on occasion of International Women's Day and Mahashivratri, 08ᵗʰ March, 2024 with online presence of Padma Shri recipient Smt. Gulabo Sapera ji, a legendary folk artist.

|| ॐ ||

शब्दों का समंदर है यह,

बस डूबकर पढ़ते जाना है।

इंतजार करो किताब का अगली,

हमें काफिला बड़ा बनाना है ।।

रेनू – अभिषेक

॥ ॐ ॥

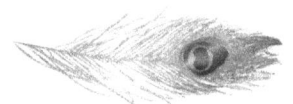

E-mail : ankakshrmiracless@gmail.com
Whatsapp # +91-9368746306

Notes

शब्दों का समंदर है यह,

बस डूबकर पढ़ते जाना है।

इंतजार करो किताब का अगली,

हमें काफिला बड़ा बनाना है ॥

रेनू – अभिषेक

॥ ॐ ॥

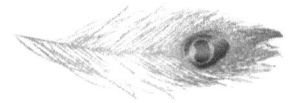

E-mail : ankakshrmiracless@gmail.com
Whatsapp # +91-9368746306

Notes

www.ingramcontent.com/pod-product-compliance
Lightning Source LLC
LaVergne TN
LVHW070538070526
838199LV00076B/6801